# Linguistic Investigations of Aphasia

# LESSER

# LINGUISTIC INVESTIGATIONS OF APHASIA

STUDIES IN DISORDERS OF COMMUNICATION

SECOND EDITION

# W

WHURR PUBLISHERS
LONDON   JERSEY CITY

© Whurr Publishers Limited 1989

First published 1978, reprinted 1981, by
Edward Arnold (Publishers) Ltd
Second edition 1989 published by
Cole and Whurr Limited
Reprinted 1990 and 1991 by Whurr Publishers Ltd.
19b Compton Terrace, London N1 2UN


**British Library Cataloguing in Publication Data**

Lesser, Ruth
   Linguistic investigations of aphasia.–2nd ed.
   1. Man. Aphasia. Linguistic aspects
   I. Title II. Series
   616.85'52

ISBN 1 870332 77 6

Printed and bound in Great Britain by Athenaeum Press Ltd, Newcastle upon Tyne

# Contents

# General preface

This series is the first to approach the problem of language disability as a single field. It attempts to bring together areas of study which have traditionally been treated under separate headings, and to focus on the common problems of analysis, assessment and treatment which characterize them. Its scope therefore includes the specifically linguistic aspects of the work of such areas as speech therapy, remedial teaching, teaching of the deaf and educational psychology, as well as those aspects of mother-tongue and foreign-language teaching which pose similar problems. The research findings and practical techniques from each of these fields can inform the others, and we hope one of the main functions of this series will be to put people from one profession into contact with the analogous situations found in others.

It is therefore not a series about specific syndromes or educationally narrow problems. While the orientation of a volume is naturally towards a single main area, and reflects an author's background, it is editorial policy to ask authors to consider the implications of what they say for the fields with which they have not been primarily concerned. Nor is this a series about disability in general. The medical, social, educational and other factors which enter into a comprehensive evaluation of any problems will not be studied as ends in themselves, but only in so far as they bear directly on the understanding of the nature of the language behaviour involved. The aim is to provide a much needed emphasis on the description and analysis of language as such, and on the provision of specific techniques of therapy or remediation. In this way, we hope to bridge the gap between the theoretical discussion of 'causes' and the practical tasks of treatment—two sides of language disability which it is uncommon to see systematically related.

Despite restricting the area of disability to specifically linguistic matters—and in particular emphasizing problems of the production and comprehension of spoken language—it should be clear that the series' scope goes considerably beyond this. For the first books, we have selected topics which have been particularly neglected in recent years, and which seem most able to benefit from contemporary research in linguistics and its related disciplines, English studies, psychology, sociology and education. Each volume will put its subject matter in perspective, and will provide an introductory slant to its presentation. In this way, we hope to provide specialized studies which can be used as texts for components of teaching courses, as well as material that is directly applicable to the needs of professional workers. It is also hoped that this orientation will place the series within the reach of the interested layman—in particular, the parents or family of the linguistically disabled.

David Crystal
Jean Cooper

# Preface

The study of how brain damage can disrupt the use and system of language in adults (aphasiology) has a fourfold fascination. It offers unique opportunities to find out more about the anatomo-physiological organization of the human brain; it gives scope for the distinguishing of psychologically separate components in mental operations, particularly in the mental operations of language; it provides a testing ground and inspiration for linguistic theory; and, perhaps most rewardingly, its findings have a direct application in the rehabilitation of sufferers from aphasia.

If ever there was a study where several disciplines ought to meet, it is aphasiology. It includes within its sphere some rich complexities, notably the physiology of the human brain, the psychology of the individual, and linguistic science. Yet, perhaps because of the largeness of its aims and because of an awareness of how limited is our present knowledge of the interrelationships amongst mind, matter and words, most followers of these disciplines have shied away from aphasiology. Sadly enough, too, the challenging topic of the language of the human mind disordered by brain damage is barely touched upon in many undergraduate medical courses.

But aphasiology cannot be ignored. Year after year thousands of people become aphasic after a stroke or other cerebral damage, and they or their relatives insist, and society must require, that something be done to help them in their tragic impairment of a supreme and essentially human faculty.

What fills the gap? In many places the rehabilitation of aphasic adults is undertaken heuristically within a medical tradition which emphasizes physical improvement, diagnostic labelling and the perpetuation of simplistic formulae for language disorders. In other places the foundations of a truly interdisciplinary study have been laid, both in aphasia research centres and in the components of undergraduate courses in speech (language) pathology and therapy. In particular the recent interest in aphasia by some linguists and psychologists, working either from their separate departments or from these research centres, has resulted in a spate of linguistically-orientated investigations which have been reported in journals but are not otherwise readily available. A review of these investigations seems timely. It should provide an accessible account of this new approach to the study of aphasia, which will prove useful to students and practitioners of speech pathology, psychology, linguistics, neurology, medicine, rehabilitation and therapy.

The present book includes such a review. As it is, to the best of my knowledge, the first such review (rather than collection of papers), it runs the hazard of two possible shortcomings: firstly, that I have imposed too idiosyncratic an interpretation, and, secondly, that with the acceleration of interest which is now taking place in this field of study fresh evidence is likely to supersede parts of it. The first danger I have tried to reduce by being comprehensive; the second is unavoidable, and indeed its very existence is encouraging.

To set this review in perspective, I have devoted the first two chapters of the book to background description: chapter 1 outlines, for the sake of students of linguistics, the medical and clinical background to aphasia, and chapter 2 gives, for the sake of non-linguistically minded clinicians, an account of some of the notions from linguistic theory which are relevant to aphasia.

I am indebted to many people for help with the book: researchers from many parts of the world, who sent me copies of their papers and pre-prints, and whose work forms the main body of the book; my father, Joseph Hird, who translated many of these papers; and Jean Cooper, David Crystal and John Pellowe, whose comments improved an earlier draft. During the incubation of the book, the University of Newcastle upon Tyne gave me facilities and support for three years as Ridley Fellow in Psychology. I am grateful also to Joyce Mitchell, of the Royal Victoria Infirmary, Newcastle upon Tyne, who introduced me to aphasiology, and to Marianne Watt for her help with book proofs.

Not least have my husband, David, and our children, Piers, Tristram, Giles, Juliet and Tamsin, shared in this book by giving me encouragement and time to write.

R. L.
May 1977

# Preface to the Second Edition

A decade ago the first edition of this book reported on the revolution which had occurred in the investigation and analysis of aphasia through the application of ideas from linguistics. It described this revolution as "accelerating", and acknowledged that it was offering a review of the state of the art in the mid seventies, the character of which was certain to change as this newly developing study grew. The additions which have been made for the present text attempt to take stock of the position ten years later, and to look at the impact achieved by the ideas which were then becoming disseminated.

As part of this it is necessary to restate some of these ideas, and the central chapters of this text, which discuss the key ideas introduced into aphasiology by linguistics (such as its description of language in terms of the levels or domains of phonology, syntax and semantics), are reproduced here with little change. These ideas have now become so germane to the study of aphasia by speech pathologists and psychologists as well as linguists that it is difficult to remember that a decade ago they were innovatory for many clinical investigators: indeed it was only in 1974 that linguistics became a compulsory subject of study in courses in Britain which lead to the professional qualification to work as a speech pathologist/therapist (Crystal, 1988). They have penetrated less well into the medical world, however, and into routine clinical practice. All the popular published tests of aphasia, for example, still use what is essentially a behaviourist framework for their assessment, in which each subtest focusses on an aspect of language behaviour such as repetition or following spoken instructions, with no sustained attempt to relate the design to a coherent proposal about the nature of language. The impact of two applied branches of linguistics, psycholinguistics and sociolinguistics, is currently changing this, and Chapter 9 describes these recent applications in assessment.

Also still incorporated in the book, for its historical value, is the brief review of the earlier application in aphasiology of the linguistic dichotomies of selection/combination and competence/performance, although these notions are no longer central in theoretical linguistics (see, for example, Milroy, 1985). I have also retained the survey of extralinguistic performance in aphasia, which anticipated much recent work, particularly in respect of serial processing and the distinction between functional levels of availability. The former notion has been productively applied to aphasia over the last decade, in examining whether problems with word order may be related to difficulty in mapping thematic roles onto syntactic structure, and the relationship between syntactic and semantic processing. The second notion concerned with the difference between automatic and voluntary processing, continues to fascinate psychologists and philosophers, and the progress which has been made in applying it to the study of aphasia is reviewed. The application to aphasia of two more recent elaborations of theories of grammar (Lexical Functional Grammar, and Government-Binding Theory) is one of the additions made to the book.

The major change of focus in the book, however, is in its discussion of the contribution which applied branches of linguistics are making to aphasiology. Sociolinguistics, extending the study of language in aphasia beyond semantics to pragmatics and discourse, is making a promising contribution through conversational analysis, and Chapter 9 describes the relevance of this to our understanding of aphasia as a basis for therapy. Neurolinguistics, developing as a new discipline which examines the relationship between brain and language, is drawing on dual advances in brain imaging and in computer modelling, and a brief review of these developments is included in Chapter 1. Unquestionably, however, the major advance of the decade has been the application of psycholinguistic models to the study of aphasia by cognitive psychologists, now sufficiently developed to have formed the cornerstone of a further new specialism, cognitive neuropsychology.

Cognitive psychologists initially took a restricted perspective on linguistics, using language as an incidental means of investigating such aspects of mental function as memory, perception and intelligence, particularly through use of single words and through reading. Consequently the psycholinguistic models which were the first to be applied to aphasia have been of the processes which intervene between seeing a word in print and pronouncing its name. Cognitive neuropsychology is now sufficiently well developed, however, to be able to offer a sophisticated linguistic framework for the analysis of many phenomena of aphasia. It has particular implications for speech therapists' interventions with aphasic people, and these important fruits of the application of linguistic investigations to aphasia are described near the end of this book.

R.L.
April 1988

# Glossary

Agnosia: inability to associate meaning with sensation, even though elementary sensation is intact.

Agraphia: acquired difficulty in writing.

Alexia: acquired difficulty in reading.

Allophones: different realizations of the same phoneme which do not change its contrastive role (e.g. in English, aspirated and unaspirated /p/).

Anomia: reduction in the ability to recall names (of objects etc.) for use in speech.

Apraxia: impairment of voluntary and purposive movements which cannot be attributed to muscular weakness or defects.

Asymbolia: inability to associate meaning with one or more classes of symbols.

Cerebral cortex: the outer layers of the cerebral hemispheres of the brain, consisting of nerve cells, their interconnections and supporting cells.

Connotation: emotional and affective meaning.

Corpus callosum: the major band of nerve fibres which connects the two cerebral hemispheres of the brain.

Denotation: referential meaning.

Dichotic listening: a technique used in psycholinguistic experiments, in which sounds or words are presented competitively to each ear.

Distinctive features: those features in terms of which the differences between phonemes can be defined (e.g. place of articulation, voicing).

Dysarthria: difficulty in the articulation of speech sounds, attributable to muscular or neuromuscular defects.

Echolalia: the pathological repetition of heard words or phrases.

Emic: a term abstracted from such words as *phonemic* and *morphemic* to refer to the system and distribution of contrastive linguistic units.

Etic: a term abstracted from such words as *phonetic* and *graphetic* to refer to the description of physical phenomena in speech and writing without explicit reference to their function.

Grammatical words: words which do not carry full lexical meaning but have grammatical significance (e.g. articles, prepositions, auxiliary verbs).

Hemianopia: blindness in one half of the visual field.

Hemifield viewing: a technique used in psycholinguistic experiments, in which material is shown rapidly to one visual field (right or left) and is thus registered by one cerebral hemisphere.

Hemiplegia: paralysis of one side of the body.

Infarct: an area of dead tissue due to obstruction of a terminal artery.

Inflection: affix added to the root of a word to determine its grammatical significance (e.g. the inflection -ed on walk, in walked).

Lexeme: the common semantic element which underlies the variant forms of a
word (e.g. the commonality underlying sing, sings, sang, sung).

Morpheme: the smallest meaningful contrastive unit of grammar, further distinguished as free morpheme (e.g. house, bake) or as bound morpheme (e.g. the
plural inflection realized in its different phonological forms as /s/, /z/, /əz/).

Neologism: a novel word which does not appear in a dictionary of the language.

Neurolinguistics: the study of the relationship between language and its neural
basis in the brain.

Paradigmatic: pertaining to the relationship amongst forms which might occupy
the same place in a linguistic structure (e.g. the contrast between /tap/ and
/map/, or Horses sweat, Gentlemen perspire, Ladies glow).

Paraphasia: misproductions of words, or productions of inappropriate words (see
table 10, p. 187, for subclasses of paraphasia and examples).

Perseveration: the pathological repetition of an earlier response.

Phoneme: the minimal contrastive unit of sound in a language (e.g. /pit/ consists
of three phonemes which can individually be contrasted by comparison with
/bit/, /pat/, /pip/ etc.).

Phonetics: the study of the movement of speech organs, the acoustic properties
of speech sounds and their perception.

Semantics: the study of the system of meaning in language.

Substantive words: words which carry the main lexical meaning in a sentence
(nouns, verbs, adjectives, adverbs).

Syntagm: a syntactic unit, a phrase.

Syntagmatic: pertaining to the relationship between linguistic units which form
linear sequences (e.g. the contrast between /tap/ and /pat/ is syntagmatic).

Syntax: the study of the arrangement of and relationships amongst words in sentences.

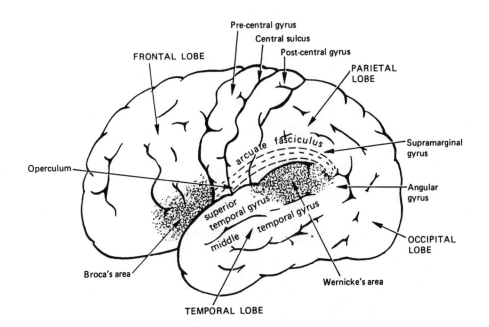

# 1

# Interpretations of aphasia

A working definition of aphasia is that it is a disorder of language resulting from brain damage. The simplicity of this definition is deceptive. The meaning of the term "aphasia" (or "dysphasia", with which it is taken to be synonymous) like all other open-class words, provides "a relatively simple semantic framework that can be enriched by inferences based on knowledge" (Johnson-Laird, 1987;p197). Johnson-Laird was emphasising particularly the influence of sentence and situational context upon the meaning given to a specific instantiation of a word. In respect of the term "aphasia", there are broader contexts to consider; the term has different enrichments to different disciplines, and shifting boundaries according to its application. As understanding grows of the nature of language and of mind and brain, the inferences about aphasia based on knowledge will also result in an amplification of the core of meaning of this word.

The situational context of this book specifies a particular focus on the understanding of the meaning of aphasia. The context is one in which the focus is on the application of linguistics to aphasia, rather than on the neurological consequences of brain damage (although advances in neurolinguistics will be touched upon later). Similarly the social consequences of aphasia are not a central theme, except in as much as they arise in a discussion of the sociolinguistic examination of this disorder. In this book, the definition is also restricted to a disorder of language due to brain damage after verbal skills have become established, thus excluding from our frame of reference developmental aphasia (or dysphasia). The latter applies to a failure to achieve an age-appropriate language system, possibly due to pre-natal or infantile damage or to unknown developmental factors.

Within acquired aphasia, we shall also focus on adults, although, like adults, children can also acquire aphasia from road accidents, tumours, strokes, infections etc. In fact acquired aphasia may be more frequent in children than in adults. Satz and Bullard-Bates (1981) have made a comparison of children and adults in respect of the incidence of aphasia after brain damage, and report 57% in children in contrast to 36% in adults. Lebrun (1987) attributes this to three factors: the greater vulnerability of neural structures which are still developing; the fact that linguistic skills are not yet as consolidated as they are in adults; and the greater proportion of head-injuries in children compared with strokes in adults, with the implication of more bilateral damage. (This last hypothesis is not supported, however, by Loonen and Van Dongen's 1988 study of 28 children showing that, although bilaterality of damage was a critical parameter in recovery, children with head injury recovered better than those with strokes).

Despite its higher incidence, however, acquired aphasia in children brings special problems of study. With the exception of the language disorder in the Landau-Kleffner syndrome, of which epilepsy is a symptom, children who acquire aphasia are generally considered to recover more quickly and more extensively than do adults. It has been suggested in fact that, if the damage had occurred before speech was acquired, no aphasia may result (Bishop, 1988), although language may be delayed (Byrne and Gates, 1987). The traditional picture of total eventual recovery from aphasia (other than due to the Landau-Kleffner syndrome) acquired in children who were formerly competent users of language has had to be modified, however, since children have been examined by more penetrating tests of their language and educational status (Woods and Carey, 1979; Cooper and Flowers, 1987; Loonen and Van Dongen, 1988). Residual problems with word-retrieval, syntax, verbal memory, spelling and acquiring foreign languages have been reported, despite apparent "clinical" recovery. Nevertheless, we shall restrict the description of acquired aphasia in this book to adults because the study of aphasia in children brings in further complicating factors which cloud an already complex picture, factors of stage of education, effects of social deprivation on the development of language and a changing neuronal substrate.

For simplification also, let us follow the school which restricts the definition of aphasia to a disorder acquired after a focal lesion to the brain (e.g. Damasio, 1981). This will exclude discussion of the slowly progressive aphasias reported in a number of papers in connection with a possible relationship to dementia (Mesulam, 1982; Benson, Cummings and Tsai, 1982; Poeck and Luzzatti, 1988). Dementia, and other conditions such as schizophrenia, can result in consequences for the language system which are sometimes described as aphasic. The 1987 meeting of the Aphasia Committee of the International Association of Logopedics and Phoniatrics focussed on the theme of whether or not the language disorder which is associated with dementia could legitimately be described as aphasia. The arguments for including it within aphasia were that it was the result of brain damage and that the speech of some such patients was characterised by word-retrieval, semantic and verbal memory problems which bore resemblances to the language of some kinds of aphasic patients; it was argued that it was better to include the language disorders of dementia within the overall domain of aphasia, so that a complete picture of language processing in the brain could be built up, despite the co-ocurrence in dementia of other deficits of cognition. The arguments against were twofold. Introducing yet another element into the as yet unresolved and complex picture of aphasia could confuse rather than clarify; there was also a fear that extending the term aphasia to dementia could prejudice reactions to 'truly' aphasic patients, for whom it is socially important to reiterate that theirs is not an intellectual disorder, but one which is restricted to the language system. One of the aims of students of aphasia, it was argued, is to assist in the differential diagnosis between aphasia and other disorders with which it may be confused in clinical practice. The balance of opinion was that it was better not to refer to the language disorder in dementia as aphasia, and this verdict will be followed here (but see the discussion in Au, Albert and Obler, 1988, arguing that "the language disorders which accompany dementia be viewed as if they were variations of classical aphasic syndromes" (p. 171)).

We will admit also a further restriction, in order to limit the scope of this survey, i.e. that the language disorder must be persisting rather than transient. This will exclude from our theme the temporary effects on language of short-lasting interruptions to the brain's blood supply (transient ischaemic attacks) or by epilepsy (but for reviews of the latter see Racy, Osborn, Vern and Molinari, 1980, and Rosenbaum, Siegel, Barr and Rowan, 1986).

It is evident, too, that "language disorder" is also an inadequate component of our definition, and that "complex of language disorders" might accommodate our needs better. An aim of this book is to help discuss how a linguistic perspective has helped us to determine what this complex of language disorders may be. Our working definition of aphasia, therefore, restricted for the purposes of simplification in this book, has become: a complex of persisting language disorders, acquired after focal lesions to brains which previously had a mature language system. Before we begin this review of linguistic investigations of the nature of aphasia, thus defined, let us first outline its basic neurology, and then briefly review some historic and contemporary clinical analyses of aphasia.

## The basic neurological background

In some cases the focal injury we have referred to can be extensive. It can, for example, be as extensive an injury as the cutting out of the entire cortex of one hemisphere of the brain in an attempt to extirpate tumour or to diminish severe epilepsy. Or it can be widespread focal damage as in one type of aphasia, *isolation of the speech area*, the best known example of which occurred following carbon monoxide poisoning (Geschwind and Kaplan 1962). The justification for describing this as focal damage is that deprivation of oxygen first affects those areas of brain where the branches of the main cerebral arteries end, in the border zones or 'watersheds' between the arteries. Consequently a general reduction in oxygen supply can result in focal areas of damage in these zones.

The most common causes of the focal damage which leads to aphasia, however, are cerebro-vascular accidents (*CVA*s or *strokes*), head injury from external trauma (as in falls, road-accidents, or war wounds) and the surgery required to remove tumours. Within these causes it is common practice to make further distinctions. In head injuries, a broad classification is between those which are *closed*, in which the impact may have produced as much or more damage on the opposite side of the brain, due to rebound, as on the impact side, and *open* injuries where the site of injury is clearer. Strokes can be distinguished according to whether the vascular accident or accidents occurred in the part of the brain supplied by one of the two carotid arteries or by the vertebral-basilar artery system. Lasting aphasia results from strokes which arise from blockages of an artery (due to an accumulation of fatty tissue on the wall and/or to the lodging of a circulating clot) and those which arise from the bursting of an artery. With present-day techniques the diagnosis of whether the damage is due to blockage or bursting usually cannot be made with absolute certainty except in a few patients (see Held 1975; Oxbury 1976). The clearest aphasic symptoms—clearest in the sense of affecting selective aspects of language rather than producing a gross overall impairment—are probably the result of embolic (clot) strokes occurring in youngish patients who have otherwise healthy brains except for the area supplied by that part of the branch of an artery whose supply has been blocked. But such patients are in a minority, and it has been the practice to base theories of aphasia on studies of groups which not only include different kinds of strokes, but even several other etiologies. One interpretation of aphasia is an exception: Luria's classification (described on pp. 16-17) was based principally on examinations of Russian soldiers with head wounds, and other patients who had had surgery.

It is not known with any degree of certainty to what extent etiology is a significant factor in the nature of an aphasia. When groups of patients are studied together, etiology is compounded with age: patients with language disorders after stroke tend to be older than those who have head injury or who have recovered from tumour, and age is an important factor in the nature of the aphasia and in the pattern of its recovery, because age affects the capacity of the surviving brain tissue to compensate for the damage. But there are some indications that different etiologies may result in different types of aphasia in their own right. A group of people who had become aphasic after closed head injury were found to have only the kinds of aphasia described as Wernicke's aphasia and amnesic aphasia, and not to have motor aphasia (these terms will be discussed shortly) (Heilman, Safran and Geschwind 1971). Geschwind (1974, pp. 502-3) has pointed out that some syndromes do not occur with the missile wound injuries which Luria studied; *pure word-deafness* occurs only with a deep lesion which has spared the surface of the brain; *pure alexia* (reading difficulties without writing difficulties) follows an interruption of the blood supply of the left posterior cerebral artery that has disconnected areas of the brain; and *isolation of the speech area* results from the particular damage already referred to. Moreover Green (1969a) has observed that phonetic cues to the beginning of a word are helpful to patients with what Luria describes as *semantic aphasia* only if the damage is due to tumour and not to vascular disease. There is consequently a growing tendency for investigators to distinguish between etiologies, and to restrict their observations at any one time to one kind of patient.

However it is not only different causes of aphasia and the age of the patient which may complicate the findings. There are other factors influencing the nature of the aphasia. Of particular importance is the degree to which speech is lateralized in one hemisphere of the brain. Many studies have shown that, in most individuals, one half of the brain, usually the left, is much more involved with the control of speech than the other. This has some correlation with hand preference, but not a clear enough one to be definitive in any individual: some 98 per cent of right-handed people have left hemisphere dominance for speech, but only about 60 per cent of left-handed people. Consequently the great majority of aphasic patients have focal lesions in the left hemisphere. Though left-handed people can become aphasic more often after right-hemisphere brain damage than do right-handed people, they are more likely to recover quickly, perhaps because speech is not as strongly lateralized. The situation is complicated by the fact that handedness is not an all-or-none affair in terms of left and right. There are degrees of preferential use of one hand; and language experiments by psychologists who have compared people who have left-handers in their family with those who have not suggest that there may be concealed genetic traits which affect language lateralization. It is probably more realistic to think of lateralization as being a continuum (Liberman 1974). This is one of the many reasons why an injury in the same part of the brain in two people can have quite different effects on language.

Besides age, etiology and lateralization, other proposed influences on the nature of aphasic symptoms are intelligence, educational level and degree of pre-traumatic linguistic skills. We also need to add to this list the possible influence of gender. The study of sex differences in aphasia is relatively recent. Pizzamiglio, Mammucar and Razzano's 1985 study of recovery from global aphasia found that women showed better recovery than men on tests which required lexical-semantic, phonemic or sentence comprehension, concordant with McGlone's (1983) hypothesis that women have more bilateral representation of language com-prehension than men. Cappa and Vignolo (1988) found corroboratory support for sex differences in their CT scan study of 53 men and 32 women with global aphasia; they found an overwhelming preponderance of women in the group with anterior lesions, and concluded that either language is more focally organized in the left hemisphere in women, or that there is a greater 'distance' effect of anterior damage on the posterior language zones in women. Contradictory results, however, have also been reported. Basso, Capitani and Moraschini's 1982 study of a large group of aphasic men and women found the women's recovery of spoken language superior to the men's, but not their comprehension, while Sarno, Buanaguro and Levita (1985) failed to find significant differences between 37 men and 23 women in recovery from aphasia after stroke.

A further factor which needs to be considered is whether the site of the aphasia-causing lesion is cortical, subcortical or implicates both regions of the brain. Over the last few years a variety of subcortical aphasias have been described, implicating a particular role for the thalamus in the neural organization of language (Wallesch and Wyke, 1983; Alexander, Naeser and Palumbo, 1987; Naeser, 1988). Although tentatively associated in particular with the phenomenon of perseveration, these subcortical aphasias have generally been described, however, in the same terms as the cortical, or have been used to account for aphasic symptoms which do not conform with the classical cortical syndromes.

The neurological analysis of aphasia is likely to become increasingly sophisticated in the future due to two developments: the rapid advances which have been made in brain imaging, and the incorporation of ideas from computational linguistics. Computers working in parallel to imitate neural networks have shown a capacity to learn some aspects of language through self modification of their hidden units (Schneider, 1987), and it is possible that this 'connectionism' may feed back into greater understanding of how the brain may cope with language. Already computational linguistics has been applied to the study of aphasia, though in a pre-connectionist paradigm (Arbib, Caplan and Marshall, 1982). "Lesions" introduced into computer models of language have mimicked the lexical and syntactic disorders associated with some syndromes of aphasia. This work is still at an early stage, however, and of greater immediate clinical application are the new methods of imaging the brain.

The greatest advance has been in the development of techniques which can demonstrate not only anatomical sites of lesions, but functions of the living brain, including malfunctionings after damage. This has been achieved through monitoring the flow of radioactively tagged blood through the brain, indicating which regions are active when certain language tasks are performed. Positron emission tomography of this kind has been used both with brain-damaged people and with normal volunteers (Metter, 1987; Petersen, Fox, Posner, Mintun and Raichle, 1988); we shall return to its application to the psycholinguistic modelling of aphasia in Chapter 9. A less invasive method of establishing sites of functional lesions is also becoming available in the shape of magnetic resonance imaging. This too can be sensitive to metabolic changes in the brain, by using difference sequences of pulses to tune the resonance and thus detect the concentrations of phosphorus atoms which are associated with regions of the greatest metabolic activity. Other non-invasive techniques are also being used to examine the living brain, such as magnetoencephalography, many of which may have applications in neurolinguistics and aphasiology (see Lesser, in press a, for a review of the application of brain imaging and other technniques to the study of aphasia).

## The clinical interpretation of 'language' in the 1960s and 1970s

Definitions of aphasia in the 1970s are revealing as to current conception of the nature of language. Halpern (1972, p. 3) defined aphasia as 'a multi-modality language disturbance due to brain injury. It is a linguistic deficit that causes the individual to have difficulty in the comprehension and/or formulation of language symbols'. Eisenson (1973), after reviewing a number of definitions of aphasia from over the nineteenth and twentieth centuries, extracts from them two areas of consensus: that aphasic persons show evidence at some stage of impairment in intake of sequential verbal events as well as for sequential verbal output, and that aphasic involvements are best expressed in terms of reduced probability of output or comprehension rather than in absolute terms. The definition Eisenson finally proposes is: 'Aphasia is an impairment of language functioning of persons who have incurred localized cerebral damage that results in a reduced likelihood that an individual involved in a communicative situation will understand or produce appropriate verbal formulations' (p. 26). Both Halpern's and Eisenson's definitions illustrate one of the basic problems in defining aphasia—whether it is to be considered as an impairment of speech *and* comprehension or as an impairment of speech *or* comprehension. The history of the study of aphasia has produced a situation where on the one hand aphasia, as we shall see, needs to be defined as multi-modal (i.e. affecting all the four modalities of language behaviour; speech, auditory comprehension, writing and reading) and yet has been described in terms of speech *or* auditory comprehension being impaired. It is not surprising that those who come to the study of aphasia with fresh eyes from another discipline find this situation anomalous, and that linguistically-minded aphasiologists are devoting some time to the resolution of the anomaly.

To see how this situation has arisen, we must observe that until recently there has been only one framework for the description of aphasia—that of the language modalities. Neurological data about the anatomy and dynamics of brain function are not secure enough at present for a complete description of aphasia in neurodynamic terms to be possible. Similarly, psychological models of the mental organization of language are as yet inadequately developed. Consequently the only framework for analysis on which aphasiologists have been able to rely has been the obvious one of behaviour in the different language modalities. In some respects this is a very suitable framework. It can be observed that some brain lesions apparently seletively affect the ability to speak (*dysarthria*, or to read (*pure alexia* or *alexia without agraphia*) although other language modalities seem to be intact. There is near universal agreement that dysarthria impairs only 'the actualization or realization of the phonological component' of language (Whitaker 1976, p. 430), in other words that it is an articulatory disorder of speech which does not involve other aspects of language. Most classifications of the dysarthrias distinguish them by the site of the brain lesion (in the cerebellum, in the basal ganglia, in the nuclei of the cranial nerves and their axons to the articulatory musculature, or in the innervation of these nuclei from the cortical motor zones)—see Darley, Aronson and Brown (1975) and Whitaker (1976). But there is also universal agreement that, because only one modality of language, speech, is impaired, dysarthria is best considered as distinct from aphasia. Pure alexia, on the other hand, is commonly described as a 'pure aphasia' (Goodglass and Kaplan 1972; Goodglass and Geschwind 1976), even though those who use this label interpret it as a disconnection of the visual input of reading from the language zone of the left hemisphere, the language zone itself being intact (Geschwind 1965). Other isolated disorders which affect only auditory verbal comprehension (*pure word-deafness*) or writing (*pure agraphia*) are much less well documented and their existence is controversial (but see Hécaen 1972).

Because of the primacy in language of the two modalities of auditory comprehension and speech, some aphasiologists have questioned whether disorders in these modalities can occur without secondary consequences for other language modalities. In some of the few reported cases of pure word-deafness it has been acknowledged that the patient had earlier shown signs of a more generalized language disorder; in other studies the 'purity' of the syndrome is questionable because the methods of examination of the disorder have not been penetrating. Luria (1970) and Hécaen (1972) both describe aphasias where the deficit in auditory comprehension is attributed to an impairment in the analysis of speech sounds and where there are additional deficits in the other modalities. Other theories of aphasia, to be described shortly, make impairment of comprehension the key factor in all aphasia, rejecting additional sensori-motor complications which affect the mechanisms required for speech, reading and writing as essentially non-aphasic in character.

There is particular controversy about whether or not some articulatory disorders after cortical lesions can be distinguished from aphasia. Although lesions in the primary motor cortex may result in non-aphasic dysarthria, other cortical lesions in adjacent zones may result in disturbances in the production of speech which are of a different nature from those of dysarthria, and which have been given the names *apraxia of speech* or *verbal apraxia* or *verbal dyspraxia*. In this condition the speech disorder cannot be atttributed to an elementary difficulty in controlling the muscles which are used in articulation, as these muscles function normally when required for purposes other than speech, such as reflex swallowing, blowing, and coughing. The difficulty appears to be at a higher level, in the purposive coordination of movement peculiarly for speech. Opinion is divided as to whether apraxia of speech should be regarded as an aphasia or not. Some argue that it is a disorder which affects a medium of language exclusively, and a medium which is of central importance to the primary system, and that apraxia of speech patterns according to linguistic regularities, making this indisputably a form of aphasia. Others argue that it is essentially a problem of neuromuscular incoordination, albeit one at a high level, and that no other aspect of language is involved: it responds to a different kind of therapy from aphasia and it therefore should not be classified as an aphasia. We shall return to this controversy later, in chapter 8.

Many of the difficulties of defining aphasia arise from the inherent anomaly of needing to characterize aphasia as a central disorder of language which has repercussions on all the modalities of language, while yet having no other framework of analysis by which to describe it except these modalities. If this is the only framework of analysis that is available, various kinds of aphasia can only be distinguished by degrees of relative impairment in each modality. The key contrast in the aphasias therefore resolves itself into one between speech and auditory comprehension. This has resulted in an unsatisfactory impasse for interpretations of aphasia. On the one hand it is acknowledged that aphasic patients have a central disorder of language, while on the other hand some classifications are based on the necessity of assuming that speech and auditory comprehension are diametrically opposed. Patients are either *expressive* with a restricted flow of speech and good comprehension, or they are *receptive* with an unrestricted flow of speech and poor comprehension. There are variants on this terminology: motor/sensory, emissive/impressive, encoding/decoding. This kind of classification is fostered by many of the formal clinical batteries of aphasia tests, which systematically put the patient through his paces in the modalities of speaking, reading for comprehension, writing and auditory comprehension. In the majority of these assessments the search is not for commonalities of behaviour regardless of modality as indications of a central disorder, but is rather for signs of different degrees of impairment in the different modalities. There is a consequent tendency for the therapy which derives from these batteries to emphasize a modality approach with an emphasis perhaps on writing or on comprehension exercises.

It has long been acknowledged that the strict opposition of aphasias into expressive and receptive is untenable, if we exclude from the definition of aphasia the pure disorders which affect only one modality. Aphasia is primarily recognized in an individual through the speech disorder; without this sign to attract attention aphasia would remain undiagnosed. Indeed Wernicke, and Geschwind a century later, have deplored the fact that some kinds of aphasic patients are often misdiagnosed because, on superficial acquaintance, their speech appears to be adequate. Consequently it is readily acknowledged that aphasic patients diagnosed as 'receptive' have an abnormality in their speech. It is not so immediately obvious whether or not 'expressive' patients have a deficit in their auditory comprehension, because it is much more difficult to examine auditory comprehension reliably than to observe speech. Speech can be tape-recorded: auditory comprehension cannot. Linguistic aspects of comprehension are often difficult to distinguish from extra-linguistic aspects, i.e. from intellectual comprehension and from non-verbal gestural and social cues to the content of the language. Examination of auditory linguistic comprehension for these reasons necessarily has to be structured and formal and to involve another speaker, whereas speech can be analysed at a variety of different gradations of spontaneity and formality.

There is also the problem of whether or not to include in expressive aphasia those patients with apraxia of speech who on formal testing cannot be shown to have any impairment in auditory comprehension. Depending on one's theoretical preference one can argue that this demonstrates that some expressive aphasics do not have any problems in comprehension, or alternatively that these patients are not aphasic because their comprehension is intact.

The pros and cons of the division of aphasia into modality-based syndromes have been argued for a century. The earliest detailed descriptions of aphasia (that is to say of aphasia in a number of patients, rather than anecdotal descriptions of individuals) such as those of Broca in France in the 1860s and Jackson in England in the 1890s commented on the preservation of comprehension and intellect, despite an aphasia so severe as to make the patients virtually speechless. It was proposed that it was the faculty of 'articulated language' (speech) which was in the left hemisphere but that comprehension, being more automatic, was the province of the right hemisphere or perhaps of both hemispheres. When Wernicke observed that there were some patients who after left hemisphere damage made inappropriate responses to questions although the faculty of articulated language was apparently preserved and speech flowed easily, he deduced that they had a loss of auditory comprehension due to destruction of the sound-images of words. From this there arose the dichotomy of aphasia with comprehension difficulties and aphasia without.

Such a dichotomization of aphasia was not universally accepted. One of Broca's compatriots, Marie (1906), stated firmly that all aphasics have a disorder of comprehension, which he recognized as being at a central level and not limited simply to auditory comprehension. Aphasia in fact was a disorder of intellect. 'If I for my part were to give a definition of aphasia the factor which I would be compelled to stress would be the diminution of intelligence' (1906, translation 1971, p. 54). He illustrated his claim by describing a professional cook, who, some years after becoming aphasic, attempted to poach an egg by putting the butter on top of the awkwardly cracked egg, instead of first melting the butter and then adding the egg. It was not articulation difficulties in speech that made an aphasia, but comprehension difficulties, and the true aphasia was therefore the kind described by Wernicke. Articulation difficulties could be experienced with or without aphasia, and Broca's aphasia was a combination of these articulation difficulties with aphasia. As Marie neatly put it in his famous formula:

Broca's aphasia = Wernicke's aphasia + anarthria

A belief that aphasia necessarily implicates intelligence has not been without its supporters throughout the century of aphasiology. In the *sensualistic/spiritualistic* controversy in the late nineteenth century, the interdependence of language and of thought was hotly disputed, the sensualists taking the view that wihtout language thought was impossible, and the spiritualists that thought could have an independent spirit-like existence. When an eminent physiologist, Lordat, had what was probably a mild stroke and temporarily lost both the power of speech and of rapid comprehension of speech, he seized on his retained capacity to analyze his disorder, and to think, as evidence for the spiritual nature of thought and its independence from language. But there were others (even as late as 1969, in a paper by Bay) who argued that Lordat's disorder could not have been a true aphasia because there is necessarily a disruption of conceptual thinking in aphasia. Goldstein (1948) was one of the best known proponents of the belief that aphasia, whatever its superficially different forms, is unified by a common intellectual loss. He saw this loss in terms of an incapacity for abstract thinking, and a reliance on the concrete here-and-now. But, without holding that aphasia is an intellectual disorder and that comprehension in this sense is impaired, other aphasiologists have argued the case that all aphasic adults share a common disability which is described as impairment of verbal comprehension rather than of intellectual comprehension. While recognizing the current opposition of speech and comprehension in the contemporary classifications, Head (1926, p. 547) protested at its inadequacy: 'Although the defects produced by an organic lesion of the brain fall naturally into disorders of verbal formulation and defective recognition of meaning, we cannot divide the manifestations of aphasia according to these categories into two mutually exclusive groups. For the use of language as a whole is more or less affected . . .' A later enthusiastic advocate of this unitary nature of aphasia was Schuell (Schuell, Jenkins and Jiminez-Pabón 1964). She concluded, from her observations and examinations of a large number of patients referred for assessment and treatment in Minnesota, that sensori-motor diffi- culties related to specific modalities were essentially extraneous to the disorder which was common to all aphasic adults. The quality of this disorder was shown in the reduction in verbal comprehension, in vocabulary and in verbal memory which all patients have. The superficially different syndromes of the aphasias could be accounted for by whether or not a 'simple' aphasia was or was not accompanied by these additional complications of sensori-motor disturbances in speech and writing or by visual disturbances.

Despite the attempts to emphasize the essentially unitary nature of aphasia, and the essentially extraneous quality of the articulatory disorder which sometimes accompanied aphasia and sometimes could occur on its own, the division of the aphasias into two main classes maintained its attraction. The terminology of expressive and receptive had a convenience which it was hard to shake off. Weisenberg and McBride (1935, p. 465), in the first study to use standard tests with a relatively large number of aphasic patients (over 60), came to the conclusion, as Head had done, that expressive aphasias are 'language disorders which involve far more than verbal formulation and expression', but they nevertheless described the terminology of expressive and receptive as 'on the whole extremely satisfactory'. If there is no alternative framework except the language modalities which is available for the analysis of aphasia, such terminology and its associated conceptualizations of aphasia are likely to persist.

The development of more rigorous and standardized clinical investigations of aphasia following Weisenberg and McBride's precedent has led to a more sophisticated variant of the modality framework. This makes additional distinctions within the modality of speech in terms of the nature of the stimuli by which the speech is elicited. It distinguishes speech which consists of the naming of objects (or pictures), speech which is imitative of the examiner's speech (repetition) and speech which is 'spontaneous', i.e. is elicited in conversation or in the description of events (often the description of events which can be inferred from a picture). It thus offers additional dimensions by which to distinguish different classes of aphasia, but once again they are behavioural dimensions of the modalities rather than ones which might in themselves show up qualitative differences within a central disorder.

## Clinical examinations of aphasia

All the leading batteries of tests used in the diagnosis of aphasia are based on the modality framework. The Minnesota Test for the Differential Diagnosis of Aphasia (Schuell 1965) and the Boston Diagnostic Aphasia Examination (Goodglass and Kaplan, 1972, 1983) and its derivative the Western Aphasia Battery (Kertesz, 1982) are divided into subsections which examine each modality, with the subtests within these sections increasing in difficulty and with mostly pass-fail scoring, though sometimes with acknowledgement of delays in responding. The Boston examination covers the widest range of kinds of speech, from conversational through automatic speech to repetition and reading aloud. The Porch Index of Communicative Abilities (PICA) (Porch, 1967) uses subsections divided according to three methods of response — speech, writing and gesture (reading subtests being classed as gestural because they require the patient to arrange cards): auditory comprehension is assessed through the patient's incidental comprehension of the test instructions and the characteristics of the responses made. Porch's major contributions to the examination of aphasia were his multidimensional scoring and his application of more rigorous psychometric methods than had hitherto been thought practical. But his attitude to the content of aphasia batteries and the framework for analysis of aphasia was uncritical and perhaps fairly representative of the feeling at the time when his index was being developed; 'The problem of constructing such a battery is not so much one of selecting valid tasks as these have been fairly well agreed on' (p. 10) but one of producing a more sensitive and reliable system for scoring these agreed tasks. The development of the cognitive neuropsychological assessment of aphasia in the 1980s has revealed the naivety of such a confident statement of the 1960s.

With the exception of some aspects of Luria's examinations of aphasia, which did not become readily available till Christensen's (1974) version was published, and which have consequently not been widely promulgated in the western world, surprisingly little of modern linguistics has yet permeated into formal assessments of aphasia. When linguistic variables are controlled in these tests they are the variables of word frequency in the language, part of speech and sentence length. With one or two exceptions, variables such as semantic class, phonetic similarity and syntactic structure are not acknowledged.

It is against this background that linguistic science can offer a framework for analysis, and a multiplicity of distinctions within one language, which are in principle independent of the modality in which the language happens to be realized. The framework and the distinctions are suitable for the analysis of language as a central system, and provide a much needed complement to the inherently limited dimension of the modalities for the examination of aphasia. This framework is described in chapter 2. It is not the only dimension additional to the modalities which is useful in the examination of aphasia; a third one is tentatively suggested in chapter 4, as well as the processing and conversation models described in chapter 9.

## Terms in classifications

Before we turn from clinical aphasiology to linguistic theories, however, it is necessary to be aware of the different meanings of terms which have been used in the study of aphasia. Some aspects of the differences in defining the term *aphasia* itself have already been described; but when it comes to defining different types of aphasia, difficulties with terminology become even more rife. The terms which are used derive from the analysts' theories, and as several disciplines have an interest in aphasia the terms reflect an assortment of neuroanatomical, neurophysio-logical, psychological and linguistic concepts coupled with attempts to be objectively non-committal (e.g. 'Type A'); table 1 lists some terms which have been used in classifications of aphasia.

The multiplicity of labels in the table provides but a small sample of those which have been used to describe different aphasias: MacMahon (1927b) has reported at least 113 in the literature on aphasia. The table also excludes the 'pure aphasias' (in

# TABLE 1

### *Classifications of aphasia*

(excluding 'mixed', 'global' and 'pure' forms—see p. 10)

---

**I** APHASIA IS ONE-DIMENSIONAL, and can properly only be classified by severity and by whether or not it is accompanied by other symptoms, e.g. sensori-motor deficits or visual deficits.

| | Reference |
|---|---|
| | Schuell et al. 1964 |
| | Bay 1966 |

---

**II** OBJECTIVE MEASURES DISTINGUISH A MAJOR DIVISION IN APHASIA

| (predominantly expressive) | (predominantly receptive) | Reference |
|---|---|---|
| Non-fluent | Fluent | Goodglass et al. 1964 |
| Type A | Type B | Howes 1964 |
| Anterior | Posterior | Benson 1967 |

---

**II** IN PRACTICE IT IS USEFUL TO DISTINGUISH THREE CLASSES OF APHASIA

| | | | Reference |
|---|---|---|---|
| Predominantly expressive | Predominantly receptive | Amnesic | Eisenson 1954 (after Weisenberg and McBride) |

---

**IV** THERE ARE SEVERAL APHASIAS

| 1 | 2 | 3 | 4 | 5 | 6 | 7 | 8 | Reference |
|---|---|---|---|---|---|---|---|---|
| | Syntactic | | | *Jargon (severe pragmatic)* | Pragmatic | | Semantic | Wepman and Jones 1961 |
| Dynamic | Efferent motor | Afferent motor | | Sensory (acoustic-agnosic) | | *Semantic* | Acoustic-amnesic (and other Nominative) | Luria 1964, 1976; Jakobson 1964 |
| | Word-dumb | | | Word-deaf | Central | | Nominal | Brain 1965 |
| Transcortical motor | Broca | | Conduction | | Wernicke | *Isolation syndrome (transcortical sensory)* | Anomic | Geschwind 1965; Goodglass and Kaplan 1972 |
| *Expressive 2 (agrammatic without dysarthria)* | Expressive 1 | | *Expressive 3 (conduction)* | Sensory 1 | Sensory 2 | *Sensory 3 (attentional disorder)* | Amnesic | Hécaen and Dubois 1971 |
| | Broca 1 | Broca 2 (mild, with dysarthria) | Conduction | | Wernicke 1 | *Wernicke 2 (isolation syndrome)* | Amnesic (mild Wernicke) / Nominal | Lecours 1974 |
| Transcortical motor | Agrammatic | Anarthric | Phonemic | | Semantic | | Nominal | Brown 1977 |

Classes of aphasia which are not represented approximately in at least one other classification are printed in italics. With these exceptions, similarity in classifications is indicated by their vertical alignment.

Goodglass and Kaplan's 1972 terminology) of alexia, agraphia and alexia-with-agraphia (reading and writing disorders). Aphasias are also sometimes identified as *mixed* or as *global* or *total*. Predictably there is not even unanimous agreement about what constitutes global aphasia. For some it is a convenient term to describe the severely handicapped patient who neither speaks intelligibly nor appears to comprehend language which is not supported by a non-verbal context. Others suggest that global aphasia conceals a disturbance of language which is either primarily of the expressive or Broca type or primarily of the receptive or Wernicke type. It is also disputed whether there can ever be such a condition as total aphasia; it can be argued that the human brain, whilst consciousness is retained, always retains at least some capacity for the comprehension of language.

The table shows how classifications have been concerned with improving on the first dichotomization of aphasia into the two oppositions of expressive and receptive. Eisenson (1954), for his test of aphasia, followed Weisenberg and McBride's modification of the terms by 'predominantly' and by the isolation of a third group of patients who had fluent speech and good comprehension but conspicuous difficulties in naming objects (amnesic aphasia or anomia). Another reaction was the attempt to provide objective distinctions within the one modality, speech, about the impairment of which there was common agreement. One objective measure which was suggested was to calculate the ratio of nouns to pronouns in the patient's speech (Wepman and Jones 1966). The expressive aphasic adult would be expected to have a much higher proportion of nouns than of pronouns in his speech. Goodglass, Quadfasel and Timberlake (1964) preferred a different measure, phrase-length, which could be more readily calculated. They observed that some aphasic speakers never, or rarely, put more than two or three words together, while other speakers characteristically utter phrases of normal length (though not necessarily of non-deviant structure). The distinction broadly aligns with that previously made between expressive and receptive aphasias, but is non-committal about whether there are comprehension difficulties in the one or the other. The group of aphasics with short phrases (the non-fluent) can therefore include people who have comprehension difficulties; whereas the group with normal phrase-length (the fluent) can include people with a mild aphasia or with a recovered non-fluent aphasia who have minimal comprehension difficulties. Although the classification has an inherent attractiveness in its objectivity it is therefore felt by some people that it confuses within the same groups some qualitatively different kinds of disorders. Nevetherless it has received empirical support from a study by Benson (1967). He used fluency ratings devised from Goodglass's study but included an additional cluster of speech characteristics such as the number of words uttered per minute, and confirmed that it was possible to dichotomize the majority of patients into two groups in terms of these speech characteristics. Moreover these two groups could be anatomically distinguished. When brain scans were used to ascertain the approximate size of these lesions, those with non-fluent aphasia were found to have lesions which were anterior to the Rolandic fissure, which separates the frontal lobe from the other lobes of the left hemisphere, while those with fluent aphasia were found to have lesions posterior to this.

A third range of objective measures was used by Howes (1967) with very similar results. From nine measures of the statistical characteristics of aphasic speech and responses to word-association tests he also concluded that there was an essential dichotomy in the aphasias, distinguishing two groups which he labelled Type A and Type B. Type A is characterized by a reduced rate in the emission of words but by relatively normal word associations produced after delay and by a proportionately more frequent use of the common substantive words in the language than occurs in normal speech; these patients can nevertheless make use of some rarer words showing that the normal pattern of word frequency distribution in speech has shifted but has not lost its essential shape. Type B patients retain a normal rate of emitting speech or may show an accelerated one; where word associations are possible, they are bizarre. Howes related these two types of aphasis to two hypothetical mechanisms in speech behaviour. One mechanism—the *alpha system*—receives neurally coded representations of the information a speaker wishes to express, and outputs it in a form which can be used by the speech musculature: words become shaped in their phonic forms and sentences are given structure. The *beta system* provides the neurally coded representations for the alpha system. These coded representations are of anything which can be expressed verbally, i.e. propositions, feelings, memories, attitudes, perceptions and thoughts. From 'the enormous wealth of potential information that can be expressed verbally' the beta system has to select what is necessary for a particular topic and inhibit others. In Type A aphasia it is the alpha system which is damaged, and in Type B the beta. Although Howes derived most of his evidence from taped interviews with some 60 patients, each of about 5,000 words of conversational speech, his division of them into two classes was corroborated by the additional experimental measures he used supplementary to the analysis of this spontaneous speech. In addition to the word-association test which requires aural comprehension, a word-perception test showed that the perceptual thresholds of words were strikingly elevated in Type B patients and also showed great variability, whereas in Type A patients there were only very slight rises in thresholds. Because of the differences in the proportions of the number of patients who had paralysis of arm and limb (70 per cent in Type A and 20 per cent in Type B) and therefore in whom the site of injury probably included the pre-Rolandic area, Howes considered that his evidence supported that of others in indicating that two different areas are implicated in the two types of aphasia. Type A aphasia is associated with an anterior region centred in the third frontal convolution (Broca's area) and Type B with a posterior region centred in the superior temporal convolution (Wernicke's area).

As table 1 shows, this broad division into two types which these objective measures of differences in speech suggested has been further elaborated into some four to seven types of aphasias. These classifications do not divide aphasia along exactly the same lines. Nor is the terminology consistent. Different terms are used for what can be broadly classified as the same syndrome in different classifications (e.g. nominal, amnesic, anomic, semantic aphasia), while the same term can be used to describe different syndromes (e.g. for Wepman and Jones *semantic* corresponds approximately with *anomic*; for Brown it describes disturbances in thought-speech transition at a prior stage to that resulting in anomia; and for Luria it is characterized by a disturbance of the ability to synthesize logical grammatical constructions into a whole). However, types of aphasia in different classifications have a fair degree of uniformity as is indicated in the table by their vertical alignment, although the emphasis given in their descriptions often varies. Hécaen and Dubois have drawn attention in their classification to two types of aphasia which others do not distinguish. The first is the linguistically significant distinction between an expressive aphasia which follows the usual Broca type pattern of impairment in speech both in articulation and grammar, and another type in which grammatical impairment occurs without articulatory difficulties. The second type unique to the French classification is *sensory aphasia with attentional disorganization*. In this syndrome speech is disjointed and characterized by perseverations and reiterations, and, although syntactic structure is apparently preserved, sentences are not completed due to the patient's distractability (Hécaen and Goldblum 1972). In some ways this resembles the syndrome of transcortical sensory aphasia in Goodglass and Kaplan's classification, in the tendency for the patient to echo back what he has just heard.

There are three of these classifications which are of particular relevance to linguistic investigations. One is Luria's, which provided a confirmation for the first application of linguistic theories to the classification of aphasia by Jakobson. Another is that of Goodglass and Kaplan, following Geschwind, the classification used at the Boston Aphasia Research Center which has been used in a large number of linguistic investigations of aphasic disorders in the English language. The third is a classification developed by Brown which relates different types of aphasia to different stages in the microgenesis of language in individual speakers.

Luria (1964; 1966; 1970) has distinguished six main types of aphasia. By a careful mapping of the sites of injury in the wounded soldiers whom he examined and by accompanying these with a detailed examination of their language disorder, he was able to establish with some confidence the correlations between the syndromes he identified and the territory in the brain which had been destroyed. He also distinguished between disorders which were temporary and those which were lasting. The syndrome of *acoustic-agnosic aphasia* (also referred to by L uria as *sensory* aphasia) can be related to a lesion in the upper gyrus of the temporal lobe— the area which has been given the name of Wernicke's area (see figure 1). According to Luria the primary difficulty is in phonemic hearing, i.e. in discriminating speech sounds. There are secondary effects on the system of word meanings; the collection of speech sounds which forms the word becomes vague and undifferentiated. The patient has difficulty in distinguishing syllables or words which sound similar and finds it hard to analyse words into their component sounds or to re-synthesize them. Because of the effect on word meanings he has naming difficulties and cannot be helped by prompting with the initial sound. The second kind of temporal-lobe aphasia occurs with lesions in the middle gyrus, *acoustic-amnesic* aphasia. The most conspicuous feature of this is the inability to retain the meaning of series of words. There is instability of retention of traces, so that one word inhibits the next. These patients, while retaining phonemic hearing, have naming difficulties, particularly with series, but these are different from those of other nominative aphasias, i.e. the visual and the associative (Luria 1976). With lesions in the area where the temporal, parietal and occipital lobes meet, the disturbance of *semantic aphasia* is likely to occur. Phonemic hearing is preserved and so is the understanding of single words. What is disturbed is the system of simultaneous connections that lie beyond the limits of the immediate meaning of the word, and the relationships which words take on when they are associated in phrases and sentences. The significance of a phrase or sentence exceeds the significances of its component words and this kind of patient cannot extract this kind of meaning which depends on simultaneous synthesis. The patient can find it impossible to distinguish between phrases such as 'the wife's uncle' and 'the uncle's wife' because he cannot extract the composite meaning. The same applies even when the relationship is expressed explicitly with a locative preposition or a conjunction: 'The mountain rose above the cloud' cannot be contrasted in meaning with 'The cloud rose above the mountain'. Similarly, comparatives pose particular difficulties because of the need for simultaneity; a question like 'Mary is blonde, Susan is brunette, so who is less fair?' proves impossible to answer.

In none of these three aphasias are there articulation difficulties but these are prominent in two of the motor aphasias, *efferent motor* aphasia and *afferent motor* aphasia. In efferent aphasia there is a pathological inertia in the motor system (referred to by Luria in Pavlovian terminology as the *motor analyzer*). Consequently, the patient has difficulty in initiating speech movements and in the rapid transfer from one articulation to another: a separate effort is required for each sound and the flowing movement of speech is drastically disrupted. At the grammatical level the same difficulty shows itself in the disintegration of the dynamic scheme of the expression as a whole. In afferent motor aphasia, in contrast, there is no primary difficulty in initiating speech but the disorder lies in the kinaesthetic feedback of the motor patterns of speech. Feedback has become diffuse and lost its specificity, so that there is difficulty in assuming the correct positions of articulatory organs. The most conspicuous sign may be that there are substitutions for individual articulemes, for example within /b/ /p/ /m/, sounds which have in common that they require movement of the lips but which also need further differentiation for clarity (in terms of voicing, continuation and nasality). Because reading, writing and auditory comprehension are also dependent on inner speech there are secondary effects on these modalities. The sixth kind of aphasia is given the label *dynamic* because, like efferent aphasia, it is a disorder in the dynamic prcesses of neural excitation. In fact it may be a stage of recovery from efferent aphasia, or an independent form from a more anteriorly placed lesion. The difficulty in initiating and in transitions occurs not at the articulatory level but chiefly at the level of phrases and sentences, so that this kind of patient cannot produce a sequence of sentences to describe episodes in a story. Because of the initiatory difficulty he tends to echo something which another speaker has initiated for him and to resort to habitual phrases. Jakobson's linguistic interpretation of Luria's syndromes is described in chapter 3.

The Boston classification uses a framework of component deficits rather than neurodynamics and the Pavlovian system of analyzers as does Luria's. The areas of deficit are articulation, fluency, word-finding, repetition, seriatim speech, grammar, paraphasia, auditory comprehension, reading and writing. This approach is exemplified in a book by Gardner (1976) on his work at the Boston Aphasia Research Center. He writes (p. 57): 'After my work with nearly two hundred aphasics, bolstered by discussions with colleagues who have together seen several thousand. I can safely affirm that the various language capacities can be and usually are differentially affected in aphasia. It is far more common, that is, to see patients whose ability to speak is significantly more or noticeably less impaired than their ability to comprehend; or whose repetition capacity is significantly superior or inferior to their spontaneous speech; or whose writing is far worse or whose reading is far better than could have been expected in a random distribution of these capacities.' Consequently it is possible to describe the five main syndromes which are distinguished in this classification (excluding the pure one-modality 'aphasias') in terms of a matrix headed by the language behaviours (see table 2).

TABLE 2

*Boston classification of aphasias*
(based on Green 1969a)

| Type of aphasia | Fluency in spontaneous speech | Repetition | Naming | Comprehension |
|---|---|---|---|---|
| Broca's | − | = | = | + |
| Wernicke's | + | − | − | − |
| Conduction | + | − | − | + |
| Anomic | + | + | − | + |
| Isolation syndrome (transcortical sensory) | = | + | − | − |

*Key:*   + intact   − impaired   = limited, in proportion to other impairments

According to Goodglass and Kaplan (1972) the essential characteristics of *Broca's* aphasia, which they equate with Luria's efferent motor aphasia, are awkward articulation, restricted vocabulary, restriction of grammar to the simplest most overlearned forms, and relative preservation of auditory comprehension. Writing is at least as impaired as speech but reading is only mildly affected. In *Wernicke's* aphasia the critical features are impaired auditory comprehension—evident even at the one-word level—and fluently articulated but paraphasic speech, i.e. with an inappropriate use of words (*semantic paraphasia*) and/or with words produced with omitted or missequenced or extraneous or duplicated sounds (*phonemic paraphasia*). The major feature of *anomic* aphasia is word-finding difficulty predominantly for nouns in a context of fluent grammatically well-formed speech with very little paraphasia though some circumlocutions and virtually intact comprehension. The oustanding difficulty in speech is phonemic paraphasia. The *isolation syndrome* is rare and is characterized by the retention of the ability to repeat fluently despite a major loss of other language skills, comprehension, naming and spontaneous propositional speech. If the feature of disproportionate ability in repetition appears together with relatively spared comprehension and with little spontaneous speech the disorder is described as *transcortical motor aphasia* (sometimes equated with Luria's dynamic aphasia).

As in Luria's classification these syndromes are related to lesions in certain areas of the left hemisphere (see figure 1, p. xiii). Anomic aphasia may relate to a recovering or partly damaged Wernicke's area or to damage to the supramarginal gyrus (the 'association area of the association areas' where, Geschwind suggests, occur the abstraction and integration of sensory information which are necessary for naming). Conduction aphasia is attributed to a lesion in the arcuate fasciculus, a tract of fibres which links Broca's area and Wernicke's area. Because each of these two areas is intact, the patient can both speak and understand spoken language, but because information cannot be relayed from one area to the other he cannot repeat what he hears. This anatomical explanation for conduction aphasia has been disputed, as indeed has the validity of singling out repetition as a special performance (Brown 1975a). The concept of disconnection on which the syndrome is based (disconnection of one brain area from another), although it provides a plausible explanation for impairments which affect only one sensory modality (such as alexia), runs into some difficulty within the general syndrome of aphasia if this is thought of as a central disorder which affects, to some degree, all language behaviours. The disconnection of Broca's and Wernicke's areas would not explain the paraphasic difficulties which occur in conduction aphasia nor the influence of different parts of speech on ability to repeat. Freud (1891) argued against the disconnection model which Wernicke proposed and of which Geschwind's model is a revival, on the grounds that it implies brain centres for different activities. Fibres in themselves cannot carry out any modifying activity but simply transfer an identical message from one nerve cell to another, the integration occurring in the areas to which the fibres relay. It has also been pointed out that the arcuate fasciculus consists of short fibres rather than long ones, which implies that the connections it makes may be predominantly cortical-subcortical rather than cortical-cortical. Moreover Pribram's (1971) holograph model of neural action, although speculative, offers an account of how associations may take place within a system rather than through tracts linking systems to systems. Geschwind, however, was careful to point out that he did not wish to imply that there are brain centres for specific language activities, and he proposed that the very simplicity of his model is advantageous in clarifying ideas about aphasia and that in essentials it is supported by anatomical evidence when that can be obtained from post-mortems. Some doubts, however, about the anatomical basis for Broca's aphasia have been expressed by Mohr (1976), as well as for conduction aphasia by Brown, although Whitaker and Selnes (1975) have pointed out that in view of the known anatomic variations in individuals the degree of agreement on localization which has been reported is highly suggestive. Ojemann (1983) has also reported considerable variability in individuals in the cortical locations which evoked changes in naming when electrical stimulation was applied. Stimulation through subdurally implanted electrodes has confirmed that interference with Wernicke's area can be associated with impaired comprehension, but also results in an arrest of speech which varies between patients (Lesser, Lüders, Morris, Dinner, Klem, Hahn and Harrison, 1986). The studies of blood flow referred to earlier have shown metabolic activity during language processing in brain areas not associated with language in Geschwind's model, i.e. the right hemipshere and superior aspects of the frontal lobe.

Brown (1975b) in a development of the ideas expressed in his book in 1972 conceives of aphasic syndromes as representing breakdowns at different stages of the microgenesis of language in normal speakers. He accepts the broad distinction between anterior and posterior aphasias. His conceptualization is that in the early stages of language organization bilateral brain structures are involved: unilateral structures and increasing specificity of certain structures within the left hemisphere become more important as the genesis of language progresses from deep to surface levels. In the anterior disorders these stages of progression from bilateral to specialized unilateral functions are revealed in mutism (at the deepest level), transcortical motor aphasia, agrammatism and finally anarthric (Broca's) aphasia. Like Hécaen, therefore, Brown makes a distinction between disturbances of grammatical and articulatory organization. In the posterior disorders, the deepest level of language, semantic evocation, is disturbed in three kinds of semantic disorders, all of which are frequently associated with bilateral pathology. They are *semantic aphasia*, characterized by circumlocutory tangential speech; *speech paraphasia*, characterized by difficulties in referential naming; and *semantic jargon*, which displays both features. After the developing linguistic content has more or less successfully traversed this semantic stage, a disruption produces either nominal disorders or phonemic disorders at further stages. Within the nominal disorders, verbal paraphasias may be produced—i.e. within-category misnamings such as 'red' for 'green'—or there may be blockage of these incorrect responses and hence failure to produce the name, as in anomia. After the lexical item has been correctly selected, a disruption at the stage of phonemic formulation results in the phonemic paraphasias of conduction aphasia.

The majority of the linguistic investigations of aphasia (involving more than one subject) have used, as reference, one of the classifications of aphasia given in table 1. But, apart from the objective classification into fluent and non-fluent, which as we have seen has inherent limitations, it would be a mistake to give the impression that these syndromes are easily recognized in a clinical population.

Despite the fact that research studies often report that groups were used which comprised numbers of certain types of aphasics (perhaps ten Broca's, ten Wernicke's and ten conduction aphasics were compared) the speech therapist in clinical practice seems to have considerably more difficulty in coming across clear-cut cases of these syndromes. Her patients with repetition difficulties are perhaps not fluent enough for them to fit into the conduction syndrome. Other patients with what might approach a Broca's aphasia are discovered to have considerable difficulty on a test of auditory comprehension like the Token Test (De Renzi and Vignolo, 1962) although their everyday comprehension would not have led this to be suspected. Other patients with comprehension deficits do not qualify as Wernicke's aphasics because their speech though occurring in fluent bursts does show some signs of articulation difficulties, a condition which according to the old textbooks just should not occur. Over and over again the therapist is obliged to classify her patients as 'mixed' or to make more compromises than is desirable.

Nor is it possible to turn to the formal assessments of aphasia for objective confirmation of the placement of a patient into a category. Of those classifications which are specifically related to formal tests, Schuell's classification does not offer dimensions within the aphasias, but only makes the practical distinction of aphasia with or without different accompanying deficits. Wepman and Jones's battery requires categorical scoring judgements from the examiner about the nature of the responses so that a patient can only be categorized as 'syntactic', 'pragmatic' etc. if the examiner has already decided that he is making 'syntactic', 'pragmatic' etc. types of responses. The Boston Diagnostic Aphasia Examination makes the placement of patients into diagnostic categories one of its principal aims. However, even here, it is notable that despite the sophisticated nature of the test, the placement of a patient into a category is based not primarily on test results but on the subjective ratings of six features of his spontaneous speech together with one objective measure, that is, his score on the subtests of auditory comprehension. As Goodglass and Kaplan admit (1972, p. 2): "The scores do not objectively and automatically classify the patient nor point to the optimum approach to therapy. The greater the experience of the examiner, the more useful the interpretations that can be made from the test record". The Western Aphasia Battery attempted to rescue the test from the first criticism, by tabulating the scores in such a way that every patient is forced into a category, although still retaining an element of subjectiveness in the qualitative scoring of elicited connected speech. The German Aachen Aphasia Test (Willmes, Poeck, Weniger and Huber, 1983) has tackled the problem in a different way by computerising the results so that the statistical probability of the patient's falling within a certain syndrome can be read out.

The real stumbling-block, however, is that every battery for aphasia necessarily reflects the theoretical preconceptions of its authors, and that all current batteries are based on the preconception that the medical notion of a syndrome is valid for aphasia. With the rise of a specialism stemming from a psychological rather than a medical root, i.e. cognitive neuropsychology, this notion has come under serious criticism. The arguments against using syndromes to cluster the symptoms of brain-damaged people are summarized in Ellis (1987). The cognitive neuropsychological proposal is that mental processes are organized in cognitively distinct modules, forming a 'functional architecture' which is generally illustrated in the form of boxes connected by arrows. It is argued that modular organization is an efficient method for the brain's structuring of mental activity, and that these independent but co-operating modules can be selectively put out of action. A currently proposed architecture is described in Chapter 9, but here it is sufficient to note how this observation has been used to argue against syndromes. Models of aphasia at the end of the last century also used boxes and arrows, but these boxes had labels like 'comprehension' and 'speech', and the allied syndromes were 'sensory' and 'motor'. Drawing partly on linguistic theory, cognitive neuropsychology has split these modules into a variety of components, and will continue to do so as new patients are studied who show disturbances which do not accommodate themselves to the proposed architecture. One solution would be to continually refine syndromes into subsets of syndromes, which then become syndromes in their own right, which are further divided as knowledge increases. As Ellis points out, this is a *reductio ad absurdam*, as pure cases of each sub-type will become progressively harder to find. Present-day syndromes are polytypic; they list a number of behaviours some of which, but not all, are associated with each patient included in the syndrome. Each person labelled as having Broca's aphasia, therefore, may differ in important ways from all other patients with this label. As Ellis writes, therefore (p. 404): 'It has not proved possible to give a unified account of *any* of the putative syndromes thus far identified'. The only viable alternative, he argues, is to study each aphasic patient in detail, in order to give as precise a description as possible of the patient's symptons, and evaluate the implication of the results of this investigation for the theoretical understanding of language processing.

The conventional classifications of aphasia may have a limited use, in areas where patients need to be grouped by some standard, such as gross approximation of syndrome with anatomical lesion site. In their implications for theory-based rehabilitation they have much less potential for the speech therapist than does the cognitive neuropsychological approach. Indeed, even advocates of syndrome classification, Goodglass and Kaplan (1972) and Duffy and Ulrich (1976), have pointed out that, in speech therapy clinics, the selectively impaired patients in whom distinct symptoms are clear enough to be recognized are far outnumbered by patients with extensive lesions in whom differences in symptoms are masked by severity.

It is essential to make distinctions by which aphasia can be analysed, but the analysis is limited by the distinctions it can make. It is clear that, if each patient's symptoms are to be precisely described, a solely behavioural framework is grossly inadequate. The linguistic framework which underpins the newer methods of analysis, including the cognitive neuropsychological, is described in the next chapters. After discussions of how the linguistic levels of lexical semantics, syntax and phonology have been applied to the study of aphasia, the analysis is extended to the supra-sentence level of discourse and conversation, with examples of how this aspect of linguistics is also providing insights into the nature of aphasia.

# 2

# Linguistics and aphasia

Although the systematic study of aphasia began over a century ago, it is only relatively recently that it was first formally proposed that linguistics was the appropriate discipline within which this study should be undertaken.

Before the 1950s a few eminent doctors had acknowledged the potential usefulness of linguistics in investigations of aphasia—Luria in 1947, Goldstein in 1948, Grewel in 1949, Ombredane in 1951—and one major study of phonetic disintegration in aphasia had been undertaken by two doctors working with a linguist, Alajouanine, Ombredane and Durand in 1939. From the other side, two forefathers of modern linguistics, de Courtenay in 1885 and de Saussure two decades later, had suggested that a study of the genesis and pathology of language could be rewarding for linguistic theory. But the beginning of the current era of interest in aphasia for its own sake can probably be dated from the formal proposal of the linguist Roman Jakobson (1955) that, as aphasia is a disorder of language, its study should be a matter for the discipline which concerns itself with language, linguistics. More recently Jakobson has written: 'Aphasia is first and foremost a disintegration of language and as linguists deal with language it is linguists who have to tell us what the exact nature of these diverse disintegrations is' (in press).

Jakobson's proposal fell at first on unreceptive ears in the linguistic schools. In 1963 Osgood and Miron reported that he was still the 'only linguist who has written at all systematically about aphasic phenomena'. One reason why Jakobson's proposal did not spark off immediate interest (and this lies more in circumstance than in intention) is that barriers have existed between professions. Because 'brain damage' is a necessary part of its definition, aphasia is a medical term. Brain damage almost invariably produces other neurological symptoms besides the aphasia which can result, and there are not only other cognitive changes but conspicuous physical ones. Aphasia is often accompanied by hemiplegia and hemianaesthesia (paralysis and loss of sensation of the limbs on one side of the body). Sometimes there is a visual field defect obliterating vision of what the patient should see on the right side of his environment (hemianopia). The damage which has instigated the aphasia often has persisting correlates—high blood pressure, diabetes, epilepsy, heart disorders. Although aphasia may be a linguistic problem, the aphasic patient is a medical problem.

The result is that many of the early studies of aphasia by linguists were either undertaken from reported data (as was Jakobson's) or were investigations of only one or two patients to whom a sympathetic therapist had given them access. Consequently the first patients studied by linguists were not representative of the average clinical population. They tended to be more robust, better educated, less severely impaired and more likely to produce a sufficient flow of speech to provide the linguist with adequate material for analysis.

There is a second reason for the dilatory response of linguists to Jakobson's appeal: we must recognize the relative remoteness of abnormal language at this time from the principal interests of most linguists. Whereas in the linguistic analysis of 'a language' a single speaker's behaviour is of little consequence, in the study of abnormal language individual differences are emphasized. It is therefore necessary, for the productive examination of abnormal language and its possible amelioration, to conceive of linguistic systems in terms which can be translated into psychologically real mental processes which operate in the individual speaker. When Jakobson wrote, the main constructive proposals that had been made in this direction were those of de Saussure in the early decades of the century. But although de Saussure emphasized that language must be related to brain, the insights into language organization that he provided have been used, by Jakobson and Sabouraud, to provide not so much models of language processes which might be disordered in aphasia but the general principles on which such models might be constructed. One of these principles was the distinction between the abstraction of 'a language' (*langue*), the common system deducible from all its speakers, and the act of speaking by individuals, which is what the linguist actually observes (*parole*); the distinction is similar in essence to that between *competence* and *performance* made later by Chomsky (see chapter 3) which has been one focus of interest in aphasiology. A second principle of de Saussure's was that language can be dissected along two axes, *successivity* (the *syntagmatic* axis) and *simultaneity* (the *associative* axis, later called by Hjelmslev the *paradigmatic* axis to avoid the ambiguity which 'associative' had acquired). It was this principle which Jakobson made the foundation for the first linguistic typology of the aphasias (see chapter 3).

But it was not until the first formulation of generative transformational grammar by Chomsky in 1957 and its revision in 1965 that there was an upsurge of interest in what could for the first time be presented as a possible psychology of language as a mental process. This model of language was couched in detailed enough terms to make it possible to test out the extent to which a linguistic grammar was a 'mental grammar', engendering so much experimentation that a new discipline of *psycholinguistics* evolved. As it turned out, in many respects these standard and extended transformational grammars have proved to be inadequate explanations for what people do in psycholinguistic experiments (see Greene 1972 for a review). Nevertheless the hunt for an acceptable model of the mental organization of language is on and aphasia is playing an increasingly important part in this search. Interest has also been renewed in how far the facets of such a mental organization as can be pieced together will prove to be related to brain organization, resulting in a new body of study under the rubric of *neurolinguistics*. At the present time, neurolinguistics, in the Western world (though less so in Eastern Europe), has been almost entirely concerned with the anatomical correlates of language and the localization of its systems in the brain, rather than with its possible physiological and dynamic correlates (Lenneberg, 1973, 1975, provided an exception). Though neurolinguistics derives some of its data from a variety of sources (e.g. electrical stimulation of the brain, event-related potentials, dichotic listening, hemifield viewing, studies of patients with the two hemispheres surgically separated) its major source of localizing information is aphasia. The increasing interest of some linguists in the psychology of language in individuals has therefore met up with an increasing recognition by some neurologists that linguistic science can make an indispensible contribution to the study of mental and brain processes.

At present, therefore, the situation between linguistics and aphasiology is not so much that linguistics has included the study of disordered language after brain damage within its scope, as Jakobson's proposal seemed to invite: nor is it correct to represent linguistics as entering the hospitals like a Florence Nightingale with a light, bringing order into confusion. A more realistic picture of the situation today would show the development of communication amongst the several disciplines concerned with the study of aphasia. Over the last decade two multidisciplinary centres have established international reputations (and there may be others which are equally advanced though less well known). At the Centre for Neuropsychological and Neurolinguistic Research in Paris and the Aphasia Research Center in Boston, linguistic theories have been blended with neurological skills and psychological techniques. These multidisciplinary centres are associated with hospitals in city conurbations where a large number of patients can be drawn upon for the experimental application of linguistic theories. From many other clinics in various parts of the world, important linguistically-orientated studies have been published in international English-language journals or books in addition to the USA and France, notably Belgium, Britain, Canada, East Germany, Italy, Japan, Poland, Romania, Russia, South Africa and West Germany. In Britain the importance of linguistics in the study and treatment of language disorders has been recently acknowledged by its compulsory inclusion in the training of speech therapists and by the setting up of a qualifying undergraduate course for speech therapists within a university department of linguistics. Although in many countries, even in advanced ones, there is still no provision for organized aphasia therapy or for the training of therapists, in those countries where aphasiology has developed, there has been the increasing recognition of the importance of linguistics which Jakobson and his predecessors envisaged.

## Linguistic approaches

What, then, is this 'linguistically-orientated approach'? It would be more accurate to refer to linguistically-orientated approaches, for, as with aphasiology, linguistics is an umbrella term for a collection of related and developing theories. It also shares with aphasiology a certain lack of common agreement about terminology (though fortunately not quite to the same extent), and it is therefore often a wise precaution to define the particular way in which a term is used. In part the linguistically-orientated approach has consisted of picking up some particular theory from pure linguistics and looking for evidence in the speech of an aphasic speaker that the distinctions it makes do correspond with differences in difficulty for him. If this was all that had been done, the influence of linguistics on aphasia would have been limited to infiltration rather than revolution. But in fact linguistics has achieved a revolution in aphasiology in two unobtrusive ways.

The first one is through an idea which seems so simple that it is hard to remember that it has not always been obvious: it is that language is not a uniform mass from which any one sample is as good as any other of the same size (size being reducible to the single dimension of temporal length). It is still not unknown in psychological experiments concerned with mental operations for material to be classed as *non-verbal* or *verbal* and for generalizations to be made about language regardless of the particular nature of the verbal material used. But the most elementary acquaintance with linguistics makes it clear that language differs along other dimensions besides length, and that even adding frequency of usage and part of speech as other variables to be controlled comes nowhere near to accounting fully for differences in language. Language (according to most current theories) has structure, a structure which is probably hierarchical in nature, and from this structure systems can be derived in terms of basic but abstract units (some of which will be described shortly, such as distinctive features, phonemes, and morphemes). Many linguistic theories therefore offer quite complicated systems in terms of which language can be analysed. The linguistically-oriented student of aphasia would not be satisfied with a statement such as 'This patient has difficulty in repetition' or 'This patient has reading problems' but would wish to analyse the difficulties in terms of the structures and systemic features which were disrupted or retained. For example in assessing difficulties in repetition it is not sufficient to devise a set of sentences of increasing length so as to be able to say that a patient could not cope with sentences of so many letters, syllables or words in length. Whitaker and Whitaker (1972) took some sentences for repetition from a modified version of the Minnesota Test for the Differential Diagnosis for Aphasia, of which two were

(1)  I ordered a ham sandwich, a glass of milk, and a piece of apple pie.
(2)  The office is on the twenty-fourth floor of the Merchant's Bank Building.

They pointed out that linguistically these two sentences make quite different demands on the language mechanism. The first sentence has a coordinated structure, and is analogous to three separate propositions concatenated together— 'I ordered a ham sandwich, I ordered a glass of milk, I ordered a piece of apple pie.' The second sentence, in contrast, is relativized. It too consists of a set of propositions—'The office is on the floor, the floor is the twenty-fourth, the floor is part of the building, the building is a bank, the bank is named Merchant'—but these propositions are not presented as a coordinated list but as an integrated structure in which some parts are subordinate to others. Although on a simple count of letters, syllables or words the two sentences are not dissimilar, the second sentence is structurally more complex. Some aphasic patients, who are assisted by the integration of propositions into a unified structure, find the second sentence easier to repeat than the first; a smaller number of aphasic patients, perhaps because they have less difficulty in coping with a chain sequence but more with coding structure, find the first sentence easier to repeat than the second. A simple comparison of sentences for repetition in terms of some measure of length therefore fails to reveal the possibility that there may be two different brain mechanisms underlying the processing of the different sentence types of coordination and relativization. Language samples of the same size, in fact, are usually far from homogeneous.

The second major contribution from linguistics follows from the first and is also one which it is by now easy to take for granted. It is the idea that language can be described in terms of different levels of organization. It is through these levels that linguistics provides a basic framework for the analysis of language which cuts across the conventional one outlined in chapter 1 of behaviours in the modalities, and which opens the way for the analysis of aphasia as a central disorder rather than as a disorder of contrasting behaviour in modalities of language use. The number of linguistic levels which are distinguished varies according to the theory: but it is common practice to make a working distinction of three main levels. The separation of these levels has sometimes been objected to as a misleading avoidance of the complexities of the interwoven fabric of language, but nevertheless (on the old principle of divide and conquer) this notion of separable levels is proving a productive one in aphasiology, and it has even been claimed that there is evidence for the empirical validity of their separation in brain mechanisms (some of this evidence is outlined at the end of this chapter). These three main levels are the level of the system of the sounds of speech (phonology), the level of the structural arrangement of sentences (syntax) and the level of the system of meaning (semantics). In this book, as is more usual in aphasiology, the term *syntax* will be used to include morphology as well as sentence structure (see below), though for this combined study some linguists prefer the term *grammar* (others include in grammar an entire description of a language). In the account given below of the three levels, a much simplified version is given of some ideas from linguistics as they have been adapted in the study of aphasia. What follows is therefore not a 'potted' general account of linguistics, but some highly selected extracts as modified for practical use by some aphasiologists. For those who wish to put these extracts in the perspective of a general account of linguistics, several introductions are available (for example Lyons 1969; Crystal 1971).

The subdivisions which have been made in the linguistic levels may therefore be described as follows. Descriptions of the sounds used in language can be made either in terms of articulatory or acoustic events (phonetics) or in terms of the system and distribution of the sounds (phonemics): they can also be described in terms of suprasegmental features—intonation, stress, rhythm, juncture, etc., for which Monrad-Krohn (1947b) suggested the term *prosody* was preferable to the then current term in neurology of 'speech melody'. Syntactic descriptions sometimes focus on structure, sometimes on morphology, the realization of this structure through grammatical inflections. Within semantics there are two kinds of descriptions, those which describe the meaning relations amongst individual words in the vocabulary or lexicon (lexical-semantics or paradigmatic sense relations) and those which describe the meaning relationships amongst words in sentences (syntagmatic sense relations). The division between these two kinds of description is essentially one of convenience rather than necessarily reflecting a natural division of language. So little is known about the organization of meaning that it is convenient to simplify the problem by studying it first through the relationship of words considered in isolation from the context in which they occur in natural situations.

The table below summarizes the divisions in language which have been applied

TABLE 3

*Some linguistic divisions as used in the analysis of aphasic language*

| Level | Description | Examples of terms |
|---|---|---|
| Phonology | Prosodic | Intonation, Stress |
| | Phonetic | Aspiration, Fronting |
| | Phonemic | Distinctive features |
| Syntax (grammar) | Morphemic | Inflections |
| | Syntactic structure (surface) | Noun phrase, Verb, Clause |
| | Transformation | Passive, Interrogative |
| | Syntactic structure (deep) | Subject, Object |
| | Case relations/ Deep relations | Agent, Instrument, Functions |
| Semantics | Syntagmatic sense relations | Selectional restrictions Collocational restrictions |
| | Paradigmatic sense relations (lexical-semantics) | Fields, Features, Networks |
| Communication | Discourse (structure and sense relationships across sentences) | Intersentential anaphoric pronouns, Presuppositions |
| | Verbal structure of communication | Assertion, Stream analysis Support elements |
| | Non-verbal communication | Kinesics, Proxemics, Eye-contact, Social role |

or are being applied in the analysis of aphasic language. In addition to the three main levels which have been the central focus of linguistics, and which are to be discussed below, it includes a fourth area of language to which linguistics has only recently turned its attention, the study of communicative exchanges in their social setting. This includes the linguistic analysis of meaning relationships across sentences, analysis of the elements in conversations between two or more people, and the quantification of the non-verbal behaviours which accompany language. It is an area of particular concern to aphasiology because it leads to the question of the functional use of language, which is the ultimate standard by which an aphasic patient's recovery is measured. To date, however, there have been but few sporadic forays into it as an area of scientific investigation for aphasia.

## Phonology

Phonology is the description of the systems and patterns of sounds that occur in a language. There are two basic approaches in phonology—structuralist phonemics and generative phonology—and of these structuralist phonemics has been more applied in investigations of aphasia and will be outlined before the generative approach. It is first necessary to distinguish phonetic and phonemic descriptions of speech.

Phonetic descriptions are in terms of the elementary components of speech sounds without reference to meaning, and (except in the branch of phonetics which deals with acoustics) the terms describe articulatory or auditory rather than acoustic events. A phonemic description, on the other hand, applies the concept of a system of simultaneous combinations of phonetic features into phonemes which are capable of changing meaning in words. According to one theory phonemes are not so much classes of speech sounds which share common phonetic features, but are abstractions which exist only in terms of oppositions of distinctive features rather than themselves having any physical reality. We shall return to this question of distinctive features shortly; for the moment it is more convenient to assume for the purposes of analysing aphasic language that the phoneme has a physical reality as a class of sounds. Languages have their own individual systems of, usually, thirty to forty phonemes, and these systems only partly coincide across languages. Each phoneme has phonetic variations in its realization in speech which do not change meaning (allophones). For example the initial clear "l" in 'lead' is phonetically distinct from the final dark 'l' in 'deal', though both are identified as the same phoneme. Such details of pronunciation are predictable by phonological rules and can often be omitted in making transcriptions of speech—such transcriptions are known as *broad* transcriptions while ones in which these details are included are called *narrow* transcriptions. It is customary for phonetic transcriptions to be written in square brackets, and for phonemic transcriptions to be written between slashes; so a phonetic transcription of 'deal' is [dił] and a phonemic transcription is /dil/. Distinctions which are phonemic in one language, as between /s/ and /z/ in English, may be allophonic variations in another, as in Spanish where using the unvoiced fricative in some words does not change meaning but simply makes the word sound rather odd.

The phonetic–phonemic distinction (which has incidentally acted as a master model for a whole lot of other *etic/emic* distinctions in language) has been fruitfully applied in the description of aphasic speech and in demarcating aphasic syndromes. Some Broca's aphasics are said to evidence what Alajouanine, Ombredane and Durand in 1939 called *phonetic disintegration* (Lecours and Lhermitte 1966; Poncet, Degos, Deloche and Lecours 1972), an articulatory failure to realize the sounds of speech with the correct precision needed of tongue and mouth movements. On the other hand the kind of fluent speech which is characterized by phonemic (literal) paraphasias shows intact phonetic realization of each phoneme but misplanning of the patterning or selection of phonemes in a word or combination of words. Unfortunately this neat differentiation between phonetic and phonemic deviations in aphasic speech is complicated by two facts. Firstly, deviations which may be articulatory in nature can distort the realization of the phoneme in such a way that it is recognized by a hearer as a different phoneme, e.g. /daɪd/ *died* as /taɪt/ *tight*, the kind of phenomenon by which phonemic paraphasia is defined. Secondly Broca's aphasia (unlike dysarthria) seems to be characterized by 'genuine' phonemic disorders of patterning as well as by phonetic distortions. This topic is discussed in chapter 8. In practice, therefore, *phonetic disintegration* includes phonemic paraphasias, although phonemic paraphasias often occur in other speakers without evidence of phonetic disintegration.

When we describe aphasic errors in terms of the mispatternings of phonemes we are implicitly accepting the view that phonemes have some psychological reality, and are real elements in the planning of utterances. But it has also been proposed (by the group of linguists who formed the Prague School in the 1920s and 1930s) that phonemes are not themselves real or absolute units but that they exist only in terms of oppositions of distinctive features: it is the difference between *pin* and *bin* which is part of the network of relationships in the sound-system of English, rather than the entities *p* and *b* in isolation. The difference can be described in terms of binary contrasts and it was proposed at one stage that there were twelve which could be derived from acoustic analysis by spectrogram. Some were contrasts of sonority (e.g. vocalic/non-vocalic), others of protensity (tense/lax) and others of tonality (e.g. grave/acute).

The extended system of distinctive features which have been proposed in generative phonology, however, includes besides the major class features of sonorant/non-sonorant and vocalic/non-vocalic, articulatory cavity features (such as coronal/non-coronal, anterior/non-anterior), features of manner of articulation (such as continuant/non-continuant, tense/lax) and source features (voiced/voiceless, strident/mellow). It is this formulation of distinctive features which has been used in the analysis of aphasic speech by Blumstein (1973) and Martin and Rigrodsky (1974).

In generative phonology it is postulated that abstract phonemic sequences are mapped onto phonetic sequences by a set of transformational rules which change features within segments. For example a final /t/ in a word like *digest* becomes /ʧ/ in *digestion*. Although both phonemic and phonetic segments can be defined in terms of distinctive features, it is only at the phonetic level that these features represent the acoustic and articulatory aspects of speech sounds: at the phonemic level, because they are abstract, they are free from any such constraints. Because transformations mediate between the abstract level and the articulatory level, the distinctive feature values of the two levels do not need to be the same, and categorizations can be proposed at the phonemic level which do not need to take articulatory possibilities into consideration. Fodor, Bever and Garrett (1974) give as illustration of this the classification of /r/ and /l/ as both consonant and vowel at the systematic phonemic level, although by articulatory criteria of degree of constriction of the air-stream they are consonantal. At the systematic phonemic level these two function as consonants in that they can stand alone with a vowel to form a syllable, while true vowels cannot; yet they also function as vowels in that they can follow two consonants (e.g. in *straw* and *splash*). Aphasia has been used as a testing-ground for the reality of the systematic phonemic level and the transformational rules proposed in generative phonology: Schnitzer (1971) has concluded from the misreadings of an aphasic woman that many of the transformations and derivational rules proposed in generative phonology can be considered to have psychological validity (see chapter 8).

Walsh (1974) has pointed out certain practical difficulties in using, in speech pathology, systems of distinctive features which are based on acoustic properties derived from spectrograms and which are motivated by linguists' concern for notational economy. For example, the concern with using a binary notation to express opposition means that place of articulation, which is organically linear from lips to tongue tip and tongue back, has to be divided up arbitrarily (in one system of distinctive features), with /p/ and /t/ sometimes aligned together as diffuse in contrast to /k/ as grave, or with /p/ and /k/ sometimes aligned together as grave in contrast to /t/ as acute. Nevertheless, a notation based on subphonemic features is preferable to one which trivially enumerates misarticulated phonemes and Walsh has proposed that for speech pathology a system would be more useful which is based entirely on articulation. The one he proposes distinguishes vocal tract configuration features, lower and upper consonant placement features, tongue positions for vowels, manner of release and supplementary features such as voice, aspiration, and lip rounding. Features based on articulation provide a better account of misarticulations: substitution of /j/ (pronounced as 'y') for /l/ may then be explained as retracted articulation rendering a lateral release impossible, or of /θ/ ('th') for /s/ as a forward shift in articulation impeding the production of sibilance. In France, the scheme of distinctive features used by Lecours and Lhermitte (1969) in their analyses of phonemic paraphasias in aphasia is based entirely on articulatory features (see chapter 8). When distinctive features have been used in the examination of the ability of aphasic patients to make auditory phonemic discriminations in listening, a simple scheme has been used for English consonants which also does not emphasize binary oppositions but has reverted to the earlier terminology of phonetics. It distinguishes manner of articulation, place of articulation and presence or absence of voicing.

There is another sublevel of phonology which is acknowledged as of some interest in the study of aphasia, and that is the analysis of language in suprasegmental terms rather than in phonemic segments. In fact language is still described in terms of segments, but these segments are the large ones of tone-groups in which the intonation pattern changes and one element receives major stress. It is a part of language which has received less attention in linguistic theories than have other units of analysis, perhaps because it is the part which we are used to missing out when we write language down, or representing inadequately in terms of commas, question marks and so on. Recent discussions of prosody, and of intonation in particular, include those of Crystal (1969; 1975). Disturbance of 'melodic line' is one of the identifying features of Broca's aphasia in the Boston classification, and Goodglass and his colleagues have drawn attention particularly to the importance of stress in agrammatic aphasia as part of their construct of *saliency* (see chapter 8). However, although agrammatic patients typically speak in short phrases of one or two words in length, thus giving little scope for the exercise of the normal tone-group patterns of the language, the emotional use of intonation within the units they produce is usually not impaired. Patients who are without functional speech, whose repertoire consists of repeated stereotypes or of vocal gestures, often become skilled in using them with a range of different intonation patterns to communicate. One explanation which has been suggested for this retention of the use of intonation to express emotion is that the intact right hemisphere may be dominant for musical abilities. However, the relationship between musical abilities and prosody is complicated. Monrad-Krohn (1963) has commented that people can demonstrate a profound dysprosody in fluent speech after cerebral injury, and yet retain their musical faculties. Similarly, and more easily observed, is the ability which unmusical people can have to express themselves in prosodically rich language. An experimental study has shown that changes of pitch which affect meaning, as in the tone-language of Thai, are processed by the left, language-dominant hemisphere, rather than by the right, perhaps music-dominant, hemisphere (Van Lanckner and Fromkin 1973). Yet a system of therapy is being developed, called *Melodic Intonation Therapy*, which assists the severely aphasic patient to recover some speech by getting him to intone phrases and then weaning him away from melody to speech only (Sparks, Helm and Albert 1973; Sparks and Holland 1976). To some extent, therefore, melody and speech intonation patterns seem to be able to act as releasers for other aspects of language, even in patients who have suffered major damage to the language zone of the left hemisphere.

Monrad-Krohn considers that on the whole dysprosody is rare in (fluent) aphasia, but such a comment relates to an *etic* concept of prosody as related to articulatory performance rather than to the linguistically structured notions of tone-group, tonicity etc. It may be particularly crucial also, however, to discover how much an individual patient relies on intonation in auditory comprehension, a task which necessarily poses *emic* problems. There is a growing interest in the difficulties that patients have in the speed of comprehension and the rate at which they can process auditory information. But if severely handicapped patients rely more than most on intonation patterns for delimiting the units in which they process language and for grasping meaning, it may be that some kinds of sloweddown speech can add to their difficulties rather than assist them, if these critical tone-group patterns have become distorted.

## Syntax

At the syntactic level, the earliest descriptions of aphasic speech have been in terms of parts of speech or of morphological inflections rather than of structure. Morphology, as a linguistic term, concerns the study of morphemes, the smallest unit of language capable of carrying meaning. Morphemes may be either free, i.e. standing on their own as words such as *hat* and *go*, or bound, i.e. always occurring in conjunction with another morpheme. For example there is a bound plural morpheme which can be realized phonologically as one of several allomorphs, /s/ in *hats*, /z/ in *boys*, /ız/ in *boxes*, as well as a vowel change in *men*, *mice* etc. The morpheme is therefore the smallest unit of syntactic analysis, as in the examples just given where the distinction is between singular and plural. Descriptions of aphasia in terms of parts of speech have usually made a broad distinction between *substantive words* (nouns, verbs, adjectives, adverbs) and *grammatical words*. These latter have also been called function words, form words, functors, operators, interstitial words, or filler words, and include prepositions, verb auxiliaries (*is, can, did, has*, etc.) and articles (*a, the, that*, etc.). There is some empirical justification for classing inflections and grammatical words together in that many languages use inflections to denote the relationships which other languages expand into separate grammatical words; it seems possible, therefore, that both may prove to be linked in psychological models of language. At all events descriptions of aphasic syndromes associate the reduction or preservation of use of inflections with similar behaviour with grammatical words. However, grammatical words form a heterogeneous class which cannot always be assumed to use the same mechanisms. For example pronouns are often classed as grammatical words, though the case could be made that anaphoric pronouns (ones which refer back to a previously named item), when used intersententially, are features which are essentially dependent on discourse rather than on sentence as are most other grammatical words. On similar grounds a distinction would be justified between one use of the definite article *the*, where the item has already been referred to and the indefinite articles *a, an*, where the item is introduced for the first time.

In syntax, as in phonology, there are two main linguistic approaches: the generative transformational grammars, which attempt to explain the non-finite nature of language in terms of a finite set of rules, and the non-generative which, although also departing from the structuralist tradition in many ways, retain its empirical emphasis on the description of structure. One such non-generative grammar which has been used as the reference for the analysis of aphasic language is the *Grammar of Contemporary English* of Quirk, Greenbaum, Leech and Svartvik (1972), which describes the grammar used in 'educated English current in the second half of the twentieth century in the world's majcr English-speaking communities'. Because generative transformational grammars have aimed at being explanatory as well as descriptive they have stimulated hypotheses about the mental organization underlying language (even though such grammars were designed as grammars of competence rather than of language use); they have therefore had a greater appeal in aphasiology, and the discussion below relates primarily to them. But, also because in many respects these hypotheses have proved misleading, many aphasiologists have fallen back upon the classical terminology of schoolbook grammars, without relating their investigations to any specific linguistic theory of syntax.

A key notion in most formulations of syntax, generative as well as non-generative, is that sentences are not composed simply of strings of elements which have a chain relationship with each other, but that they are made up of layers of constituents which form groups. The grammar of Quirk and his colleagues, as well as that of another British linguist, Halliday (Halliday's Systemic Grammar (Muir 1972)), uses as units sentences, clauses, phrases and words. Generative transformational grammars use phrases as the first constituents of sentences and frequently employ *tree-diagrams* to express the relationships amongst elements in a sentence. For example the tree-diagram for the sentence 'Britain faces new crisis' would be represented as

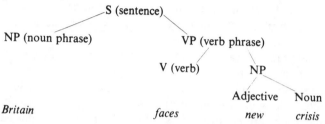

The phrase structure demonstrates that there are more intimate links between *new* and *crisis* than between *new* and *faces*. In aphasia research the hypothesis has been tested that agrammatic subjects should find it harder to bridge breaks between the higher constituents of a structure (as between NP and VP) than between words at a lower level (as between adjective and noun) (see chapter 7). Older grammatical terminology would use the terms *subject* and *predicate* as the highest level constituents of the sentence. The construct of transformations in generative grammars allows for the description of the relationship between such sentences as *The union is calling out the miners* and *The miners are called out by the union*. Although they have different surface structures it is proposed that they derive from the same deep structure, through different transformations. Transformations have a further explanatory value. They account for the fact that some sentences which have the same surface structure (and which would therefore not be distinguished by a simple tree-diagram) are in fact derived from different base structures. Chomsky's oft-quoted example is *John is easy to please* and *John is eager to please*. In the first case John is in the passive role, and contained in the deep structure must be the elements 'Someone pleases John', while in the second case John is in the active role and the deep structure must contain the elements for 'John pleases someone'. The notion of deep and surface levels of structure therefore appears to have some explanatory value for intuitions about language.

Transformational grammar gives a centrality to syntax which has been disputed by some theorists. In transformational grammar the syntactic component provides the input for the semantic component which specifies the meaning, and for the phonological component which specifies the sound; hence this grammar has acquired the label *interpretive*, as the semantic component provides the interpretation for the syntactic. An alternative conceptualization proposes that it is the semantic component which is generative rather than the syntactic. The critical issue is the extent to which deep structure is conceived of as being syntactic or semantic. Advocates of the theory known as Generative Semantics have suggested that to have a deep semantic level and a deep syntactic level is an unnecessary duplication, especially if it is admitted (Chomsky 1965) that the deep syntactic level does not have an ordered structure which can be expressed in terms of an active sentence. Fillmore (1968) also observed that the roles of subject and object which form key elements in the conceptualization of deep structure are not in fact adequate representations of grammatical roles at this level. The surface structure role of the subject can be related at the deep level to a number of different *cases*, such as Agent, Instrument, Recipient, Goal, and even Object. For example in

John opened the door

the surface subject is in the agentive case; in

The key opened the door

it is instrumental; while in

The door opened

it is objective. These case roles in deep structure remain constant whatever changes we make in the surface structure of the sentence and the criteria by which they are distinguished are more easily classed as semantic than syntactic.

The weaknesses of case grammar have recently been pointed out by, amongst others, Palmer (1976). He draws attention, for example, to the blurring of the case relations of agent and instrument in 'The wind broke the window' or 'John broke the window, as a result of someone pushing him'. Case grammar has been mentioned in this section because the number and nature of the underlying cases in sentences which use verbs like *touch* have been offered by Whitaker and Noll (1972) as explanations of the relative difficulty of sentences in the Token Test, a test of auditory comprehension in aphasia devised by De Renzi and Vignolo (1962). Two other notions have been proposed as explanations for the different psychological difficulties of classes of words. One is that of functions used in an account of the noun facilitation effect in aphasia (see chapter 7). Functions refer to the conceptual relationships which link lexical items (such as that *gift* or *give* imply a donor, a recipient and an object). Another proposal is that lexical items have in their specification syntactic features which determine the deep structures into which they can enter. For example the verb *make* has the feature of transitivity, and the verb *expect* has the feature of complement structure, so that sentences like 'They make machines' and 'They expect Rangers to win' are well formed. Chomsky (1965) refers to these features as determining *strict subcategorizations* and violation of them results in ungrammatical sentences. Psycholinguistic experiments with normal subjects have generally supported the hypothesis that verbs which can enter into a relatively large number of deep structures are more difficult to interpret quickly (see the review by Fodor, Bever and Garrett 1974, p. 348). Aphasic patients' sensitivity to violations of strict subcategorization is one aspect of their linguistic knowledge which has been examined by Bliss (see chapter 7).

The controversy about the nature of deep structure continues. One form it has taken is the issue of whether the deep relations of a sentence are to be conceived of as ordered into a linear sequence or not. At some point in the formulation of some sentences sequence is critical in English, or else a sentence such as 'The car followed the van' could be realized as 'The van followed the car'. Some theorists therefore argue that linear order must be built into the language base (which may therefore be truly described as syntactic); others claim that these preliminaries take the form of a configuration of relationships which is better described in terms of a simultaneous pattern rather than a linear sequence, with linear sequence being imposed at a later stage in the genesis of the sentence. (For a review, see Bach 1975, who comes down in favour of there being linear order in deep structure.) This theoretical dispute has some practical implications for aphasia because of the dissociation which has been proposed between semantic and syntactic disorders (Whitaker 1971a; Von Stockert 1972, 1974; Buckingham, Avakian-Whitaker and Whitaker 1975). If deep relations are semantic, recognition of them should be preserved in syntactic disorders and disturbed in semantic disorders. If they are syntactic the opposite would be predicted. Some pilot experimental work (Lesser, in preparation) suggests that the aural comprehension of sentences where deep relations are not made explicit in surface structure (as in the *easy/eager to please* model) is not as difficult for aphasic adults (taken as a group) as would be predicted from their relative difficulty for children and for normal adults. This group of aphasics had more difficulty with the aural comprehension of sentences when surface structure sequence could be confused. This suggests that possibly the distinction between a surface level of processing and a deeper level of processing may be valid for aphasia, though it would only throw light on the controversy as to whether the deeper level were syntactic or semantic if patients with 'semantic' or 'syntactic' disorders (defined in terms of surface structure) were found to behave differently at the deep structure level.

## Semantics

This hazy borderline between syntax and semantics is one where aphasia research as well as linguistic theory becomes particularly hesitant. Another route which has been attempted in its exploration is through the concept of *selectional* restrictions. Selectional restrictions were proposed in generative transformational grammar to account for the fact that the grammar did not generate semantically or grammatically anomalous sentences such as 'The idea cut the tree' or 'He frightened that he was coming'. Part of the specification of the verb was the environment in which it could occur, so that *cut* requires a concrete subject and *frighten* does not occur with a following *that*-clause. Palmer (1976) suggests that it is useful to make a distinction between grammatical and lexical (semantic) selectional restrictions, on the grounds that the hearer can usually make allowance for infringement of grammatical selectional restrictions and correct the sentence, whereas when lexical selectional restrictions are broken he tries to make sense of the sentence by seeking a context in which it would be appropriate. The investigation of aphasia by Bliss (to be described in chapter 7) corroborates this distinction, as does Whitaker's (1971a) analysis of syntactic and semantic violations in aphasic speech. In discussing lexical selectional restrictions, Palmer uses a term proposed by Firth, *collocation*, the 'mutual expectancy of words' derived from their habitual use together in sentences. For instance a 'residence' is likely to be 'desirable', 'a gentleman's', or 'detached', because we find these words often associated with it, but we would not expect it to be 'cosy'. Palmer postulates three kinds of collocational restriction: one based wholly on the meaning of the item (so that 'green cow' is unlikely), another based on knowledge of range of usage (so that rhododendrons die but do not 'pass away') and a third based strictly on co-occurrence (so that only eggs and brains may be 'addled').

A proposal in the generative tradition which relates to the first kind of restriction is that words are, in part, bundles of semantic features or components of meaning, and that some of these features must be compatible between related words. For example the verb *break*, in one of its senses, must be followed by an object with the features + *Physical Object* and + *Rigid*; we can break glass, but we cannot break paper. The notion of semantic features has been applied to the study of single words in aphasia (see chapter 5), but its application to aphasia research in the area of selectional restrictions in sentences is not without difficulties, because, as Palmer has pointed out, people make sense out of sentences which do not conform to selectional rules. Although it apparently does not observe the selectional restriction of *break*, a sentence like 'Peter broke the dog' is perfectly intelligible. Weinreich (1966) suggests that features can become transferred, so that in such a sentence we presume that the dog is rigid—a china dog, perhaps, or even a frozen one. Although *rust* lacks the feature + *Animate*, it can still 'eat'. Although *promises* are not + *Physical Object* they have enough rigidity to be 'broken'. Because of this creativity of language it becomes difficult to compose sentences where infringement of selectional restrictions results in meaninglessness.

Whitaker (1971b, p. 217) gives an example of the difficulty of assuming that there is common agreement about when selectional restrictions are infringed. A Wernicke-type patient was given a set of sentences to judge which were anomalous and which were not, and accepted as satisfactory the sentence 'I ate some buildings for breakfast.' When pushed to account for this, he came up with the explanation: 'Well, maybe you're King Kong or something.' If acid can eat metal, and bulldozers can eat buildings, and people can eat their words, patients' 'errors' on tasks where they are asked to make judgements about sentences which are anomalous because selectional restrictions are not observed may be more revealing of their inability to read between the lines about what the examiner wants of them rather than of a blurring of word meaning as such. This is not to say that there may not be a blurring of word meaning in aphasia, but only that it is at present easier to study it in terms of single words rather than in terms of contextual relationships in sentences. There have also been some speculations that the lexical-semantic organization of language may be more bilaterally represented in the brain than the syntactic (Brown 1976; Lesser 1976b): if this does indeed prove to be so, we have a psychologically valid reason for investigating meaning in single words as well as in sentence propositions, in addition to the practical justification of its convenience.

The study of single words has been of particular interest to aphasiologists because of the problems in naming which can occur after brain damage. Difficulty in naming objects is the outstanding characteristic of anomic aphasia, but there also seems to be a general reduction in this capacity in all kinds of aphasias; in milder cases it is revealed only in words of lower frequency in the language or in less familiar, perhaps metaphoric, uses of words such as the 'teeth' of a comb. Consequently linguists' analyses of lexical meaning and psycholinguists' suggestions about the organization of the lexicon are of particular interest in the study of aphasia. Several dimensions of lexical meaning have been proposed: Leech (1974), for example, lists seven: conceptual, connotative, stylistic, affective, reflected, collocative and thematic. The majority of the studies of lexical meaning in aphasia have been concerned with denotative meaning (approximating to Leech's 'conceptual'). Denotative meaning has been defined as having two aspects; *reference*, concerning the relationship of the word with the object or event which it describes, and *sense*, the interrelationships amongst words themselves, such as synonymy and antonymy (having the same sense or the opposite sense). A few studies have been concerned with connotative meaning. Definitions such as Leech's include in connotative meaning all those residual aspects of meaning which are not part of the dictionary definition (such as that cats are soft to touch and that elephants never forget). As used in aphasia research connotative meaning has been defined as emotional or affective meaning. It has been measured by a technique known as Osgood's Semantic Differential. Subjects are asked to rate words on (usually) three seven-point scales. The poles of the scales are labelled good and bad, strong and weak, and active and passive, respectively. Amongst normal subjects there is a consistent agreement about the placing of words on these affective dimensions: *farm*, for example, is almost always rated towards the good, strong and active poles. Osgood and Miron (1963) report some speculations about whether or not connotative meaning should be spared or impaired in aphasia. Is it more abstract than denotative meaning and therefore more vulnerable to brain damage? Is it more basic and primitive and therefore less vulnerable in brain damage? Or is it an essential part of meaning interdependent with denotative meaning and therefore necessarily impaired to the same degree? Some studies of connotative meaning in aphasia are outlined in chapter 6.

In chapters 5 and 6 we shall look also at the five principal ways in which the organization of denotative meaning in the lexicon has been conceptualized, which have been applied in aphasia research. One proposal is that words are clustered into categories such as number names and colour names, and the question has been asked whether or not different categories of words may be selectively spared or impaired by brain damage. A second model describes words as having around them a field of related words; 'violin' for example would have in its field 'orchestra', 'viola', 'music', 'bow', etc. For aphasia the especial interests are firstly the extent to which this field may have become distorted and secondly to what extent priming with related words can assist the anomic patient to find the word he is seeking.

A model arising from this second one conceives of the related words as forming a network of associations, the distance of one word from another in the network being empirically verifiable. A fourth proposal for the organization of the lexicon uses the idea of semantic features already mentioned. Words are related to each other, perhaps hierarchically, by the number of features they share. Finally another approach stresses the referential aspect of meaning and that the lexicon must include cross-modal complexes for which the simultaneous synthesis of perceptual impressions is necessary. None of these models is incompatible with any of the others, and none claims to be a complete model for the psychological organization of meaning in the lexicon.

One problem about proposing models for the mental organization of the lexicon is that it is not at all certain whether we are justified in talking about meaning as if it could be dissociated from the phonological and syntactic components of the lexicon. For a word to be a word, it has to take a phonological shape, and, sometimes, a commitment to a certain syntactic role. Meaning can only be expressed through its realization in a specific form. Yet one of the experiments described in chapter 5 can be interpreted as showing that the semantic field of a word can exist psychologically and be accessed without the word being nameable. Experimenters in psychology have recently been interested in the 'feeling of knowing' that people get when they are trying to remember a word when someone gives them a definition for it. It is possible to have a strong subjective impression that one knows the word, and yet to be unable to recall anything about its phonological shape. Under such circumstances if one is then provided with the word it can often be immediately recognized. Sometimes more information is available—the 'tip of the tongue' feeling—and in such a case one can frequently access the initial letter, the number of syllables and the stress pattern, but still frustratingly not be able to produce the whole phonological form. So we are faced with the difficulty that there may indeed be a level of semantic organization which is psychologically valid, but that we are unable to access it overtly without drawing on another level of language organization, phonological form. Consequently models which have been put forward of how words are retrieved from the lexicon (as opposed to how meaning is organized in the lexicon) include all its components, phonological and syntactic as well as semantic. One such model, which is being applied in aphasia research at Cambridge, England, is Morton's logogen model (Morton 1970). *Logogens* are memorial representations of words, that part of the nervous system where a specific event takes place every time a particular word becomes available as a response. Each logogen has a threshold for its 'firing': when the level of activation exceeds the threshold, the logogen fires. Inputs which can activate or contribute to the activation of the logogen are visual inputs of the written word, auditory inputs of the heard word, contextual influences from associated words, or contextual influences from preceding words in a sentence or from situations, or from a cognitive store through which words can be self-activated rather than passively activated from external input. In addition to the logogens, which are conceived of as having phonological shape, there are higher-order nodes called *ideogens* which form an abstract memory system, the major concern of which is semantic analysis. Morton's model can therefore accommodate the notion that semantic components of the lexicon may be partially dissociable from the form-taking components which are necessary for the actualization of words in speech or writing; in this respect it lends itself to the differential analysis of word-finding disorders in aphasia.

Linguistic investigations of aphasia have generally focused on one or other of the three linguistic levels of phonology, syntax and semantics whose definitions by linguistically-minded aphasiologists have just been described, although some studies have been made of the relationships amongst the levels. Chapters 5 to 8 review some of these investigations at the lexical-semantic, syntactic and phonological levels.

Whitaker (1971a) proposes that there is neurological evidence from aphasia that the levels of organization shown in table 4 below have some autonomy. There is clearest evidence for the independence of the physical phonetic level in that this is impaired in dysarthric patients who have no other language disorder. Morpheme-structure rules specify the segmental and sequential redundancies in a

TABLE 4

*Levels of organization of language proposed as having functional neurological validity*

(based on Whitaker 1971a)

---

1.  Physical phonetic: neuromuscular coding
2.  Phonological representations
    a) Morpheme-structure rules and low-level phonetic Phonological Rules
    b) Abstract Phonological Rules
3.  Lexical representations: conceptual units without neuromuscular specification
4.  Syntactic component (concerned with e.g. strict subcategorization)
5.  Semantic component (concerned with e.g. semantically based selectional restrictions)

---

language (for example, in English, that no words begin with a velar nasal /ŋ/) and, according to Whitaker, as well as Lecours and Caplan (1975), aphasic speakers who are not dysarthric show observance of these rules even though their utterances may contain unintelligible sequences of neologisms (other investigators, however, have commented that morpheme-structure rules may not be invariably observed, for example MacMahon 1972b; Poeck and Huber 1977). Whitaker therefore proposes that morpheme-structure rules are better considered as part of the neuromuscular habits associated with a language than as a facet of the central language system. He comes to the same conclusion about low-level phonetic rules in the phonological component of grammar (taking as his model transformational generative grammar), which can be illustrated by the rule that in English voiceless stop consonants are aspirated before stressed vowels but not if they are preceded by /s/, e.g. /pʰɪt/ but /spɪt/. Non-dysarthric aphasic speakers observe these rules, whereas the more abstract phonological rules, such as the rules for stress placement in a word may not be observed. It seems therefore that the phonological representations of words can be disrupted as an autonomous level, though whether this disruption is one of the rule-system itself, or of the actualization of it through neural control circuits is questionable.

Some patients who have difficulty in uttering the phonological representation of a word even when they have just heard it are able to do this when the word is provided for them to read. Others are not so assisted. From this, Whitaker argues that another level may be distinguished, that of lexical representations, or conceptual units which exist without neuromuscular specification. In the patients in whom phonological representations of (some) words cannot be accessed either through hearing or reading, it would seem that this level of lexical representation, the conceptual phonological form of the word, may itself be impaired. The speech of patients who use recognizable clearly articulated words, but in a context which is not meaningful because they only occasionally have syntactic and semantic relationships with each other, suggests moreover that the phonological-representation level can be intact even though syntactic and/or semantic levels are not.

The remaining dissociation which may be proposed, then, is the separation of syntactic and semantic levels. Whitaker argues that the speech of some patients shows a systematic deviance which indicates a loss or impairment of a semantic nature, while that of others shows deficits of a syntactic nature. Semantically deviant utterances (violating, for example, selectional restrictions which are semantically based) may maintain correct syntactic categorization (for example in the use of *that*-complements). Despite the difficulty of deciding whether a syntactically deviant utterance is semantically anomalous or not, Whitaker argues that the semantic and syntactic aspects of language are functionally separable. It is interesting to note that the observations from which he drew this conclusion were made primarily from patients who produced a fair quantity of speech in conversation or in set tasks, and that the syntactic deviancies he describes fall under the heading of what is usually classed as *paragrammatism* rather than *agrammatism* (see chapter 7). Other aphasiologists have looked to contrasts between the agrammatic and the fluent for evidence of the separation of syntactic and semantic components (e.g. Von Stockert and Bader 1976, described in chapter 7).

But although there is this tentative evidence that often in an individual patient one level is more impaired than the others, and that certain parts of the brain may contain mechanisms which are more important for one kind of linguistic organization than the others, the linguistic levels are closely interrelated, and impairment of one level must have repercussions on others. In normal speaker-hearers they are so intermeshed that they cannot be separated as different functional levels of organization but only of description. One of the exciting contributions which the study of language after brain damage has made is this partial teasing out of the levels within the complex system of interrelationships.

# 3

# Linguistic dichotomies

In the last chapter we saw how linguistics can offer two radical contributions to the study of aphasia—the elementary notion that language must be differentiated in terms of structure rather than simply by surface measures of length and word frequency, and the basic conceptualization of this differentiation in terms of different levels of description. In this chapter we shall be concerned with two fundamental dichotomies that have been proposed for language, both of which for the study of aphasia have been in turn taken up enthusiastically and in turn modified because they have proved to be oversimplifications.

One is the distinction between competence and performance, which Chomsky proposed in 1965; the other is the Saussurian distinction between selection and combination. The latter distinction has been used as the basis for two typologies of aphasia, one by Jakobson, the other by Sabouraud and his colleagues (1965). Although Jakobson's was the earlier typology, Sabouraud's provides a closer link with the topic of the last chapter, linguistic levels, and will be outlined first.

## Selection and combination

Sabouraud used de Saussure's two linguistic planes, the semiological (symbolic) and the phonological, with the axes of selection and combination applied to both of these. On the semiological level the units are words, the selection is from the lexicon and the combination is into a text. On the phonological level the units are phonemes, the selection is from the stock of phonemes and the combination is into a chain which forms a word. Thus language can be represented by a dual system of coordinates, as, vertically, the lexical and phoneme-stock axes on the semiological and phonological planes respectively, and horizontally, the text and word axes on the semiological and phonological planes respectively.

Broca's aphasics are characterized by disturbances along the horizontal axes, and Wernicke's aphasics by disturbances along the vertical axes. These two main types can be further distinguished by the particular plane which is disturbed, the semiological or the phonological. Thus this typology distinguishes four kinds of aphasia, by criteria which are applied primarily to one modality, speech. The semiological Broca's aphasia is characterized by difficulties in establishing contrasts of text with, theoretically, the preservation of selection from the lexicon. In fact because of the interaction between the two axes there are lexical disturbances in speech, and the deficit is not simply one which can be summed up as agrammatism.

When a selection of a word is made from the lexicon it is never made from the entire lexicon; for every utterance there are contextual constraints which limit the possible choice. For this kind of Broca's aphasic these contextual constraints are no longer operative: he selects instead in terms of the similarity of words within their own categories. An example from Jaffrain (1968) may help to make this clearer. Given an incomplete sentence like *The general opens....* with a multiple choice of words to complete it, *the coffee, the door, the telephone, the victory*, this kind of patient is likely to choose the word *victory* because of its semantic association with *general*. Secondary to the contextual disorder there is therefore what can appear to be a lack of observance of selectional restrictions. Phonological Broca's aphasia is characterized by a breakdown in the chaining of phonemes,

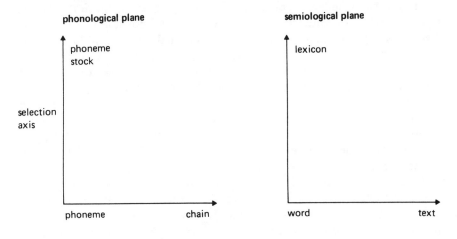

Fig. 2   De Saussure's linguistic planes and axes

although the oppositions of phonemes in the stock are preserved. The patient does not use any phoneme for any other at random, but tends rather to unify the chain and to simplify the process by omitting more contrasts than he can cope with. In semiological Wernicke's aphasia it is the lexical selection axis which is impaired, so that the patient's problem is in the definition of words in contrast to each other, but he has no problems in composing text. His speech is therefore full of vague words, incorrectly selected words, and circumlocutions, and he resorts to the frequent use of pronouns rather than nouns which require clearer definition. In its mildest form, it is anomic aphasia, in which the patient is no longer content with using vague words, but makes an active search for the precise one. The final type of aphasia, phonological Wernicke's aphasia, is manifested in an apparently random selection of phonemes from the stock. In an extreme form speech consists of meaningless chains of phonemes (but articulated without difficulty); at a milder stage the patient strings syllables together which have some resemblance to the intended word, and, when he becomes aware of his errors, makes several attempts at self-correction (other classifications have identified this as characteristic of conduction aphasia). In its mildest form the speech of such an aphasic is characterized by hesitancies, with some stuttering.

Jakobson's first analysis of aphasia also used the two axes of selection and combination, but without making an orthogonal separation as well in terms of different linguistic levels. He considered that there were two qualitatively different types of aphasia so opposite to each other, that, in their pure forms, they could be described as polar. In one, the ability to make a selection from the entities which are linked by similarity is impaired: this faculty of selection has to be employed in naming or in making a lexical choice at every point in a sentence. Jakobson gives as example the sentence *Father is sick*: in order to utter such a sentence a choice has to be made from a number of similar alternatives for *father—parent, papa, dad, daddy*, etc.—and from the number of similar possibilities for *sick—ill, indisposed, ailing, not well*, etc. Selection is an internal relation, in that the range of possibilities is not made overt. In contrast, combination is overt, an external relation of contiguity in its various forms of neighbourhood—proximity, remoteness, subordination, coordination, etc. In the other type of aphasia it is this external relation of contiguity and hence the capacity for combination which is affected.

After Jakobson had published this dichotomous typology of the aphasias, it was observed that there was a close analogy between this typology and the traditional division of the aphasias into *motor* and *sensory*. In an attempt to escape the undesirable implication of these terms, i.e. that the impairment is purely in the mechanics of execution or purely in the mechanics of comprehension, Jakobson suggested the terms *encoding* and *decoding*. These terms still give the impression of a division in central coding abilities which is related to whether or not the patient is speaking or listening, but by aligning them with the dichotomy of selection and combination Jakobson was able to justify their use, he believed, by showing that they were essentially fundamental disruptions of central language, which happen to have disparate effects on production and reception. Combination disturbances hamper the construction of a context and affect primarily the encoding activity of the patient, while selection disturbances affect primarily his decoding activity. Jakobson suggests that, in encoding, the speaker makes the selection of the elements before combining them into a whole, and that it is this secondary process of combination which is impaired in encoding aphasias. In comprehending speech, on the other hand, the first operation is to grasp the whole, and the second to identify its constituents. The secondary process in this case requires the ability to select from the number of possibilities, as from the various meanings of words which are heard as homonyms, like *bank* of a river or *bank* for money; as a secondary process is more vulnerable than a primary process, a disintegration of the ability to select affects decoding.

Jakobson was intrigued by Luria's classification of the aphasias into six major types, which he had derived from observation of head-injured soldiers and had therefore been able to relate with some exactness to the locus of the injury. By using two other dichotomies Jakobson was able to give a theoretical account of the distinctions amongst all these aphasias. The two other dichotomies were between disintegration and limitation (though, as Green (1969a), has pointed out, as this is partly a distinction of degree of severity, it is stretching matters somewhat to describe this as a dichotomy) and between sequence and concurrence. Figure 3 shows schematically how Jakobson's dichotomies are superimposed on Luria's types of aphasias with their approximate localizations.

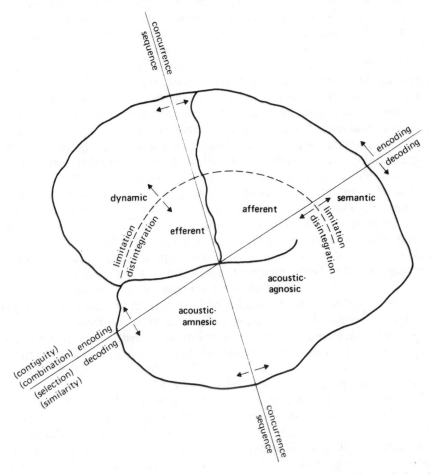

Fig. 3   Schematic representation of Luria's syndromes of aphasia in relation to lesion sites in the left cerebral cortex and to Jakobson's three dichotomies of encoding–decoding, concurrence–sequence and limitation–disintegration

To simplify the distinction, Jakobson's identification of contiguity-combination disorders with encoding and of selection-similarity disorders with decoding is used. There are therefore three encoding disorders, efferent motor, afferent motor and dynamic, and three decoding disorders, acoustic-amnesic, acoustic-agnosic (or sensory) and semantic. The distintegration/limitation dichotomy applies only to distinguish efferent motor from dynamic aphasia and semantic from acoustic-agnosic aphasia, but is not relevant to the other two aphasias. The distinction between efferent motor and dynamic aphasia appears to be one of degree in that the dynamic aphasic has difficulty only with the larger units of language, the sequencing and combination of sentences. The distinction between acoustic-agnosic and semantic is, however, qualitative, in that the first centres on auditory phonemic discrimination and the second on logico-grammatical relations.

The dichotomy between sequencing and concurrence disorders separates three aphasias in which sequencing is impaired—efferent motor, dynamic and acoustic-amnesic—from three aphasias in which concurrence of *simultaneous synthesis* is impaired—afferent motor, semantic and acoustic-agnosic. In afferent motor aphasia, the disorder of concurrence which shows itself in encoding, there is difficulty in the simultaneous combination of phonological distinctive features into the phoneme in speaking, whereas in the other encoding disorder which affects the phonological level of language (efferent motor) the disorder is in the combination of phonemes into sequences. In efferent motor aphasia, at the syntactic level of organization, sequential relationships which depend on contiguity are particularly vulnerable: the government of one word by another one which is contiguous to it is therefore likely to be a difficult construct (government refers to the necessity for nouns or pronouns to take specific cases according to the verb or preposition on which they depend, as in Latin where the preposition *ad* takes the accusative—government is less important in an uninflected language like English). On the other hand, in this kind of aphasia, sequential relationships which do not depend entirely on contiguity will be better preserved; agreement of a verb and its noun ('This book_. These book_s') will therefore be better preserved, as they reflect the coordinated inflection of two words by a higher-order feature (in this case singular–plural number). A disorder of sequencing is germane to only one decoding aphasia—acoustic-amnesia. Here again it is only those syntactic constructs which are formed of concatenated elements which are difficult to decode (e.g. There are John and Mary and Bill), while those which are held together by an internal syntactic structure present no problems (e.g. John advised Mary against Bill).

It is easy to criticize attempts to make large generalizations about aphasia as oversimplifications and no one would claim that the generalizations Jakobson and Sabouraud have made in their typologies are meant to be complete descriptions of the nature of different disturbances. They are, rather, proposals from which hypotheses can be generated. But the question is not so much whether or not the typology is an oversimplification, which is admitted, but whether the principles on which it is based are sound. There are a number of problems in this respect. Firstly there is the inherent problem of taking fundamental dichotomies in language as demarcators of aphasic syndromes, because, of necessity, the fundamentals which they use—sequence, concurrence, selection, combination, simultaneity, contiguity—are common to all language including every aphasic utterance. Linguistic levels may have a certain autonomy if they are psychologically distinct, but theoretical notions like these fundamentals of language are not so likely to prove separable. The terms are basic ones which must be applicable to all brain processes, and it is a large assumption to make that in some syndromes an elementary capacity of the brain is impaired (even if it is assumed to be only in its application to language) and that in other syndromes that elementary capacity is preserved and a different basic one has disintegrated. Defining a syndrome in terms of selective impairment of one basic facet rather than another seems somewhat like expecting one side of a wall to fall down while the other stands up. The processes of sequence and concurrence, for example, operate interactively in language. Luria and Jakobson identify the peculiar nature of the disorder in semantic aphasia as one of simultaneous synthesis of logico-grammatical constructions, as exemplified by an inability to distinguish terms such as *father's brother* and *brother's father*. This is classed by Jakobson amongst his disorders of concurrence; yet it is an inability to abstract by means of inflections a concurrence from a sequence.

Secondly there are some ways in which other people's observations do not agree with Jakobson's divisions. Whitaker and Whitaker's (1972) observations that the majority of patients find relativized sentences easier to repeat than sentences which contain coordinated lists suggest that the condition Jakobson specified as characteristic of acoustic-amnesic aphasia is the one typical of aphasics. Afferent motor aphasia, a disorder of concurrence according to Jakobson, is aligned by Goodglass and Kaplan (1972) with conduction aphasia, an aphasia in which difficulty in sequencing phonemes (or distinctive features, if these are regarded as the basic unit) is prominent.

Thirdly there is a certain surface incompatibility between Jakobson's insistence on the clear differentiation of types of aphasia and another major proposal he made, the *regression hypothesis* (1968; 1971). This hypothesis is that the aphasic adult loses first those distinctions and constructs in language which are acquired last in children. The mildest aphasias are regressions to an older stage in children and the severest to the youngest stage. Wepman and Jones (1964) took up this proposal with some enthusiasm, and drew a parallel between the stages of acquisition of language in children and the five aphasias they identified. Global aphasia was the equivalent of speechlessness in the youngest children, while the stage of babbling and cooing corresponded with jargon aphasia; the next stage in the child's progress, 'fortuitous' speech, was the equivalent of pragmatic aphasia, while the following stage of 'substantive symbols' in children corresponded with semantic aphasia. Finally the acquisition of grammar in children, the last stage of language acquisition in Wepman and Jones's scheme, has its equivalence to the aphasia in which functional independence is least impaired, syntactic aphasia. A direct implication of the regression hypothesis, interpreted in this way, is that 'a patient in process of recovery of speech will move progressively through stages of aphasia above his lowest aphasic level', thus repeating the stages of acquisition in children. If this is what the regression hypothesis implies, then aphasias are essentially distinguished by degrees of impairment, and are, as Schuell claimed, unitary in nature; this proposal cannot be reconciled with Jakobson's formulation of the aphasias in terms of radically different disruptions of elemental facets of language. In his formulation, syntactic aphasia (efferent motor aphasia), for example, does not represent the highest point of the scale of the aphasias, but a disintegration of sequence and combination, which makes it qualitatively distinct from the disintegrations which characterize other aphasias.

However, the regression hypothesis can be reconciled, at least partially, with Jakobson's separations of the aphasias, if it is interpreted as applying, not to the whole disorder, but within subdivisions of language. Within the kind of impairment each type of aphasia displays, there may be a breakdown of those particular skills which corresponds with an inherent gradation of difficulty in language, as measured by the age at which these skills are acquired. In fact at the microlevel of analysis, within the linguistic levels, there is some evidence in support of Jakobson's hypothesis. Some of the experimental studies described in chapters 5 to 8 have been concerned with examining this hypothesis. At the lexical level, Rochford and Williams have found a correspondence between difficulty in naming for aphasics and the age at which names are acquired by children. At the phonological level Blumstein found a partial correspondence between the age at which phonemic contrasts are acquired and their difficulty for aphasic adults. At the syntactic level, Goodglass and Berko demonstrated that in aphasic speech the inflection /-s/ for the verb third person is prone to be lost before the same suffix for the possessive, which in turn is lost before the same suffix used as a nominal plural: this mirrors the acquisition of these suffixes in children. Jakobson suggests that the explanation lies in the hierarchy of the structures involved. The plural form (John has dreams) is a single word which has no implication of syntactic sequence: the possessive-form (John's dream) implies the phrase level where *John's* is a modifier dependent on the headword *dream*; the third person verb form requires a clause (John dreams) with subject and predicate. For both children and adult therefore these represent inherent differences of complexity in language, which are revealed both in acquisition and in disintegration. The comparison of the acquisition of language and its disintegration in aphasia forms the topic of a current book (Caramazza and Zurif, in press) and it is not proposed to discuss the regression hypothesis more at this point. We shall return to it briefly in the summary given in chapter 9.

## Competence and performance

The second kind of dichotomy which has been applied to aphasia from linguistic theory is that between competence and performance. There have been mixed opinions about it, with some claiming that the distinction is useful in clarifying theoretical issues and in prognosis for individual patients, and others rejecting completely the application of such a distinction to aphasia. Amongst linguists, too, a body of criticism has built up over this distinction in linguistic theory.

Competence, as Chomsky defined it in 1965, is the intuitive knowledge which an idealized speaker-hearer may be presumed to have of his own language, enabling him to recognize as grammatical and non-anomalous utterances he has never heard before and to produce such utterances. Performance is the use of this competence by an individual speaker or hearer (and therefore includes the auditory comprehension of speech as well as the production of speech). Performance is therefore clouded by 'such grammatically irrelevant conditions as memory limitations, distractions, shifts of attention and interest, and errors (random or characteristic)' in the application of the speaker-hearer's knowledge (1965, p. 3). For the linguist, therefore, performance (at this period) was considered something of a nuisance; Chomsky went on to say (p. 4) 'Observed use of language ... surely cannot constitute the actual subject matter of linguistics, if this is to be a serious discipline.'

Despite Chomsky's firm rejection of the observed use of language for linguistics, there was an inherent appeal to students of aphasia in the distinction between competence and performance. The question was to find out how far an individual patient's intuitive knowledge was lost, and how far his disabilities were gross exaggerations of the performance difficulties of normal subjects which Chomsky had listed. One way was to examine every modality in which language could be used; clearly if the patient could perform a linguistic task in any one modality, competence must be retained. Whitaker in 1970 suggested that some parts of the linguistic system could indeed be lost in aphasia, and therefore constitute a loss of competence while other aspects of aphasic behaviour indicated simply an impairment, a quantitative reduction of normal verbal behaviour, an extreme on some scale of performance errors. A candidate for loss of competence which he offered was agrammatism, for which there seems to be no obvious parallel in normal speech. Whitaker saw aphasia as providing evidence for linguistics of the nature of competence: 'The loss of X due to lesion can be considered evidence that X is part of the competence of a normal native speaker' (p. 47).

At the same time Weigl and Bierwisch (1970, p. 4) were proposing that there was no evidence to suggest that competence was ever lost in aphasia: instead they saw the various types of deficit displayed in aphasia as reflecting the various components of performance, offering the hypothesis that 'aphasic syndromes in general are to be understood as disturbances of complexes of components or subcomponents of the system of performance, while the underlying competence remains intact'. They discussed two possible exceptions to this—the agrammatism which Whitaker was also singling out, and global aphasia. Of the first they suggested that an agrammatism which occurs in both speech and comprehension (the only kind which makes a possible candidate for a loss of competence) may in fact reflect a general disturbance of cognitive strategies such as underlie, for example, serial ordering, which are preconditions for the normal syntactic processes. Tacit knowledge of syntax may therefore be intact, as part of linguistic grammar, but inaccessible because of an essentially non-linguistic disturbance. The second possible exception, global aphasia, could also, in Weigl and Bierwisch's eyes, not be used as evidence for a loss of competence: it provides no evidence for or against if the patient does not recover some language, while if he does make some recovery of language skills that in itself is evidence that competence was not lost. Weigl and Bierwisch continued: 'If this hypothesis is correct, as it seems to be, then obviously competence and performance must be psychologically different aspects of the general phenomenon of speech behaviour. In other words, the distinction between competence and performance is not merely a heuristic or methodological assumption but reflects a fact that can be established neuropsychologically.' They rejected as absurd the notion that each form of performance behaviour which can be selectively impaired (e.g. repetition, writing to dictation, reading aloud) can be connected to its own competence. They draw attention to the day-to-day fluctuation of abilities and to the possibility of *deblocking* a disturbed ability by generalization from a retained ability as both evidencing that the underlying knowledge of language must be retained.

A year later Whitaker had modified his position. He pointed out that, as aphasia results from brain damage, to say that brain damage never produces a loss of linguistic competence is to argue that competence has no neural representation in the brain. 'If it is not a real property of the brain it cannot be investigated by any empirical techniques discussed so far, and thus such a view rejects the possibility of correlating Linguistic and Neurological theories of language' (1971, p. 16). For Whitaker this is clearly untenable. Whereas previously the practical distinction between a disorder affecting competence and one affecting performance had been made in terms of whether or not all modalities were affected, Whitaker preferred to make a distinction between deficits in a *central language system* which has a neurological substrate and deficits in one or more of the *peripheral language modalities*. Since true aphasia is distinguished from other disorders because it is a deficit in the central system rather than limited to a peripheral modality, it would have to be defined as a deficit in competence, if this were to be equated with the central language system. If aphasia is necessarily a disorder of competence as well as of performance, the distinction between competence and performance in neurolinguistics 'is no longer appropriate or useful'.

Schnitzer (in press, a), however, defends the distinction as applied to aphasia: 'one need not abandon the competence-performance distinctions (as a productive neurolinguistic notion) as Whitaker does'. He suggests that competence should be defined as knowledge of the structure of a language in the sense of *knowing that* rather than the sense of *knowing how*. This competence is the commonality of a variety of linguistic tasks; and it is the individual tasks which are different kinds of performances. Examples of the kinds of tasks to which Schnitzer refers are transforming sentences, nominalizing lexical items, describing linguistic intuitions, and correcting the speech of children and non-native speakers. The abilities involved in these performances are independent, in all probability, of the specific modality through which they are executed. This therefore frees the competence–performance distinction from its dependency on whether or not one or more modalities are involved, and substitutes a different criterion, of generality. A deficiency which affects all these modality-independent tasks 'would have to be either a remarkable coincidence or (more likely) a deficiency in the linguistic competence underlying all the abilities'. In other words Schnitzer aims for an analysis of aphasia which does not depend on modality contrasts and similarities but which is essentially modality independent.

There is, evidently, something inherently appealing in the competence–performance distinction which makes some aphasiologists (and developmental psycholinguists) prepared to redefine the terms rather than to lose the distinction it offers between what is noumenal and what is phenomenal. If a patient is unable to carry out a specific linguistic activity in any form, in any modality and at any time, it is useful to have some way of distinguishing the pervasiveness of this deficit from his other deficits which are more limited.

The problem was that Chomsky had defined competence in such a way as specifically to exclude observations of individual use, which makes his definition particularly inept for the assessment of abnormal speakers. It had carried with it into aphasiology the notion that the system of rules, the intuitive knowledge of which constituted competence, was either spared or damaged as an undifferentiated whole. Components and subcomponents were attributes of performance rather than of competence. The extension of meaning which competence has acquired in its application in the study of the acquisition and breakdown of language lies primarily in the making of distinctions within competence—in fact in the possibility that instead of *competence* there are *competences*. The amendment is derived from four observations: there are degrees of competence, there is communicative competence for social acceptability, there are separate competences for speech and for comprehension, and there are different competences for the different linguistic levels. This is, of course, very different from the competence which Chomsky defined with a rigid demarcation between competence and performance.

Firstly, when the term competence is applied to real-life speaker-hearers rather than the idealized, it becomes obvious that speech communities are not homogeneous, but that within the same community there is a range of language skills. The range is related to social class, to educational level, to age and to other individual differences (Hymes 1971). There are stages of acquisition of competence in children: at some points in this acquisition newly acquired rules may be insecure, for example when children apparently become worse at understanding the passive (Bever 1970; Maratsos 1974; Beilin 1975). There are some rules which are acquired late in childhood by some children, or which are not acquired at all. Carol Chomsky's (1969) study of children who were asked to 'tell X what to feed the doll' or to 'ask X what to feed the doll' showed that even at age 11 there were some children who had not acquired the distinction between the deep relations of such pairs of sentences (in which the deep subject of the verb infinitival complement is identical with X in one sentence but not in the other). Adults in the same community, and of the same social class, can have a good or bad 'command of language'. People of about the same educational level and intellectual standing (e.g. university students) can be sorted out on tests as being *high-verbal* or *low-verbal* (Hunt, Lunneberg and Lewis 1975). A recent study (unpublished) has shown that, in one speech community in the North of England, a proportion of a small sample of normal adults had a surprising difficulty in making the apparently simple distinction between singular and plural when the only clue lies in the verb used and is not duplicated in the noun; this happens when the auxiliaries *is* and *are* are paired with nouns like *sheep* or *deer* which take the same form in the singular as in the plural. In this community some normal adults found it difficult to decide whether 'The sheep is eating grass' was more appropriate for a picture showing one sheep or two, and some wrote 'sheep is' after having seen two toy sheep placed under a box, and used the two sheep when asked to act out a sentence with 'sheep is'. Again, in the same community, some normal adults interpreted the word *touch* in the Token Test in a way which would give them an error score on conventional marking, but which is a logical and apparently consistent interpretation. For a sentence such as 'Touch the blue square *and* the yellow circle' these subjects responded with the same gesture as they did for 'Touch the blue square *with* the yellow circle'. 'Touch' was therefore apparently interpreted as 'Cause X and Y to become in a state of touching' rather than 'Touch X and touch Y'. The same interpretation also seems to be made of 'Touch the car and the sheep'. Whitaker and Noll (1972) have suggested that in the Token Test some of the difficulties children and aphasic adults experience with the final section can be attributed to the fact that sometimes *touch* has an implied instrumental case (with your hand) and sometimes an overt one (with the yellow circle). From the findings mentioned above, it would seem that for some speakers this 'difficulty' results in two acceptable interpretations. Consequently if an aphasic adult 'misinterprets' a sentence such as 'Touch the blue square and the yellow circle', it may reflect his pre-traumatic idiolect rather than a pathological reduction in language. The same applies to the plural–singular distinction when the cue is a single one on the verb unduplicated by its noun phrase. This is not to say that an inability to make such distinctions may not be a pathological disorder, but simply that it cannot always be assumed that it must be. Even at these simple levels a norm of linguistic competence cannot be assumed for an individual. Because of these individual and dialectal differences in the 'command of language', caution must be used in deciding what is a pathological error and what not. The aphasic adult's linguistic competence is being compared not with that of an ideal speaker but, theoretically, with his linguistic competence before he became aphasic.

A second competence which has to be acquired is the knowledge of what is socially acceptable and appropriate. We make adjustments to our speech depending on whether we are, for example, talking to children or trying to make a good impression at an interview. There are also long-term changes connected with social role. Labov demonstrated in 1965 that the probability that the /r/ would be pronounced after a vowel in the speech of New Yorkers could be accurately predicted if one knew the speaker's social class, his age, the speech situation, and what Labov called his *linguistic insecurity index*—the amount of over-correction the speaker might show through his desire to improve his status. There are also certain grammatical forms which are more appropriate to a situation than others. Lakoff (1972) has pointed out that, when a hostess is offering her guests a cake, the appropriateness of the modal form of the verb she uses is in direct opposition to what might be expected from normal usage. If she says 'You must have some of this cake', she is being polite: with 'You should have some of this cake', she is less so; while with 'You may have some of this cake' she is bordering on incivility. These are distinctions which it is sometimes difficult for non-native speakers to learn, except as one-off situations. Since they are also distinctions which children usually acquire at a later age than other aspects of language because they require the ability to empathize with another speaker's point of view, there is a prima facie case that they may be lost in aphasia. Impressionistically, however, such social linguistic sensitivities usually seem to be retained in aphasia though not in disorders after generalized brain damage such as senile dementia. But there are anecdotal reports of fluent aphasics making remarks which are socially bizarre, and losing the power to join in light-hearted banter (though as Gardner, Ling, Flamm and Silverman (1975) have shown aphasia does not necessarily implicate a loss of the sense of humour). As an area of possible linguistic impairment in aphasia, the social appropriateness of language seems to have been as yet little explored (though De Ajuriaguerra and Tissot (1975) have described presenile dementia from this perspective).

The third distinction in competences which has been made is between competence for speech and competence for comprehension. In the first formulation of competence, this distinction would have been unthinkable, and indeed still is so to some linguists. When a model of language was devised for the ideal speaker–hearer all that was necessary to convert it for application to speech or to hearing was to change the direction of the arrows between the boxes (if the model did admit of sequentiality of psychological processes). But this kind of theorizing clashed head-on with the long tradition in aphasiology of regarding speech and comprehension as almost diametrically opposed, with one major class of aphasics being impaired in the flow of speech but not in comprehension and the other major class being impaired in comprehension but not in the flow of speech. We have already commented that Jakobson, dissatisfied with the transmissive terms of *motor* and *sensory*, substituted the central terms of *encoding* and *decoding*, thus carrying the split between speech and comprehension into the centre of the coding system of language. Jakobson has consolidated this distinction in his most recent statement (in press): he describes emission and reception as two basically different phenomena, and says, 'In studying aphasia, we must keep in mind the possibility of a radical separation between these two competences.' A fundamental distinction between speech and comprehension is that comprehension is probabilistic whereas speech must be at least partially pre-planned. For the speaker there are no homonyms: he knows whether when he uses the word *bank* it refers to a place where money is kept, or to a riverside slope. But not so for the hearer who may have to keep both possibilities in mind, or to keep the phonological form in some temporary store until more information later in the utterance disambiguates it. Fodor, Bever and Garrett (1974) have suggested that comprehension may not necessarily require a use of the *algorithmic* linguistic rules which must be employed in constructing a grammatical utterance: it is possible that the hearer uses *heuristic* processes (trial-and-error guessing), or that, at the very least, such processes serve to restrict the space over which he has to apply algorithmic rules. At all events there appears to be a considerable mismatch between what we can understand and what we can ourselves produce: it is much easier to extract the gist from a foreign language than to speak it ourselves.

The same has been observed in developmental studies. In general the young child's comprehension of language is said to exceed his production of language

(Fraser, Bellugi and Brown 1963). Because comprehension is assisted by non-verbal context, and because he can make use of clues beyond the lexical and syntactic information in the utterance itself, the child can perform more adequately in his role as an interpreter than as a speaker (Clark, Hutcheson and Van Buren 1974). However, comprehension in the full sense requires an ability to put oneself in the speaker's place which young children have not yet developed. When knowledge of syntactic structure as such is tested, it is also clear that production can sometimes precede comprehension. Children who are already capable of producing well-formed subject–verb–object sentences in their spontaneous speech may not yet be capable of making in comprehension the correct choice between reversible sentences, a choice for which the only cue is the precedence of one noun before the other to indicate its syntactic role as subject rather than object (Chapman and Miller 1975). Bloom (1974, p. 286) has accounted for the comprehension–production gap by the proposal that 'the two represent mutually dependent, but different, underlying processes with a resulting shifting of influence between them in the course of language development.'

There is also more specific evidence from developmental studies of phonology that production and comprehension reflect different competences. Labov (cited by Hymes 1971) has documented studies of lower-class Negro children who comprehend both standard and non-standard phonology, but produce only non-standard phonology when they speak themselves. In fact this discrepancy is commonplace: regional speakers understand received pronunciation in television broadcasts although they themselves do not use it, and American and Australian Westerns do not need to be dubbed for British viewers who would be hard pushed to mimic any accent. A dramatic example of such a discrepancy occurs characteristically with some children who are unintelligible because of a disorder at the phonological level of their speech. Under test conditions they can recognize as appropriate and meaningful phonemic contrasts which they do not themselves signal (N. V. Smith 1974). This is more than an adjustment to a different realization for each phoneme (such as occurs with the different accents as described above). Analysis of the speech sound system which these children use in speech frequently shows that the boundaries which the child has drawn in the phonological space do not coincide with those of his speech community. His disorder is not so much in the praxis of realizing the same set of phonemes as is used in his community, but is rather in the system of phonemes he employs; the distinctive oppositions which he makes which constitute this system are not the same (are perhaps more simple, or are perhaps grossly deviant) as those which his parents use. Yet he not only understands the speech of his parents, but will reject outright a mimicry of his own speech as unacceptable (Brown calls this the *fis* phenomenon where the child who says *fis* for *fish* will not accept it as meaning *fish* from an adult). It seems that his own speech played back to him from tape can be as unintelligible to him as it is to his hearers (Panagos and King 1975). It therefore appears that he has a different competence in comprehension from the competence that can be inferred from his speech. There is no reason to dismiss the discrepancy as one of performance difficulties in speech affecting the display of a central competence.

The final distinction in competence to be commented on here is that amongst competences at the different linguistic levels.

If we conceive of there being different competences for phonology, syntax and lexical organization, some part of the discrepancy between speech and comprehension in aphasia can be explained by the different demands the modalities make on syntactic and lexical competences. Syntax plays a crucial role in the construction of sentences in speech, but guessing strategies together with lexical knowledge can support a substantial degree of comprehension. Much of the evidence in support of selective linguistic competences for the linguistic levels has been sought for in aphasia. For example, Whitaker (1971a), Von Stockert (1974) and Schnitzer (1974) are amongst the researchers who have proposed that semantic and syntactic organization can be disrupted in part independently.

In contrast to the first dichotomy described—that between the selection and combination axes of language, which has proved something of a strait-jacket for classifying aphasias, however important it may be in describing language—the at first equally formal distinction between competence and performance has proved to be a stimulus to a more insightful examination of aphasic language. The aphasic's present language knowledge must be compared not with some idealization of what it ought to be (and not necessarily with the therapist's own competence) but with that of his pre-pathological condition, 'warts and all'. Competence must also include communicative competence, and in particular the knowledge of when language is appropriately used and the interpretation of what is said in terms of the particular situation and speakers. It can also be argued that differences of language behaviour in the modalities are such that they relate not to performance or transmissive malfunctions but that there are different competences for speech and comprehension. Finally, again we find it useful also to apply the distinction of the linguistic levels.

The blossoming of models of language processing in psycholinguistics, itemising, for example, the several stages which are hypothesized to intervene between seeing a word and speaking its name, can be taken as a further expansion of the notion of language competences. We shall return again to this theme, but meanwhile let us note that this expansion or redefinition of competences does not mean that the study of performance can be relegated as of less concern in aphasiology. The limitations of memory, distractability, inattentiveness and the variability of behaviour depending on the patient's interest are matters of importance to anyone concerned with experimental investigations of aphasia, and indeed are also highly relevant to those linguists (particularly sociolinguists) who devote their main attention to the description of samples of spontaneous speech rather than experimentally contrived situations. For this reason, before we describe the linguistic investigations of what may come generally under the heading of core language competences in aphasia, it is necessary to consider those aspects of behaviour which traditionally come outside the province of language; these are the subject of the next chapter.

# 4

# Performances in aphasia

It is tempting to believe that when we have identified someone as being aphasic we have identified his prime mental dysfynction, disordered language. But the observation that this is the most conspicuous symptom in an aphasic person does not mean that in all other respects his brain is functioning normally and that other psychological functions are intact. Because an underlying theme of the linguistic investigations which are described in chapters 5 to 8 is that selective aspects of linguistic disorganization can be distinguished, it is salutary to remind ourselves at this point that the aphasic subjects who are investigated frequently have other disorders of higher cortical functions, which attract less attention once the major diagnosis of aphasia has been made, but which nevertheless can have some influence on the performance of a task which is intended to be purely linguistic.

There are four kinds of other dysfunctions:

(1) disorders of primary functions, such as sight and hand motor control
(2) higher dysfunctions secondary to, or associated with, the language disorder
(3) higher dysfunctions related to lesions outside the prime language areas of the brain, and which can be identified as distinct extra-linguistic disorders
(4) a generalized reduction in efficiency after brain damage.

## Disorders of primary functions

Of these dysfunctions the first group is most easily recognized. Clearly some initial difficulties in writing following a right-sided paralysis can be attributed to elementary difficulties in control of the right hand or to the necessity for the left hand to acquire a new motor skill requiring fine coordination. Visual field defects can go unnoticed more easily by the inexperienced clinician; and even when a frank visual field defect has cleared on routine testing, there may still be a residual neglect of part of the impaired visual field when signals are presented to both hemifields simultaneously (though this may be more common after damage to the right hemisphere than to the left, according to Oxbury, Campbell and Oxbury (1974)). Consequently the linguist must exercise a little discretion if he finds a patient who reads aloud words like 'courageous, development, excitable' as 'courage, develop, excite': it is possible that a simple explanation may be that the patient has neglected to read the entire word because of inattention to the right side of the printed space. Fortunately, in the modality of hearing, it is less likely that focal unilateral cortical injury will produce an impairment which affects the aphasic's elementary perception. Each ear has bilateral projections to the auditory cortices in the temporal lobes, and it seems that bilateral damage usually has to occur (probably symmetrically in the left and right hemisphere) for the condition known as *auditory agnosia* in which the patient cannot attach meaning to sounds like the ringing of a telephone bell. It is less certain whether or not the ability to attach meaning to *verbal* sounds, the condition known as *word-deafness* or *auditory agnosia for speech* also implicates a bilateral lesion, though most studies of such patients report bilateral damage (see the review by Goldstein 1974). There is reason to believe that each hemisphere may be capable of perceiving words as meaningful, in which case a bilateral lesion would be required; but it has also been suggested that the mode of perception of each hemisphere is different (Levy 1974a; 1974b). It may be that the right hemisphere perceives words holistically and the left hemisphere perceives analytically—the auditory analogue of 'look and say' and phonic reading. At the primary acoustic level of hearing, however, there seems to be no equivalent to the cutting off or reduction of sensory input which occurs with vision after unilateral cortical lesions. Nevertheless, there is a higher than average incidental rise in hearing thresholds in many brain-damaged people, perhaps due to the complications of arteriosclerosis and high blood pressure. In any older population, too, there will be the increase in thresholds at the higher frequencies which is known as *presbycusis*, and which may particularly affect the ability to distinguish the fricatives amongst the speech sounds. In linguistic investigations of phonemic discrimination in aphasia this has to be borne in mind.

## Higher dysfunctions secondary to, or associated with, the language disorder

Another problem which the investigator meets is to know how much the aphasic patient's impaired performance in an experimental situation is related to possible secondary effects on verbal or on non-verbal aspects of intellect. The extent to which it is possible to make such a distinction was one of the topics of a recent conference on the relationship between aphasia and intelligence (Lebrun and Hoops 1974). Here again there are advantages in considering language as heterogeneous. That part of language, phonological and syntactic, which relates to form rather than content, is less likely to be relevant to the ability to use rational thought than is the semantic level of language. Consequently it is those patients who appear to have a major deficit at the semantic level (after posterior rather than anterior lesions) about whom the question is discussed of whether or not thought is impaired. Statements like Marie's that intelligence is necessarily diminished in aphasia have therefore only been made by people who consider the true aphasia to be of the Wernicke type and consequently necessarily characterized by comprehension difficulties. The disorder in aphasia has at times been described as a reduction in the ability to use symbols, of which the disorder in verbal symbols is the prime example (Duffy, Duffy and Pearson 1975). It has also been suggested, however, that different kinds of *asymbolia* occur (Leischner and Fradis 1974, p. 279, translated), such as for mathematical signs, traffic signs or Morse code, and that 'The asymbolias ... represent in every case a clinically independent syndrome, which may be present like the agnosias, the apraxias, the acalculias and the amusias with an aphasia but also outside of such.' This reflects a general trend towards sifting out the underlying components which contribute to any overt behaviour, and a belief that different locations of brain damage will affect in different ways the various factors which contribute to intellect. This not to imply the abandonment completely of the notion that aphasia may affect a general quality of intelligence, or $g$ as it is commonly abbreviated. Basso and her colleagues in Milan (1973, p. 727) have suggested that there is a region in the left hemisphere which overlaps the language area which 'subserves a superordinate intellectual ability, sharing many of the characteristics attributed to the $g$ factor by psychologists'. They have demonstrated (1976) that a proportion of aphasics, particularly global aphasics, make errors when asked to choose a colour for an object which is typically associated with one colour (like a pillar box), even though no use of language is apparently required. On top of the linguistic deficit, Basso and her colleagues suggest, there is a basic problem in some aphasic subjects in making associations which are not necessarily mediated through language—perceptual associations of objects with their colour, use, sounds and drawings. Consequently there may be an impairment which is not in the strictest sense aphasic, in that language itself is not involved, but which is nevertheless related to aphasia in that it necessarily has repercussions on a fundamental prerequisite of language, the ability to make associations, and therefore cannot occur without resulting in aphasia.

## Higher dysfunctions related to lesions outside the language areas

There are other disorders, however, which can be dissociated more clearly from language disorder as such, some of them because the specific functions which are disordered are thought to be the province of the right hemisphere. Memory for people's faces, for example, is usually attributed to the right hemisphere and is perhaps one example of the superiority of this hemisphere for visuo-spatial discriminations. Table 5 summarizes some of the suggestions which have been used based on neuropsychological evidence about different roles in higher cortical functioning which are played by the two hemispheres and more particularly by the three large lobes in each hemisphere. (This evidence has been derived mostly from psychologists' studies of brain-damaged patients or from their experiments with presenting information first to only one hemisphere in the intact brains of students by using hemifield viewing or by giving their ears competing information. The terminology used is therefore psychological rather than linguistic.) An accumulation of evidence from a multiplicity of slightly varied tasks has led to the speculative summaries of the specializations of different processes between the two hemispheres in the general terms given at the top of the table. But the distinctions are far from absolute. Besides the similarities of functions within a hemisphere, which can be broadly summarized as verbal in the left hemisphere and visuo-spatial in the right hemisphere, there are similarities across the lobes of both hemispheres.

TABLE 5

*Localization of lesions in the human brain which are associated
with impairment of higher cortical functions*

(as described in neuropsychological studies)

| | *Left cerebral hemisphere* | *Right cerebral hemisphere* |
|---|---|---|
| *General* | Serial organization | Gestalt organization |
| | Analysis | Synthesis |
| | All-or-none discrete functions | Graduated diffuse functions |
| | Conceptual, elaborative processes | Emotional, immediate processes |
| | Categorization of environmental changes | Sustaining of enviromental situation |
| | Primary vigilance | Secondary vigilance |
| | Auditory attention | Visual attention |
| | Rhythm | Music (chords) |
| | Volitional and conscious organization | Automatic and involuntary organization |
| *Associated with lobes:* | | |
| *Frontal* | Verbal fluency | Insight into errors? |
| | Regulation of behaviour by speech | Social awareness? |
| | Praxis | Recency judgements (visual patterns) |
| | Writing | |
| | Insight? Awareness | |
| | Recency judgements (verbal) | |
| *Temporal* | Verbal reasoning | Tone patterns |
| | Auditory verbal memory | Visual memory (long-term) |
| | Vocabulary | Auditory non-verbal memory |
| | | Memory for faces |
| *Parietal* | Calculation | Spatial perception |
| | Reading | Depth perception |
| | Writing | Hue discrimination |
| | Constructional praxis (ideational) | Constructional praxis (perceptual and spatial) |
| | Simultaneous synthesis and simultaneous form perception | Visual short-term memory |
| | Associative abilities (ability to associate objects with colour, use, sounds, etc.) | Visual recognition of objects and pictures |
| | Span of apprehension of sequences | |
| Sources: | | |
| | Beaumont 1974 | Luria and Simernitskaya 1977 |
| | Broadbent 1974 | McFie 1975 |
| | Cohen 1973 | Milner 1971 |
| | Diller and Weinberg 1972 | Moscovitch 1973 |
| | Gainotti 1972 | Nebes 1974 |
| | Gordon 1970 | Semmes 1968 |
| | Kimura 1973 | Sperry 1974 |
| | Levy 1974 | Warrington and Taylor 1973 |

For one thing, although one theory describes the distinction in terms of analysis (in the left hemisphere) and synthesis (in the right hemisphere), as we have seen Luria has deduced that an area in the left parietal lobe is of prime importance for simultaneous synthesis, with a lesion in this area resulting in semantic aphasia. For another example, if a patient is unfortunate enough to have such severe epilepsy or so extensive a tumour that his right cortex has to be removed, he does not immediately become translated to a two-dimensional world, although there is evidence that the right hemisphere is particularly important for depth perception. Another patient who has his left cortex ablated also is not completely removed from language, although he will probably have a profound and lasting aphasia: nevertheless comprehension of language is reported to be recovered in such patients (with, as far as can be known, a normal pattern of hemispheric lateralization of functions) so that they can perform as well as the right hemispherectomized on tests of vocabulary recognition (A. Smith 1974). In short some of the distinctions may prove to be distinctions of degree, rather than all-or-none specialization and we cannot assume that an aphasic patient may not also have dysfunctions of those abilities which are usually associated with the right hemisphere. We do not yet know how far damaged tissue in one hemisphere can interfere with the normal functioning of its undamaged homologue in the other hemisphere. Nor do we know how far these higher cortical functions, despite some specialization, require the cooperation of both hemispheres or of other areas within the same hemisphere. Weinstein (1964) has reviewed a number of studies which found aphasic patients to be impaired on tasks which are considered to be non-verbal. One such task is the recognition of outline figures when they have been crossed through by several lines (the Gottschaldt test). Another is a test of spatial orientation in which the subject is asked to walk along a path in a large room according to a route which he has previously seen on a map or traced with his finger. Both of these tasks depend upon visual or spatial abilities. Either the aphasic patients must be assumed to have had bilateral lesions, or these abilities depend on processes which can also be disturbed by left-hemisphere damage. Consequently if test material is used which relies on pictures or spatial arrays, we cannot necessarily dismiss these non-verbal factors as totally irrelevant to the aphasic's performance on the language test.

Within the left hemisphere, there can also be dysfunctions which occur frequently with aphasia but which are not aphasic. We have seen that there can be a difficulty in associating objects with their perceptual attributes including colour, but an apparently isolated naming difficulty for colours can occur in a condition which many people would class as not being aphasic, because speech and aural comprehension are not impaired—alexia without agraphia. This is the unusual condition in which someone finds that he can write but no longer read back his writing nor any other kind of print. Some seven out of every ten such people also have a right visual field defect, indicating that the site of the lesion extends into the left occipital lobe or its tracts. Geschwind (1965) suggests that in addition there must be a lesion in the fibres which connect the left and right hemispheres, in particular in the splenium of the corpus callosum; because the left hemisphere can no longer receive the visual input from the script, and because the input to the language system of the left hemisphere is also cut off by the callosal lesion from the right hemisphere which can receive the visual input, the patient cannot connect meaning with what he sees. Or, if his right hemisphere can connect meaning with printed words—and there is some evidence from split-brain studies that this is not implausible—it cannot connect the printed words with their phonological shapes for speech. But there is no impairment of the language system itself, and no disconnection from the motor control of writing. In these patients there is also a high proportion who have an apparently selective difficulty with colour naming. Greenblatt (1973) proposes from this evidence that there is an area of brain on the medial surface of the occipital lobe of the left hemisphere which is critical specifically for colour naming. This is not to say that colour names are 'stored' there but that for accurate association of this perceptual input with speech this particular area of brain may have to be intact. It seems in fact that a critical circumscribed lesion could selectively impair only colour naming, without an alexia. Again this raises questions about tests such as the Token Test (De Renzi and Vignolo 1962) or the Three Figure Test (Peuser 1976) which rely on the use of coloured shapes to investigate linguistic comprehension: it seems that not only people who are colour-blind could have non-aphasic difficulties with these tests, but so also could people with normal colour vision who have cortical lesions but who are not aphasic in speech and auditory comprehension. It is consequently difficult to sort out how much an aphasic's difficulties on such tests could be attributed to the extension of the lesion to this particular site outside the language area of the brain.

Of more importance in the practical examination of aphasia is the not infrequent accompaniment of aphasia by a gesture apraxia. In this condition the patient has difficulty in the voluntary coordination of arm and hand movements (and/or sometimes leg movement) to demonstrate symbolic actions. Hence, although he may have no problems in cleaning his teeth in the normal course of events, if he is asked to demonstrate how he does so without a toothbrush in his hand, he may make several unsuccessful attempts. He may, for example, substitute a finger for the toothbrush to help himself towards the natural reflexive situation. Goodglass and Kaplan (1963) have studied this condition and its association with aphasia, and have come to the conclusion that despite their frequent co-occurrence they can vary independently. It is possible that they are severally dependent on adjacent anatomical areas. It is also reported (Gainotti and Lemmo 1976) that the ability of aphasic patients to understand the meaning of symbolic gestures such as saluting (as tested by asking them tò select the correct picture out of three) does not correlate significantly with their ability to reproduce the same gestures. In gesture dyspraxia, therefore, it seems we have another compounding variable which can affect the behaviour of an aphasic patient on a test of language. If the language examination requires him to execute any action except the simplest reactive movement, it is open to some suspicion. It cannot always be assumed that a separate examination of the patient for gesture apraxia will obviate this difficulty. In the first place, it is not always possible to distinguish apraxic difficulties from difficulties in verbal comprehension, and in the second place, it may be that a 'sub-clinical' apraxia could interact with the language difficulty to overload the patient. It is only overt behaviour which can be directly measured, and this behaviour is the net result of the complex interactions amongst the stimulus which elicited it, the internal mental processes and the execution of the response. The linguistic share in the final product may not be as uncontaminated by extra-linguistic factors as we would wish to assume (Lesser 1976a).

## Generalized reduction in efficiency after brain damage

The final kind of dysfunction which can occur with aphasia which was listed at the beginning of this chapter is a generalized reduction in efficiency consequent upon any brain damage. When Lashley in 1929 found that the ability of rats to learn where to find food in mazes was impaired in proportion to the amount of cortical tissue which had been removed from their brains, rather than being related to where the tissue had been taken from, it seemed that the brain might prove to be equipotential for some high-level functions, learning and perhaps intelligence. It is now believed, however, that lesions in different areas interfere with learning and intelligent behaviour in different ways, and that although the net result is failure on a task, the failure can depend on selective disturbance of different critical components. There are still, nevertheless, some general headings under which it is useful to summarize the general consequences of brain damage. These include increased fatiguability, lowering of perception, decrease in reaction speed, fluctuations of attention, and inertness of neurophysiological excitation and inhibition.

The fatiguability of brain-damaged patients characteristically shows itself in a sudden deterioration of performance. Goldstein (1948) considered that fatigue is a defensive mechanism. However, there are reports of some aphasic patients being able to continue for long periods of time with non-verbal activities like drawing, suggesting that rapid fatiguability may be specific to functional systems rather than being generalized. On the other hand delays in responding seem to be general in aphasia and not restricted to responses to verbal material. Kreindler and Fradis (1971, pp. 65–6) report from a number of studies of reaction speed that 'we have been able to establish that the increase in performance latency and duration is common to all aphasics and, interestingly enough, not only in the case of verbal performances, but also in tests where both the stimulus and the response were non-verbal'. They noted two aspects of this lack of responsiveness: a delay before the response is initiated and an increase in the time the response itself takes. Tests of the time taken to react to the switching on of a light are reported to be more sensitive to the presence of brain damage in right- or left-brain-damaged people than is an intelligence test given with a time limit (De Renzi and Fagliono 1965). As regards perception in aphasia the disability seems to be more marked with auditory and with verbal material. Conrad (1954) has suggested that the patient with sensory aphasia may be compared to a healthy individual in front of a tachistoscope on which impressions are flashed at such a speed that the subject has difficulty in perceiving them. The aphasic has a higher threshold for perceiving speech, and the sensations he experiences do not reach the level of comprehension. It was on this principle that Schuell made intensive and repeated auditory stimulation a tenet of her programme of therapy for aphasia. The phenomenon of inertness of neural excitation and inhibition provides a neurophysiological explanation for these increased thresholds for perception and for the delayed and prolonged responses. It is also evidenced at a more central level by the tendency in aphasia towards perseveration in responses. Having initiated one response, the patient has difficulty in changing to another one and continues to repeat the first. Kreindler and Fradis describe perseveration as one of the most frequently noted aphasic defects. Consequently in linguistic examinations it cannot be assumed that a response is indeed a response to the particular word or sentence the examiner has used; it may be a response to a preceding word or a response which combines elements of reactions to more than one preceding stimulus. Perseveration is not only seen in reactive speech, but also occurs in spontaneous speech. It occurs both at the phonological and at the semantic level, and also it seems at the syntactic level: frequent stereotyped productions have been reported in some kinds of aphasic speech (Buckingham, Whitaker and Whitaker 1975). Though some of these stereotypes occur as exact repetitions suggesting that they are encoded as neuromuscular habits in their entirety, there is some evidence for a restricted degree of syntactic variation within them. Rochford (1974) gives some intriguing examples of perseveration at the semantic level. He asked a patient with jargon aphasia to name nineteen outline drawings of objects and found that the patient was sometimes able to give the right name but at the wrong time. Having failed to name 'skull', three items later the patient called a scarecrow a 'skull-bound'. On a later session with the same items re-ordered, having again failed to name 'skull', he called the skeleton a 'skol'. On another occasion, having failed on 'rake', four items later he called the skeleton 'rake'. The same patient also provides examples of perseveration at the phonological level. A dice was called 'black and white blice'; having called a drawing of a heart a 'draft', he then called a drawing of a candle a 'craft candlestick'.

It would seem, therefore, that the aphasic's problem in controlling the pattern of excitation and inhibition affects several kinds of language processes: the precise delimitation of word meaning because traces of previous semantic activations rise above threshold at inappropriate times; the ability to move from one type of syntactic pattern to another; and the selection of new phonological shapes, even when there is no question of an articulation difficulty as such. Although impaired mobility of excitation is, in addition, commonly associated with motor problems (as in efferent motor aphasia), it seems to be a feature which characterizes all the aphasic's operations with language. As well as applying to the patient's own attempts to initiate language, it is likely, according to Kreindler and Fradis, to 'underlie the aphasic patient's difficulty to differentiate stimuli' (p. 68).

Wepman (1972) describes the perseverative behaviour of an aphasic on a naming task, like the one Rochford gave, as due to switching off of attention. He suggests that stimuli received while the patient is working out a verbal formulation to other stimuli are inhibited, and that the patient continues to respond with whatever item was appropriate when his attention 'shutter' was open. The shutter-like behaviour of the patient, in Wepman's opinion, is probably involuntary; he can only handle incoming stimuli at his own, now reduced, speed. Schuell, Jenkins and Jiminez-Pabón (1964, p. 208) also report a similar phenomenon, an auditory imperception which has ' a marked on–off effect, as if the signal were not received'. Luria and Karasseva (1968) have also referred to a loss of auditory speech memory due to a heightening of auditory speech-trace inhibition, but suggest that there need not be any disturbance of the acoustic analysis of speech sounds as such. Arising from such observations there have been several studies of the importance of the rate at which stimuli are given to the aphasic patient. Albert and Bear (1974) describe a patient whose clinical symptoms were those of word deafness and whose auditory language comprehension could be markedly improved if the examiner considerably reduced his speaking rate. In a study with 46 aphasic men, Gardner, Albert and Weintraub (1975) compared (amongst other conditions) comprehension of words uttered at normal speed with words in sentences uttered at a rate of one word per second. They report a dramatic improvement in comprehension in the latter condition, independently of the type of aphasia. Weidner and Lasky (1976) also tested out the effect of slowing speech, using passages from various subtests of auditory comprehension in the Minnesota Test for the Differential Diagnosis of Aphasia which had been tape-recorded. They reported better scores for the slow speech, and that it was the less impaired aphasic subjects who benefited most from the reduction in speed. With all the aphasics, whatever the degree of severity, the subtests which showed most improvement with the slowed presentation were those which required the patient to execute directions or to point to series of items in a picture. The question of the relationship of aphasia to difficulties in serial processing is one of particular interest because of the suggestions which have been made that left-brain-damage disturbs this kind of processing.

## Serial processing

Aaronson's (1974) analysis of the temporal processes in auditory perception proposes five hypotheses. These are that perception is not instantaneous, and consequently that coding continues after the stimulus itself has ended; that time intervals between words in a string of words are necessary to process the words; that when these intervals are short, a backlog of delays develop which leads to errors related both to the items themselves and to the order in which they were heard; that specific listening strategies related to the instructions or to training are important additional factors; and that the retention of previously coded words competes for processing time with the perception of new words. This analysis is based on experimental studies of normal subjects (usually students) but it provides an explanation of how, if perceptual processes operate more slowly in aphasia, the patient could experience difficulties in the auditory comprehension of speech. It emphasizes that perception requires some retention in short-term memory beyond the sensory registration of the input, and indicates two particular aspects of memory which can be distinguished—memory for items and memory for the order in which the items were received.

Of particular concern to aphasia is the vulnerability of processing of order. Firstly, language, as we have seen, has been described as essentially linear in its nature, and even if this puts undue emphasis on the surface forms of utterances, it cannot be disputed that sequential order plays a role in language. Defective serial organization has been suggested as a factor in reading disorders in children (Corkin 1974). Secondly, serial organization has been specifically related to the left hemisphere, in, for example, Bosshardt and Hörmann's (1975) study of perception of serial order in dichotic listening, in Kimura and Archibald's (1974) study of the imitation of sequences of gesture, and in Cohen's (1973) study of serial and parallel processing. Kimura and Archibald have even proposed that speech disorders are simply a manifestation of an impairment in motor sequencing—an interpretation of speech which does not do justice to the complexity of language production as an interaction of the simultaneous and the sequential, as Poeck and Huber (1977) have pointed out. Nevertheless, putting one and one together, it would not be surprising if people with language disorders after left-brain-damage were to prove particularly impaired in tasks in which the distinction of sequence in verbal material was crucial. Surprisingly few studies so far have examined this particular interrelationship of language, sequence and aphasia. A seminal study was that by Efron (1963), who reported that aphasic patients were markedly impaired in reporting which of two pure tones differing in frequency had occurred first. Normal subjects can distinguish between such tones when the gap between them is about 50 or 60 milliseconds (trained listeners can even do so when the gap is only 20 milliseconds). In contrast, for some of the aphasic subjects in Efron's study, a 75 per cent correct level of responses could only be obtained when the gap between tones was over a second. Efron suggested that the temporal perception of sequence is performed by the hemisphere which is dominant for speech and that 'we should not look upon the aphasias as unique disorders of language but rather as an inevitable consequence of a primary deficit in temporal analysis' (p. 418). It seemed that the disorder in discrimination of sequence was related not so much to any left-hemisphere lesion but specifically to a lesion in the location which is associated with aphasia. Efron's study stimulated further investigations of the extent to which the difficulty in temporal discrimination of non-verbal sounds and lights which Efron had reported was related to the language disorder. It emerged that discrimination of the temporal order of flashes of light and sounds was impaired in left-brain-damaged patients who were not aphasic (Carmon and Nachshon 1971) in contrast to Efron's hypothesis, and that difficulty in the temporal discrimination of sounds does not correlate closely with clinical ratings of severity of aphasia (Brookshire 1972a). In fact, as Efron himself had commented, deficits of this kind in discriminating auditory sequence are more severe in expressive aphasics than in receptive aphasics, even though the former are clinically rated as having less difficulty in understanding speech. Receptive aphasics were more impaired in discriminating visual sequences. It therefore seems that left-brain-damage in general is associated with difficulties in the resolution of temporal order in perception (though the form it takes may differ with the location) and that although aphasics (with left-brain-damage) are consequently impaired in this respect there must be other complicating factors which contribute to the picture of clinical severity in aphasia.

Included in an examination of auditory comprehension in aphasia (Goodglass, Gleason and Hyde 1970) was a task in which the patients had to point to objects in the order in which they had been named. They found a poor performance in all types of aphasia, but that Broca's aphasics were particularly impaired. Albert (1972a; 1972b) devised a similar sequencing test. Twenty common objects were spread on the table in front of the patient, and he was asked to point to sequences of them in a certain order. Starting with two objects, the number was increased by one each time until the subject failed three times on a given number of objects. The 'average' aphasic (averaged over the group) could point to 2·41 items whereas none of the non-brain-damaged central subjects failed to point correctly to fewer than four. Albert found that on this test aphasic patients with left-brain-damage were impaired regardless of whether the damage was anterior or posterior. When the patients were asked to point to the objects in sequence following the examiner's pointing, and without the objects being named, the aphasics fared no worse than other brain-damaged subjects. Albert consequently favoured the hypothesis that it is in sequencing auditory input that aphasics have an especial difficulty, and that there is some mechanism in the left hemisphere which is specifically adapted to place in the correct order the elements of the structure of language. In two following studies (Tzortzis and Albert 1974; Albert 1976) Albert has demonstrated that defective short-term memory for sequences can be distinguished from a more general disorder of auditory verbal short-term memory. This provides experimental confirmation of the clinical observation that patients sometimes recall items but not in the correct order, and corroborates a number of studies with normal subjects in which it has been shown that, on tests of recall, order information can be distinguished from item information (Bower and Minaire 1974; Healy 1974; Detterman and Brown in press). Albert used a version of his Sequencing Test, scoring it twice according to items which were correct and items which were in the correct sequence, and sequences in which items were omitted. Sequencing-type errors accounted for a higher proportion of errors for aphasics than they did for other brain-damaged people. Only for the aphasics did the influence of defective memory for sequences become more pronounced as information load increased from two items upwards. The case could be argued that discrimination of sequences of words which are all of the same part of speech (concrete nouns) and related in category as domestic objects employs an ability which is essentially non-linguistic in character on material which happens to be linguistic. It is only when we come to the question of whether or not aphasic adults have a difficulty in discriminating sequence in reversible sentences like 'The lion killed the guard/The guard killed the lion', that the role of sequence is inextricably intermingled with syntactic structure. Although aphasic speech rarely evidences confusions of word order, some linguistic investigations which suggest that order confusions can be made in comprehension will be described in chapter 7. The prominent part sequencing plays in the motor organization of speech at the phonological level contributes to the linguistic studies described in chapter 8. The ability to organize sequence, and the ability to make perceptual discriminations and to retain them in short-term memory during processing, need not be linguistic although they are required for language.

So far we have discussed four of the main kinds of performance factors which can influence the results of linguistic investigations of aphasia. Before we discuss a final and important one, these will be summarized. They are

(1)  disorders affecting the transmission of language due to damage to the brain areas for peripheral sensory and motor mechanisms
(2)  non-linguistic difficulties in functions attributed to the left hemisphere, i.e. gesture praxis, colour–name association and general associative abilities
(3)  non-linguistic difficulties in functions attributed to the right hemisphere, but possibly also occurring in left-hemisphere damage, i.e. spatial orientation, visual figure-ground discrimination
(4)  change in dynamic neurophysiological processes which result in decrease in speed of reaction, lowered perception, and fluctuation of attention.

In particular these changes can have consequences on serial processing.

These performance factors are all related to brain mechanisms and dysfunctions. The final one to be suggested here concerns not so much the characteristics of the speaker's brain, but the characteristics of the circumstances in which language is used. It is important enough for it to be proposed as a third dimension in terms of which language can be studied, complementary to that of the linguistic levels and the modalities. As *functional* is conventionally used in aphasiology to describe the practical usage of language in everyday life, as in Taylor's Functional Communication Profile (1953; 1965), it may appropriately be described as *functional levels of availability*. This is not referring to the functions of language in the same way as Halliday does in children's acquisition of language, when he describes functions such as the instrumental 'I want' or the regulatory 'Do as I tell you' (though De Ajuriaguerra *et al.* have used a similar concept to Halliday's in describing the regression of language in presenile dementia). It is, rather, developed from two concepts, reduction of availability, as opposed to loss of a skill, and apraxia.

## Functional levels

The idea of aphasia as a reduction in availability of language rather than a loss of language has already been introduced in the context of the distinction between competence and performance. It is most clearly demonstrable at the semantic level. Howes (1964) has shown that the potential vocabulary of aphasics remains extensive, as it is in normal speakers, but that aphasics tend to use the more frequent words proportionately more frequently than do normal speakers. Infrequent words can still be accessed on occasion, so that the clinician who is adjusted to the idea that words of high frequency should be used in therapy material is sometimes surprised by the patient's use of a complicated rare word. Words which are frequent in the language are accessed by the patient more easily, but sometimes some combination of circumstances brings up to threshold other words. The examination of aphasia in terms of functional levels of availability is concerned with those circumstances which go beyond the immediate linguistic context.

From apraxia we derive the notion that a distinction can be made between the automatic and the deliberately elicited. The accessibility of patterns of motor behaviour differs according to the purpose for which that behaviour is aroused. In apraxia of speech this occurs at the level of phonetic and phonemic organization. In contrast to the dysarthric patient, the apraxic patient shows a sometimes complete absence of phonological difficulties when he is asked to speak an automatic series such as the days of the week, or when he makes automatic responses such as 'Yes', 'no', 'I can't do that', etc. Of this condition Darley (1968, p. 9) writes: 'There is evident discrepancy between certain speech performances and others. Just as in a non-language apraxia, we find a discrepancy here between volitional performance and reflex performance. We may hear a patient comment upon his poor performance in saying certain words after us, and as he comments he is fairly fluent and his articulation is good. He may be able to recite numbers or days of the week and produce such reactive expressions as greetings or curses fluently and with good articulation, but when his set is different in trying to produce a particular word, even though it is an easy one, he may have much trouble.' Whitaker (1971a) has also commented on the retention of *ictal speech automatisms* in a patient who could not carry on a conversation or do the most elementary language tasks such as naming familiar objects. The speech automatisms he cites include ones with some degree of syntactic complexity ('It just depends on whether I do or don't'). Nonetheless they appear to be coded as set whole units in the brain which are not used appropriately to convey meaning.

A combination of the notion of dissociation of the automatic and the voluntary in speech and the idea of reduction in availability of a central word store leads to the proposal that the dissociation may apply to the central language system as well as simply to coordination for speech.

Baillarger and Jackson in the late nineteenth century seem to have been the first to draw attention to the dissociation of the automatic and the voluntary in uses of language. Jackson (Taylor 1958) wrote, 'the more voluntary uses of language are more or less profoundly altered, while its more automatic uses are not only preserved but even liberated'. This was, Jackson suggested, because automatic language is initiated by the right hemisphere while the left initiates voluntary propositional language. In a footnote to his comment that 'The left half of the brain is that by which we speak, for damage of it makes us speechless; the right is the half by which we receive propositions' he adds 'The essential difference is not that betwixt the internal and the external use of words, for speech may be internal; we can speak, and constantly are speaking, to ourselves. The difference is in, or corresponds to, the voluntary and automatic use of words' p. 132). Jackson describes a woman who for the six months before she died said only, 'Yes, but you know' except when she saw a child nearly falling and cried, 'Take care'. Another patient who was virtually speechless was reported on one appropriate occasion to have asked 'How is Alice getting on?' Conseqently Jackson proposed that there were degrees of facility of automatic utterances, depending on the degree of emotion aroused. At the most automatic level there was 'non-speech' swearing, then 'inferior speech' such as 'Yes', 'No', 'Sorry', and then 'real speech' with a propositional content, such as the enquiry about Alice, and the warning to the child. Weigl (1961) as a preface to his comments on deblocking in aphasia offers further examples of the availability of automatic speech when the voluntary is unavailable: in one, a patient calls out 'Oh my poor little Jacqueline, I don't know your name any longer.' Luria and Simernitskaya (1977) have drawn attention again to this dissociation of the automatic and the voluntary: they endorse Jackson's comments on the different effects of right- and left-brain-damage on cognitive abilities, with experimental evidence from a test in which the memorizing of lists of words voluntarily as a set task was compared with incidental memorizing of them as part of another task. People with left-brain tumours or aneurysms were significantly impaired on the voluntary task but showed relatively less decrement than non-brain-damagaed students did in their incidental memorizing: this was tested by asking them to count the numbers of letters in the words or to look for words which included the letter $k$ and then unexpectedly asking them to recall the words themselves. In contrast, patients with similar lesions in the right hemisphere were relatively less impaired than the left-brain-damaged on the voluntary task but showed a catastrophic deterioration in the incidental memorizing. Luria and Simernitskaya conclude that left-sided lesions may result in a breakdown of conscious voluntary organization while right-sided lesions impair the more automatic aspects: 'In place of a sharp distinction between the verbal and the non-verbal, each assigned to its respective cerebral hemisphere, we have to think rather in terms of a variety of factors involved in the organization of psychological processes and of a hierarchy of functional levels in their cerebral representation' (p. 175).

In a community where *aye* is often used instead of *yes*, it is not uncommon to find an aphasic patient who freely uses *aye* appropriately, but who is incapable of producing the same phonetic realization to name his own eye. This is not the same distinction that Gardner and Zurif (1975) have commented on between the reading of *bee* and *be* (or *2 bee oar knot 2 bee* and *to be or not to be*). In the latter example the critical distinction is between part of speech: substantive words are available, grammatical are not. Rather it is a difference in availability related to the purpose for which the utterance is required. *Aye* is spontaneous, *eye* is elicited and self-conscious.

A similar discrepancy between the automatic and the controlled has been the subject of several studies and much debate in cognitive psychology in the 1980s (see Flores d'Arcais, in press, for a review). Automatic processes are characterized as occurring without awareness, being unavoidable, being resistant to modification, being highly efficient and having no capacity limitation (i.e. being able to run concurrently with other activities without interference). Controlled processes, in contast are in principle open to awareness, being under the control of the individual and therefore being modifiable; they are taxing of resources and of limited capacity. Some of the debate centres on whether automatic processes necessarily precede the controlled processes, or whether they operate in parallel. Applied to psycholinguistics in particular, further debate has been, for example, about whether all meanings or only one meaning of an ambiguous word are accessed automatically during the process of comprehension. One technique which is used to assess this is that of semantic priming, in which the prior presentation of a semantically related word facilitates the recognition of word. This technique has been applied in the study of comprehension of ambiguous words in aphasia. Milberg and his colleagues (Milberg, 1988) asked patients classified as Wernicke's aphasics to indicate whether the third word of three spoken words was a word or not (an auditory lexical decision task). A target word, such as 'money' was preceded by a homophone, such as 'bank', which was itself preceded by a word which either facilitated the homophone meaning which was appropriate to the target word ('coin') or one which was not ('river'). The aphasic patients, like normal subjects, were sensitive to priming by the appropriate meaning, in as much as their decisions were made faster than when the inappropriate meaning had been primed. Such patients, however, show poor comprehension of word meaning in tests where they have to match a spoken word with one of a set of pictures which include semantic distractors, or when they have to make explicit judgements of semantic relatedness. They seem to have implicit but not explicit knowledge of word meanings.

Schacter, McAndrew and Moscovitch's (1988) paper reviews several cognitive neuropsychological studies which bear on the dissociation between automatic and controlled processing, using these terms 'implicit and explicit knowledge'. Amnesic patients who have severe explicit memory deficits can nevertheless show implicit memory for new associations. People who are blind in part of their visual fields can nevertheless be sensitive to stimuli presented in these regions ('blindsight'), although they have no conscious experience of them. People with acquired reading disorders can also show implicit knowledge of words they cannot read accurately, as when they produce semantic paralexias, such as 'sepulchre' for the written word 'tomb'. The syndrome of 'pure alexia' or alexia without agraphia (also behaviourally described as letter-by-letter reading) can show a similar dissociation between what is consciously available to the would-be reader and automatic processing. Some (but not all) of these patients perform better than chance in choosing the correct item for a written word from an array of items (even though the initial letters of their names cannot be used as clues). They may also be able to categorize semantically words they cannot overtly read. In respect of Broca's aphasia, Schacter et al. point out that the fact that such patients have difficulty in reading function words (such as in the Gardner and Zurif example cited above) but not their homophonic substantive word counterparts argues for the preservation of implicit grammatical knowledge. Indeed studies such as those of Linebarger, Schwartz and Saffran (1983) show that this implicit knowledge can be drawn on in tasks where Broca's aphasics are asked to judge whether sentences are syntactically well formed or not. On first pass this may seem to be a demanding metalinguistic task, which should require conscious processing. In fact such judgements seem to be made intuitively, without explicit explanation of why the sentences are wrong, and to be no more cognitively demanding than making decisions as to whether a word is an appropriate member of a certain semantic category or not. These patients do not seem able to use their preserved intuitive knowledge of syntax in the more demanding processing required for language comprehension and production. Schacter and colleagues crystallize their survey of the dissociation between explicit and implicit knowledge with the proposal that

'(a) conscious or explicit experiences of perceiving, knowing and remembering all depend in some way on the functioning of a common mechanism, (b) this mechanism normally  accepts input from and interacts with a variety of processors or modules that handle specific types of information, and (c) in various cases of neuropsychological impairment, various specific modules are disconnected from the conscious mechanism.'

In complement to this cognitive neuropsychological perspective and in respect specifically of language, we may add to the three levels of language use which Jackson described (non-speech swearing, inferior speech and real speech). At the top of the scale is the metalinguistic use of language in the description of itself, the level at which linguists operate in their work. At another level is the act of elicited meaning. When a patient names a list of objects or pictures at the therapist's request, he is not communicating to the therapist the names, but he is communicating the information that he can (or cannot) utter the appropriate names. The communication is the act not the content. There is consequently no automatic pattern to fall back upon in naming. We have not established an automatic reaction of looking at (for example) a chair and saying 'chair' in the way that we might automatically cry 'look out' if we saw a chair breaking. It is a common observation that aphasic speakers who have difficulty in naming an object can have less difficulty in supplying the same word in completion of a sentence, a situation which can occur in normal conversation. If naming is put fairly high up in this hypothetical scale of difficulty, ranging from the automatic vocalization of swear words to the metalinguistic use of language to describe itself, it may account in part for the ubiquitous difficulty in elicited naming which is reported in all types of aphasia, in that naming is a voluntary purposive task which may therefore be one of the first uses of language to be impaired. Brain (1965) has commented that the meaning of words, as well as depending upon verbal and syntactic content, is influenced by 'the context of interest—a term which includes attention to an object in the environment or an idea, together with the feelings and intentions of the speaker and hearer with regard to it' (p. 93). When an aphasic patient is given a formal assessment of language in a clinical situation he is already partly removed from his natural context of interest. Formal assessments of language disorders based on clinical tests do not always agree with functional assessments on the Functional Communication Profile (see the study by Needham and Swisher 1972). There are patients whom, from their normal small-talk in the waiting room, one is surprised to find attending a speech therapy clinic, until the structured situation of a formal assessment shows that they cannot cope with this removed level of language unsupported by the natural context of appropriateness.

In therapy the distinction between automatic and purposive is emphasized and applied. Vignolo (1964) describes one of the main principles of therapy as the making use of automatic and semi-automatic abilities to lead the patient back to voluntary uses of language. In a further reformulation of this principle, Wepman (1976) has advocated, for some patients, the abandonment of formal language exercises in favour of *thought stimulation therapy* in which the patient is never asked in any way for the voluntary elicitation of verbal expression. Instead the patient't interest is maintained in a topic which is of central value in his life, and language arises incidentally as part of the discussion and planning around this topic. Wepman reports that this approach to therapy resulted in a dramatic improvement after two weeks in a patient who had previously reached a plateau after therapy which had consisted of directed effort aimed at improving word usage.

On the whole, therefore, although any scaling of language use is as yet speculative, a case can be made for more attention to be paid to the circumstances of language as well as to its form and content in linguistic investigations of aphasia.

In this chapter some examples have been given of the peculiar problems which face the investigator of language in the brain-damaged. Some of these apply equally to children with language disability, but many are problems which follow directly from brain damage. The brain-damaged patient's mental homeostasis is disturbed, and the margin of reserves he has for overcoming difficulties is reduced. Consequently what may seem to be subtle niceties which can be ignored in examining language in normal people can assume significant proportions. This is not to say that all the performance factors which have been proposed in this chapter must be controlled for in all investigations of aphasia. It is convenient to assume that aphasic adults' metalinguistic judgements about what is syntactically or semantically anomalous are a reliable index of their capabilities, and that using colours does not make a task more difficult or that asking aphasic patients to arrange tokens is no harder for them in principle than asking them to point to them. But nevertheless we should be aware in every investigation that we have made assumptions which may eventually prove to have been unfounded.

# 5

# Semantic relationships in aphasia: associations, fields and features

One of the most astonishing qualities of the human brain is its ability to retrieve specific items of information from its vast store of semantic memories within fractions of a second and to organize them into a shape which can be translated into the sounds of speech. We have only to listen to quiz programmes on radio and television to marvel at the speed with which contestants answer a barrage of questions like 'What name is given to the study of saints? In what species of fish does the male rear the young? Where did the dog Flush live?' At a less erudite level word retrieval at will is a facility which we take for granted. We assume that there should be no problem in calling a rose a rose when we see one, or a spade a spade, or in telling an enquirer the names of our children or our parents. Yet sometimes this facility is lost. We have almost all of us had the experience of being unable to recall the name of someone we know quite well, or of being unable to produce a word for some obscure definition although we feel certain we do know it and will be able to produce it some time later. At some stage in the process of retrieving information and matching meaning with sound the system fails: the exploration of these *feeling-of-knowing* and *tip-of-the-tongue* states has excited the interest of psychologists since Brown and McNeill (1966) began to examine just what information about the shape of the word is available in these intermediate conditions. These states are frequent in aphasia—and indeed in all types of aphasia, although they are particularly prominent in anomia. They present some fascinating problems in diagnosis to the aphasiologist. Does the patient really have the word on the tip of his tongue, or is there some lack of semantic definition which blurs the potential word before it even begins to take form? Or is it some failure to match a defined meaning with its phonological shape? And what of the not infrequent patients who, despite articulatory competence, have often to help themselves to speak a word by writing it down first and then reading it aloud to themselves, as if the graphemic form of the word can be accessed directly but not the phonemic? And the others, again with articulatory phonetic competence but with the phonological programming disorders of apraxia of speech or conduction aphasia, who write down words they wish to say and who cannot then read them back aloud? We shall return to this question of the relationship of difficulties at the phonological level to semantic retrieval in a later chapter. For the present, let us look at the studies of aphasia which are relevant to the question of whether or not there is, in all aphasias or specifically in anomic aphasia, a radical disturbance of word meaning which is traceable in both comprehension and in production and which therefore cannot be attributed entirely to difficulties in the encoding of meaning into speech sounds.

As a preliminary, let us first distinguish three uses of the term *word*. One is the word as its phonological (or orthographical) realization; another is the word as a unit of analysis of sentences (the most common usage of the term); a third is as equivalent to *lexeme* (Lyons 1969), a unit of meaning at a more abstract level which reflects, for example, the commonality amongst items such as 'sings', 'sang' and 'to sing'. Palmer (1976) points out that it is lexemes which generally provide the entries in a dictionary. The definition of *lexeme* usually restricts it to variants within the same grammatical class (as with the variants of the verb 'to sing' given above); but it is also possible to extend the definition to an even more abstract level, so that members of other grammatical classes may also be included within the same group ('song', 'singer'). Many dictionaries do in fact acknowledge the relationships amongst words of different grammatical classes by grouping them under the same heading, but only if they share a common orthographical form as well as meaning (e.g. 'boast' as a noun and 'boast' as a verb). If a unit of meaning were to be proposed which is independent not only of grammatical form but of phonological and orthographical form, such as that which is common to 'strong', 'strength', 'strongly' and 'strengthen', Palmer suggests that we should need some more general term for this basic lexical item than *word* or *lexeme*; but the term to which he draws attention, Firth's *formal scatter*, has the disadvantage of empha-sizing spread rather than cohesion in a commonality of relationships. For want of an agreed terminology we shall use *word* in this sense as well as in the other senses listed above.

In this chapter we are therefore considering essentially the semantic organiza-tion of the lexicon, the paradigmatic sense relationships amongst words, as if we can arbitrarily separate meaning from both the phonological form which an uttered word must take and from the syntactic and contextual constraints which are imposed on meaning as it is expressed in sentences and discourse. We are thus restricting the area of enquiry in this chapter to single words and their interrelation-ships at an abstract level, despite the fact that such a restriction goes against the tide of much current linguistic and philosophical theory. Even when there are dis-cussions of the lexicon as a store of words independent of actual sentence context, it is most common to find these words referred to as if they had an explicit phono-logical shape and syntactic form. For example there has been a controversy as to whether *lexicalist* or *transformational* models best account for the relationship between some nominals and verbs such as 'destruction' and 'destroy'. According to the transformationalist model the nominal form is derived from the verb form by a transformation, so that 'They decided on the destruction of the airport' is presumed to derive from a deeper structure 'They decided that they would destroy the airport'. In the transformationalist model, therefore, the lexicon is presumed to contain only the verb form ('destroy' in this case) from which the nominal form is derived. According to the lexicalist model, however, both verb and nominal are included in the lexicon as separate entries. Evidence from aphasia has been invoked in support of this model. Whitaker (1971a) asked three patients to read out a list of nouns and verbs or to formulate sentences around them. He observed a tendency for verbs to be read out or used in their nominalized forms: 'remember' was commuted into 'memory', 'decide' to 'decision', 'engage' to 'engagement'. Such an observation is not consistent with nominalized forms requiring more complex operations than the simple verb forms from which they are supposedly derived. But whatever the merits of either of these models, they both make the assumption that it is valid to conceive of the lexicon from which words are selected for insertion into sentences as being a collection of ready-made words each distinguished by its phonological shape and marked for syntactic class. Indeed it has been proposed that the lexicon is indexed by phonological criteria, in something like the way words in a dictionary are listed in alphabetical order. Homonyms like 'cricket', the game, and 'cricket', the insect, would therefore be stored together. However, there are some advantages for aphasiology in conceiving of a semantic level of language which is autonomous from phonological and syntactic form and in accepting McCawley's (1968) proposal that an individual's mental dictionary is organized semantically rather than phonologically. Such a concept allows us to include in the different stages of preparation for an utterance, at which word-finding difficulties can occur, a stage of semantic integration or selection which may be presumed to be prior to the stages of syntactic and phonological formulation. We can then ask whether anomia is a reflection of a disorder within this semantic level in which word meaning has become distorted rather than a problem in retrieval of pre-constituted words, phonological shapes and all. By ignoring for the present not only sentence context but distinctions of syntactic class (amongst substantive words) we can also draw on the many studies of word-finding difficulties in aphasia which have examined single words out of context, either by asking patients to name pictured or real objects or actions, or to read aloud lists of words. This approach has the pragmatic justification of simplifying somewhat a problem which is enormously complex, and for the reduction of which we have at present no adequate framework: Houston (1972, p. 260) comments that 'one might note that present psycholinguistic models of language are for all practical purposes quite inadequate to deal with the fact of anomia'.

A pragmatic approach, however, is only justified if there is some expectation that it does not make unrealistic assumptions. Palmer (1976, p. 41) cites Bazell as commenting: 'To seek a semantic unit within the boundaries of the word simply because these boundaries are clearer than others is like looking for a lost ball on the lawn simply because the thicket provides poor ground for such a search.' But there are some signs which encourage us to think that studying single words out of context may not be entirely inappropriate for aphasia. There are indications that some elementary preservation of the lexicon in comprehension is the norm in even a very severe aphasia provided the damage to the brain has been one-sided, and that the right hemisphere shows some capacity for the recognition and comprehension of word meaning although its capacities for syntactic and analytic phonemic decoding are minimal (Zaidel 1977a; 1977b). Such indications add up to the speculation that the semantic component of language may be much more widely distributed in the brain than the syntactic and phonological components, and that the speech zones of the left hemisphere are specialized for the transformation of this diffuse semantic knowledge into its formal shapes as uttered words in sentences and for its consequent elaboration. If such speculations are supported, the simplification of the study of semantics in aphasia, by restricting it initially to the meaning component of single words, may eventually be justified as reflecting a true division of some aspects of language organization in the brain. At present such speculations are controversial (see for example Palmer's (1976, p. 42) denial that 'we can look for meanings or relations between them divorced from the forms of language'). We should not lose sight of the essential unnaturalness of the task when we urge aphasic adults to name a series of pictures or objects. Kogan (cited by Maruszewski 1975) has drawn attention to the fact that in everyday life it is objects which are not in view which are named rather than ones which both the speaker and the hearer can see. As was pointed out in the last chapter the task of producing a specific name at will is nearer to the metalinguistic than the automatic on a scale of functional levels. Gelb and Goldstein (1924) accordingly attributed the naming disorder in amnesic aphasia to a disability in achieving the abstract attitude needed for naming in such situations. Consequently although we pool together semantic misnamings in such naming tasks, semantic paralexias and spontaneous word searchings in communicative utterances, we have to remind ourselves that we are pooling data collected from different functional levels, and that, as explorations of aphasia become more sophisticated, it may be necessary to make further distinctions.

## Central and restricted semantic disorders

To begin this account of the examination of word-finding difficulties as reflecting a disorder within the semantic level, let us look first at the extent to which naming difficulties are dependent on the modality through which they are examined.

From the neurological perspective, a broad distinction has been made between *classical anomia*, which affects all modalities and which is also evident at least to some extent in spontaneous speech, and *specific anomias* in which the naming difficulties are restricted to one particular medium of input (Geschwind 1967). In the latter cases it must also be established that the naming difficulties are not due to some peripheral disorder of perception. As examples of these restricted forms of anomia, Geschwind describes two kinds of patient. One patient examined by him and Kaplan had no difficulty in naming objects by sight or in spontaneous speech, but made bizarre misnamings when he was blindfolded and given an object to feel with his left hand. He called a ring 'eraser', a watch 'balloon', a padlock 'book of matches', and a screwdriver 'piece of paper'. It could be established, however, that he had no problems in the sensory recognition of the object, as he could pick out the object he had felt with his left hand from a selection of objects, or, when still blindfolded, could show the correct usage of the object with his left hand even while calling it by an inappropriate name. Geschwind accounts for this highly specific naming difficulty by suggesting that damage to the corpus callosum had disconnected the right hemisphere, to which the sensory information from the left hand was relayed, from the speech zones of the left hemisphere. A second type of patient who displays a restricted difficulty in naming is the patient who has colour-naming difficulties in association with reading difficulties in the syndrome of pure alexia without agraphia (though problems in naming colours occur in only about 70 per cent of patients with this syndrome). Again this is explained in terms of disconnection: this time the disconnection is of the right visual cortex from the speech area. Such patients are said to have no problems with the correct use of colour names in spontaneous speech, or in answering such questions as 'What colour is butter? What colour is a pillar box?' because, like the first patient, they have no damage to the language system itself. In both these kinds of patients it is only the attaching of a specific label to a sensory impression received through one modality which is impaired. The misnamings made under these circumstances suggest that the patient is making a wild guess. The disconnection, according to Geschwind, works both ways, affecting both the uttering of a name and the interpretation of a heard name: the patient's difficulty in naming colours is matched by a difficulty in selecting a named colour from a group. Consequently Geschwind suggests that this type of selective anomia is best characterized as an 'inability to match a stimulus to its spoken name' (p. 104). According to Geschwind it is not the same as an agnosia, however, which means an inability to recognize objects or other percepts, and which can also of course result in a failure to utter the correct name. An agnosic patient would not be able to show recognition by demonstrating the use of an object he could see (visual agnosia) or feel (tactile agnosia) or hear (auditory agnosia).

The distinction between anomia and agnosia, particularly visual agnosia, is not, however, always as clear as these labels would imply. Bender and Feldman (1972) found that all the patients they examined who had been described as having visual agnosia had perceptive or dysphasic difficulties which could have accounted for their problems. An alexic patient seen by the author has described her additional visual agnosic difficulties by saying that she did not know what a cup was until she picked it up. Interestingly enough, this happened even with a picture of a cup. Apparently she was able to extract enough information from the picture before she 'recognized' it to imagine herself picking up the object it represented, and then at that stage was able to recognize and name it. Warrington (1975) has described three patients with visual agnosia (the total number amongst the large number of patients seen over three years at a major neurological hospital), all of whom had suffered bilateral brain damage. She suggests that it is useful to distinguish two stages in visual recognition: an apperceptive stage in which a perceptual classification occurs (such as the identification of different typographical shapes as belonging to the same alphabet letter), and an associative or semantic classificatory stage in which the significance of the symbol is interpreted. Warrington proposes that this visual associative and semantic memory system may be partially distinct from the verbal semantic memory system, and she consequently retains the term *agnosia* to describe the condition in which the patient cannot identify common objects (despite retained sensory and cognitive abilities), even though it can be demonstrated that he has some partial knowledge about the objects such as the semantic categories to which they belong. She also therefore deduces that visual object agnosia cannot be satisfactorily accounted for in terms of a disconnection of different brain processes, but rather that the semantic memory system itself must be damaged, although it may be a specifically visual semantic memory.

For the classical type of anomia as part of aphasia there is common agreement that it is the language system itself which is disturbed rather than a disconnection of the system from a modality of input. The difficulty of naming on confrontation involves more or less all types of material and is more or less equal for all sensory media. According to Geschwind, the naming errors are generally related by sound or by meaning to the target word, or are circumlocutions, and occur in spontaneous speech as well, From the linguistic viewpoint rather than the neurological, it is the semantic errors made in this classical type of anomia which are the more inviting to study, as they offer some means of examining the structure of semantic memory in the lexicon. By tracing the changes and distortions in the lexicon in anomia, we may be able to gain an insight into this level of linguistic organization. If Warrington is correct, even in restricted anomias there may also be illuminating changes in a semantic system rather than the total disconnection which would not be so informative.

However, in classical anomia, if the semantic system itself is damaged, we should expect that errors would be made not only regardless of the sensory medium in which the stimulus to be named was presented, but that they would be made in comprehension as well as in speaking. Some descriptions of anomia have run counter to this expectation. Geschwind (1967) in fact makes the relative preservation of comprehension in the classical type of anomia one of the distinguishers between this and the restricted type of anomia. In classical anomia, despite the errors in speech, the patient can usually choose the correct name if it is offered to him by the examiner and can select a named object from a group. In modality-specific anomias he cannot. In the absence of comprehension deficit, classical anomia therefore, according to Geschwind, appears to differ not only in degree but also in kind from the isolated naming disorders.

More recently, however, it has been suggested that there is a comprehension deficit in the classical aphasic anomia which parallels the semantic deficit in speech. It is suggested that semantic comprehension only seems to be preserved because the tests which are used to examine it are less demanding: it is easier, if some partial awareness of the meaning of a word is retained, to make a correct choice from a limited number of words or objects than to retrieve the word for speech from a much wider range of possibilities. Some of the studies to be described shortly have had a subsidiary interest in examining the degree to which semantic disorders in speech are matched by semantic disorders in comprehension; we shall refer to these findings in their other contexts. But here it is appropriate to describe two studies, more than a decade apart, which have addressed themselves specifically to this question. Alajouanine and his co-workers in Paris (1964) suggested that patients with Wernicke-type aphasia could be distinguished according to whether they made principally phonemic paraphasias or principally semantic paraphasias, and that in each kind the specific paraphasic disorder in speech would be accompanied by a specific parallel deficit in comprehension. Amongst the many tests they gave the patients was one in which they showed them ten sets of five pictures, each set illustrating words from a semantic category. The categories were *food, writing materials, furniture, toilet materials, cutlery, smoking, clothes, sewing materials, farm animals* and *bicycle parts*. An example of a set of words for one category (*food*) was *butter, cheese, bread, chocolate, meat*. The patient heard one of the words, and pointed to his choice amongst the five pictures. There were only five patients whose speech was characterized by semantic jargon, as opposed to nineteen whose speech was characterized by phonemic jargon; but those with semantic jargon made proportionately three times as many errors on this semantic test of comprehension as did the others (18 per cent errors). Alajouanine therefore proposed that there were two distinct functional systems, an auditory-phonatory system and a system of semantic integration, which could be disturbed relatively independently. The breakdown in semantic values which characterizes semantic jargon in speech is therefore a reflection of a disturbance at a central level.

As evidence that naming difficulties in speech are necessarily paralleled by semantic difficulties in comprehension, this study is not conclusive, as it was restricted to Wernicke type patients with semantic jargon, in whom some comprehension impairment might be predicted. Anomia as the principal symptom in aphasia is typically characterized by circumlocutory rather than jargon speech and by good functional comprehension.

More recently Gainotti and his colleagues in Rome (1975; Gainotti 1976) have re-examined this hypothesis of Alajouanine's, using a test which examines simultaneously both semantic and phonemic discrimination, the 'verbal sound and meaning discrimination test'. Like Alajouanine's task, this also uses pictures. In this case there were six pictures to choose from to match to a heard word: one correct, one of a phonemically related word, one of a semantically related word and three of unrelated words. This reduced the probability of a patient's choosing a semantically or phonemically related picture by chance. They included amongst their subjects five different types of aphasics according to predominant symptoms of phonemic jargon, semantic jargon, mixed jargon, phonetic disintegration with agrammatism and reduced speech flow, and patients classed as amnesic aphasics. They found that in semantic jargon and in amnesic aphasia the prevalence of semantic over phonemic discrimination errors was significantly higher than in non-aphasic brain-damaged control subjects, thus supporting this part of Alajouanine's hypothesis; but there was not a significant association of phonemic jargon with predominantly phonemic errors in discrimination. Gainotti suggests that the high incidence of semantic discrimination errors, in amnesic aphasic as well as in semantic jargon patients, may indicate a breakdown of the semantic level of language integration in both these kinds of patient. Moreover there was an unexpectedly high incidence of semantic errors in the other aphasic groups, including those whose symptoms would put them into the category of

Broca's aphasics, raising the question of the functioning of the semantic system in aphasia in general. Gainotti suggests that the breakdown of the semantic level of language integration may be a basic trouble in most forms of aphasia. In a later discussion of these findings Gainotti (1976) comments that this breakdown at the semantic level cannot be explained in terms of disorders of performance components, as Weigl and Bierwisch's (1970) application of the competence–performance distinction to aphasia had suggested. According to Gainotti the strong correlation between the emission of semantic paraphasias and the impairment of auditory semantic discrimination seems to demonstrate that in aphasia a true level of integration of language, at the semantic level, has been affected.

This is one viewpoint which has many supporters. It is partly on the assumption that a central level of language integration is being accessed that researchers into semantic disorders in aphasia may often make no distinctions between measures of semantic comprehension which involve the patient in reading and sorting words, and measures which involve him in listening to words and making choices based on pictures. Use of pictures restricts the vocabulary which can be tested to a limited range of unambiguously picturable words, predominantly nouns, and there are obvious advantages in extending the range if printed words can be used to test semantic abilities. But another viewpoint on semantic disorders in aphasia is that the semantic structure of the lexicon is undisturbed but that the threshold for evocation of words is raised (Rochford and Williams 1962; 1965). The role of the cerebral speech areas, from this perspective, is considered to be related to the availability of words rather than to semantic storage itself. If it is the threshold for availability rather than the structure of the system which has changed, then the medium of access through which the word is made available assumes a more crucial role. To reconcile these two viewpoints we shall need a more detailed knowledge of lexical organization than can at present be derived. By hypothesizing that semantic organization can be independent of the shapes which can be called 'words', we can consider models of this organization in terms of abstract relationships amongst components of meaning. We shall look first at these relationships in terms of associations.

## Associations

Ullman (1956, p. 16) has described the relationships amongst words in the lexicon as follows: 'Words do not stand isolated within the vocabulary; the relation between name and sense must be supplemented by other relations connecting each word with its neighbours. Every word has what has been called its 'associative field': the whole vocabulary is intersected by associations between names and between senses.'

We shall look in the next section at some of the conceptual categorizations of associative fields which linguists and others have made: in this section we look at the empirical collection of data about associations which psychologists have undertaken, and which have served as a basis for studying aphasic misnamings and misinterpretations.

The beginning of word association research is generally credited to Francis Galton in the latter part of the nineteenth century (Forrest 1977), although Clark (1970) refers to the 'free association game' as being centuries old. The original purpose in asking people to say (or write down) the first word that came to mind for each word in a list (free associations) was to obtain information about their mental status or personality (Kent and Rosanoff 1910). More recently, because these responses tend to show a predictable degree of agreement, this method has been used as a way of exploring the nature of the relationships within the lexicon, rather than differences amongst individual people or groups of people. There are now several collections of *norms* of word associations, gathered chiefly from students' responses, but sometimes from other age groups and educational levels; the best known of these in the English language (principally) are probably those by Postman and Keppel (1970) and Deese's (1965) Associative Dictionary. Such norms list the number of associations given by the group of subjects for each stimulus word (often using the same list of 100 words derived from Kent and Rosanoff), and give the number of times each response word is used. In one list from 400 British students, for example (Miller 1970), the average number of different words elicited for each word was about 85 from the whole group and for each word on average 125 of the students gave the same word as their first response.

The kind of response given differs with age. Children tend to give more responses which are not of the same grammatical class as the stimulus word (competing or syntagmatic responses), whereas adults tend to make more responses of the same grammatical class (paradigmatic responses). For example, the stimulus word *dog* might elicit a response such as *barks* from a young child, but *cat* from an adult. The proportion of paradigmatic responses from adults, however, depends on what the grammatical class of the stimulus word is: adverbs and infrequent adjectives, even with adults, tend to evoke more syntagmatic responses (e.g. *auburn—hair*) than paradigmatic. In adults' association norms there is also a proportion of associations which are alliterative or rhyming (such as *lamp—light*, *salt—sea, sheep—sleep*) but almost invariably there are strong semantic links in addition to the phonological ones, unless the subjects have been pressured into producing extremely fast responses in which case these rhyming kinds of responses predominate. This suggests that (unpressurized) associations to substantive words can provide some insight into the interrelationships within the lexicon without being unduly distorted by syntactic and phonological contextual influences.

The degree of agreement from adults in their word associations can be remarkable. Kent and Rosanoff found, for example, that of the 1,000 subjects in their sample no fewer than 650 gave the response *light* to the stimulus word *lamp*. Fox (1970) showed that if a group of subjects is given the same list of words again after 60 days there is a very high agreement between the two sets of responses, even though individual subjects may show on average a change in about half their responses, usually to words which do not have a dominant first response. Subjects therefore seem to select from a finite pool of words for each stimulus word under these conditions. Lesser (1973) showed that the size of this pool was influential on the ability of an aphasic woman to find and utter associative responses. When the possible pool of responses was large, the subject had more difficulty in finding a response than when it was small; when the pool was small, with few responses given to that word in the norms (and therefore usually with one or two dominant responses), the aphasic woman was often able to find a conventional response. The proportion of less conventional and idiosyncratic responses and of failures to respond increased in linear progression as the size of the pool increased. Despite the variety of individual experience, there therefore seems to be a commonality in semantic structuring of knowledge, and word associations seem to follow laws which show that they access this structuring.

Since Noble defined the meaningfulness of a word as the number of associations it was capable of eliciting ($M$), there have been a number of associative indices proposed as measures of the degree to which words are interrelated. Marshall and Cofer (1963) reviewed ten. From these they conclude that there are non-direct associations amongst words as well as direct simple ones, and that associative indices have considerable power in predicting the outcomes in situations where words are used.

A compilation of these direct and indirect associations is the Associative Thesaurus collected by Kiss (1973) from about 9,000 students at British universities, probably the largest single collection of word-association data in existence. Kiss and his colleagues at the University of Edinburgh conceived of the structure of the thesaurus as a large network in which the nodes are words, and the connecting arcs between nodes represent the mathematical probabilities of giving those words as responses to the stimulus words they link. By starting with about 1,000 words and then eliciting responses in turn from the words which had been given as responses to this first list, they established the relationships amongst, in all, over 55,000 words. From a network of this kind it is possible to calculate not only what responses a stimulus word elicits, as can be done with normal word-association counts, but also to find out to what stimulus words a certain word is elicited as a response. The network appears to be densely interconnected near its centre with a progressive thinning out of links towards the periphery. The word *man*, for example, near the centre of the network was found to have 1,071 links with other words, while about 60 per cent of the words had only one link. A characteristic of such a network is that the flow of the associational links is directional: words which are given as responses to a stimulus word are usually not equally likely to elicit the original stimulus as a response in turn. From the network Kiss extracted two main kinds of semantic relationships: relevance and similarity. The relation of relevance, he suggested, reflects what goes on in people's mental images of the world, and the concepts on to which words are mapped. Similarity reflects the degree to which the relevance of two words overlap.

The conceptualization of semantic space as filled with a multidimensional network is to some extent forced upon the researcher by this method of collecting data through associations. Deese (1965), using factor analyses of free association data, extracted several dimensions of meaning but considered that dimensions extracted from such data are probably the results of the combined effects of all sorts of processes at work rather than pure semantic systems. Other people prefer to conceptualize the semantic associations amongst words as a hierarchical network. Collins and Quillian (1969) believed that they had found evidence which supported such a hierarchical model. They proposed that people store in semantic memory facts such as that a canary can fly, and that a robin can fly, and that a sparrow can fly, and so on, not with the words *canary*, *robin*, *sparrow*, etc. but with the category word *bird*. But information about a certain kind of bird which is peculiar to that kind of bird, such as that a canary is yellow, is stored with that particular word. They predicted that people should be faster in verifying a statement such as 'A canary is yellow' than in verifying a statement such as 'A canary can fly', for which the associative link is one step removed and is at the hierarchical level for *bird*. Although Collins and Quillian found that their predictions were supported, it has been suggested that such data on meaning comparisons reflect not the intrinsic organization of the lexicon, nor the mechanics of retrieval, but only a comparison process: if a decision has to be made about whether or not the words have different meanings it is said to be more difficult if the meanings partially overlap (Schaeffer and Wallace 1970), although the organization of the lexicon and the retrieval of each of the two words would necessarily be the same whether they overlap or not, in terms of an associative hierarchical model such as Collins and Quillin proposed. Consequently alternative conceptualizations of semantic organization have been proposed which emphasize category size and similarities of feature components in words. These are to be discussed in another section.

Whatever the relative merits of the multidimensional associational models, of the hierarchical association model or of other models, association models have the practical advantage for applied linguistics that their data are entirely empirically derived rather than being the result of the constraints of an imposed theory. The over-inclusiveness of free associations, which Deese (1970) and Miller (1969) have commented on as a weakness of this method of testing semantic relatedness, can be turned to advantage when they are used as a standard of comparison for aphasic naming errors. It has been pointed out by Schuell (1950) and again by Rinnert and Whitaker (1973) that there is a considerable resemblance between the naming errors of aphasic patients and the associations given by normal subjects.

Schuell collected examples of misnamings in speech and misreadings from 15 patients receiving speech therapy and analysed them according to the classification of word associations proposed by Jung and Riklin in 1918. Excluding idiosyncratic, residual and clang (rhyming) responses, these researchers had proposed that associations could be described as either *inner* or *outer*. Some of the *inner* associations they define are those of coadjunction (e.g. *murderer—gallows*) subordination (*tree—beech*), supraordination (*cat—animal*), contrast (*good—bad*), predication (*glass—brittle*) and causal dependence (*cut—pain*). *Outer* associations can reflect coexistence (*table—chair*), synonymy (*quarrel—dispute*), word complements (*fish—monger*) and other relationships like completion of clichés. If aphasic misreadings which could be attributed to visual confusions, such as *apple* for *able*, were classed with the clang errors, Schuell found that the aphasic errors (excluding perseverations) could be characterized as conforming in the following proportions to the categories of associations suggested by Jung and Riklin:

|          |      |
|----------|------|
| Inner    | 45%  |
| Outer    | 14%  |
| Clang    | 26%  |
| Residual | 14%  |

Schuell concluded that 'paraphasic and paralexic responses resemble word-association reactions of normal individuals; therefore there is no evidence that either paraphasic or paralexic responses represent a breakdown of the word-association process' (p. 304). The implication is that the aphasic's difficulties are similar to those which the non-aphasic individual experiences in a mild form when seeking a word.

Rinnert and Whitaker analysed the semantic confusions reported from aphasic patients in several published works, as well as those they had observed themselves. Their data in total consisted of 217 confusion pairs. For 131 of these pairs they found norms for at least one member of the pair in either Deese's Associative Dictionary or the collection of norms in Postman and Keppel. From these data there were only 37 cases in which neither of the words in the pair was an associate of the other, and, even in these cases, intuitively closely related words were often found as associates even though the exact word was not. Rinnert and Whitaker suggest that semantic confusions are more similar to word associations than dissimilar, but that in general semantic confusions are more specific than word associations. They speculate that those features which differentiate the error word from the target word may become missing from the internal representation of the items, or be overwhelmed by what the two items have in common; or alternatively it may be that the error word is somehow easier to produce or more accessible than the target word, or that perhaps the choice between items which share certain semantic features is essentially random. The tentative categorization of aphasic semantic confusions which they proffered used eleven categories: synonyms, antonyms, coordinates from the same category (coat—sweater), sub- and superordinates (vegetables—potatoes; banana—fruit), object description (water—wet), part-whole relations (children—family), action outcome (speak—discussions), spatial contiguity (glasses—eyes), item location (chair—office), instrument function (curtains—draw) and shape and size analogies (boy—small pencil).

Since the semantic confusions of aphasic speakers seem to correspond to a considerable extent to the free word associations of normal speakers, the question arises of what happens when aphasic speakers are asked to produce free associations. Wyke (1962) conducted an experiment with four predominantly expressive aphasic patients whom she compared with three non-aphasic patients with right-sided or generalized brain damage. Amongst other tasks she asked them to give free associations to 25 words from the Kent–Rosanoff list. The performance of the aphasic subjects on this task was significantly inferior to that of the other patients in that they produced a larger number of unconventional responses, i.e. responses which are not listed in the norms. These unconventional responses were of four kinds: words which sounded similar to the stimulus word (*cabbage—carriage*), nonsensical associations, egocentrisms and tangential associations. The latter kind of associations in which some indirect relationship with the stimulus word could be detected (*carpet—coat*; *sour—tasteless*) formed the majority of the aphasic patients' unconventional responses. Wyke suggests that the verbal reactions which the patients displayed were those which usually lie at the periphery of the semantic complex for the key word rather than near its nucleus. In contrast to Schuell's conclusion, she asks whether 'This may be the result of a basic breakdown of association of ideas, rather than of a simple alteration in language habits.' An unpublished study by Reynolds in 1960 (reported by Carter 1969) came to a different conclusion, however. This investigation found that the association responses of fourteen aphasic subjects to 90 words from the Kent–Rosanoff list showed significant agreement amongst themselves in terms of whether they were superordinate, coordinate or subordinate contrasts to the stimulus words: moreover the classes of responses were similar to those of non-aphasic adults. The investigation of speech characteristics by Howes and Geschwind (Howes 1964), which resulted in the Type A and Type B classification described in chapter 1, also included a word-association task given to 60 aphasic patients. Howes found that the nature of the word associations given depended on the character of the aphasia. Type A patients gave, albeit after delay, essentially normal associations; Type B failed to give associations or gave bizarre ones.

From these varied results it would seem that the semantic quality of word associations depends on the nature of the aphasic disorder and that responses to such tests could provide some insight into the degree of semantic disorder in a patient. (The picture with regard to syntactic factors, however, is somewhat different, and will be described in chapter 7.)

Word-association norms have also been used as a basis for tests of semantic comprehension in aphasia, as providing an empirically more verifiable measure of semantic relations than the intuitive guesses about semantic similarity which are used in some tests of comprehension. Pizzamiglio and Appicciafuoco (1971) selected 30 sets of four picturable words, using sets which had been found in word-association norms from Italian students to have a high degree of associative overlapping. An exact index of semantic similarity for each set of words was derived by calculating the amount of overlapping of the associations which words in it had elicited, and the word with the highest overlapping was taken as the stimulus word for that set of four pictures. Then 120 adults, including 60 people with aphasia of varying kinds and severity, were asked to listen to a list of 30 tape-recorded words, and for each to select one of the four pictures they thought best represented that word. Some of the control subjects made up to four errors on the 30 items, and this was taken as the cut-off point between aphasic and normal behaviour. Only six aphasic subjects out of the 60 scored above this cutting score. Patients classified as Broca's and amnesic aphasics made fewer errors than did patients classified as Wernicke's aphasics, but when a smaller sample of Broca's and Wernicke's aphasics was taken which was matched for severity of aphasia it was found that there was no difference between them. The semantic disorder in comprehension, therefore, appeared to be related to severity rather than to type of aphasia in this study. The order of difficulty of the stimulus words was compared with the index of similarity derived from the amount of overlapping (reported in Pizzamiglio, Parisi and Appicciafuoco 1968), but the correlation was not found to be significant, indicating that other factors than semantic similarity are influential on what makes the stimulus words in such a test difficult—the researchers suggested that one important factor was probably the frequency of the word in the language. However, it was found that the correlation between the words chosen as wrong responses and the index of semantic similarity was significant, so that it seemed that the strength of semantic similarity played a major role in the decision process, even if it did not in the patients' sensitivity to the stimulus words. An English version of this test is described by Lesser (1974).

A similar use of word-association norms has been made by Lansdell (1973), this time in exploring the effects of temporal and subcortical neurosurgical operations in men and women. He used 55 words from the Kent–Rosanoff list which had been found over the decades reliably to elicit standard responses, and accompanied each word with, besides this expected response, three less likely responses and one unlikely response. This test was presented in printed form, rather than using pictures: the stimulus word was printed in capital letters and followed by the five choices in lower-case letters. The subjects were asked to choose a word from amongst these which they thought would be the most popular associate for the word in capitals. As the 156 subjects were neurosurgical patients, it was possible to give them the test both before and after the operation. Thirty-one of the subjects had unilateral temporal lobe removals, and 41 unilateral coagulation of tissue in surgery to the thalamus, one of the subcortical nerve cell structures in the brain. A control group of normal people was also given the test twice to check on the extent to which responses might be expected to be stable. From the results with the patients Lansdell discovered that it was only with male patients who had undergone subcortical surgery on the left side of the brain that there was a significant difference in the number of errors made in selecting word associations before and after surgery. The results of the word-association test were unrelated to the traditional factor of verbal comprehension as it is measured by Wechsler–Bellevue Scale of Intelligence. It was possible, however, that this unusual result of an effect only of subcortical lesions could have been related to damage along the tracts of electrodes which had been implanted a week or so before the surgery. But it was notable that the impairment occurred only in men, supporting the theory that there are differences between the sexes in hemispheric specialization. None of the patients was described as aphasic, and it is interesting to observe that even after removal of some part of the left temporal lobe there can be no impairment of linguistic competence which a word-association test of this kind is sufficiently sensitive to detect.

## Associations as semantic fields

One way in which the word-association test is a rather crude instrument for examining lexical structure is that it takes no cognizance of the effect of list order on responses. It assumes that each response is only to that stimulus word and that there is no effect left from previous stimulus words. Experiments with associated words by Meyer and colleagues (Meyer, Schvaneveldt and Ruddy 1972; 1974; Schvaneveldt and Meyer 1973) demonstrate that activation of one word has an effect which does influence decisions about later words. In their studies of retrieval and comparison processes in semantic memory in normal adults, they asked people to decide as quickly as they could whether or not two strings of letters both represented words or whether one or both strings were not acceptable words (such as *smuke* or *reab*). For the items in which both strings were real words, the experimenters sometimes used pairs of words which were associated (*bread—butter*, *doctor—nurse*) and sometimes pairs which were not associated (*bread—doctor*, *nurse—butter*). There was a substantial facilitation when associated words were used, with subjects responding much faster. The experimenters suggested two possible models, both of which could account for such a facilitation. One was that stored information can be read out of only one location at a time, and that, as associated words are stored near to each other, the distance to be 'travelled' is less: they called this the *location-shifting model*. Alternatively, retrieving information from one location may be conceived of as producing a spread of excitation to nearby locations, making it easier to access information stored there, i.e. the *spreading-excitation* model. To test which of these models provides a better account, they carried out a further series of experiments, putting unassociated words between two associated words (e.g. *bread—star—butter*). If the unassociated word was read in between the two associated words, it would cancel out any possible facilitation of association, if the location-shift model was correct, as the path between the two associated words would be interrupted by the shift to the unassociated words. But if the spreading excitation model was correct, there would still be some facilitation of the associative effect despite the interruption of an irrelevant word. The results supported the spreading-excitation model. They also showed that the process examined was that of retrieval, not of semantic comparison, as Schaeffer and Wallace had suggested of the effects which Collins and Quillian had found in their experiments. When the three strings of letters were *not* all words, subjects recognized this fact more quickly if the strings included two associated words than if the strings included two unassociated words. Schaeffer and Wallace's observations had indicated that semantic comparison processes are slowed down if the two words share some features.

The notion of spreading excitation links with the neurophysiological interpretation of the mental operations underlying language, as requiring controlled patterns of excitation and inhibition, a model which is being developed in East European countries. A seminal study which investigated the dynamics of semantic systems through classical conditioning was that by Luria and Vinogradova (1959; see also a condensed account in Luria 1975b). The investigations, a development of Russian studies in the 1940s, were carried out with normal subjects and with mentally retarded children. Luria conceives of each word as being a multidimensional matrix of connections of sound and meaning from which the subject each time selects the appropriate meaning; the associations of each word form a *semantic field*. (This neurophysiological concept of a semantic field is different from the one used in linguistics, for a discussion of which see the beginning of chapter 6.) As he was able to demonstrate by objective methods, using semantic conditioning, this semantic field can be distinguished as having a central area near the nucleus of the word itself and a peripheral area. The technique makes use of the fact that an orienting reaction to a stimulus (the reaction when a person becomes aware of or has to attend to a stimulus) results in different physiological changes from those which result from a pain reaction to a stimulus. In an orienting reaction blood vessels in the fingers contract and blood vessels on the temples of the head dilate. With pain reaction, blood vessels in both the head and the fingers contract. The first stage in the investigation of the dynamics of semantic fields was to establish in a subject an orienting reaction to a certain word. The subject was given instructions to listen for one word recurring in a list of words (e.g. *cat*) and to press a button with his right hand each time he heard it. Each time this happened, the instruments recording the blood-pressure changes in his head and in a finger of his inactive left hand showed that the vascular orienting reaction was occurring. Then words which had associations with the key word were introduced (*kitten, mouse, dog, animal*). Even though there was a complete absence of any movement of the hand pressing the button, an orienting reaction was still evident from the changes in blood vessels in the head and other hand. Words having a close connection with the target word produced a greater effect of the orienting reaction, while words less obviously associated with the key word provoked a less evident reaction, and words which had no sense link with the key word provoked no vascular reaction, even though they had phonetic similarities with it. Luria concluded that the semantic system is dominant, and that sound resemblances are not included in this system in normal subjects, although he observed that in children with oligophrenia it seemed to be the sound links which were dominant over the semantic. In a second experiment, instead of being asked to press a button when a key word was heard, the subjects were given a painful electric shock. The orienting reaction to the word (contraction of vessels in the finger and dilation of those in the head) became replaced by the pain reaction (parallel contraction of blood vessels in head and hand). When closely associated words were introduced into the list to which the subject was listening, the pain reaction occurred also with these. If the key word was *violin*, for example, pain reactions also occurred to *violinist, string, bow* and to the names of several other stringed instruments. But when other words were introduced, which had a less close connection, the orienting rather than the pain reaction occurred: these were words like the names of stringless musical instruments, other words connected with music, and sometimes words which were only similar to the key word in sound. Again, completely neutral words produced no vascular reactions. As the experiment continued, the pain reactions to all words but the specific key word faded out, and then later the orienting reactions faded out, until the subject responded only to the key word and showed no reaction to any other word. If such an experiment is made more complicated by using phased conditioning to two words, it can be shown that each acts independently when their semantic fields are far apart (as when *cow* is included with *violin*). However, one semantic system can inhibit the periphery of another if the reactions to the first system are not yet firmly established. Such conditioning methods can elicit information, therefore, about the dynamics of semantic fields in an objective way and more accurately, Luria and Vinogradova suggest, than can conscious impressions: the subjects in their study were reported as being unaware of their re-

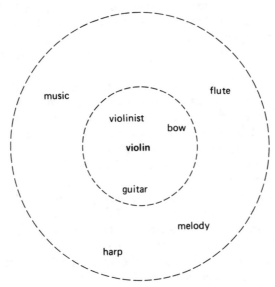

Fig. 4   Schematic representation of the central and peripheral areas of the semantic field of
*violin*

actions to the associated words, or of why different words had been included in the list.

Semantic fields, as investigated in this way, prove not to be identical with logical categories. For example, Luria reports that although the names of stringed instruments appeared to be closely associated with *violin*, the word *harp* did not elicit the strong reaction of other stringed instruments. There are clearly other relationships besides logical relationships at work in the placement of words within a semantic field and perhaps similarity in visual shape and size may be one of the important influences. This is but one example of the way it proves difficult in the application of linguistics to make the clear distinction between sense relations and knowledge-of-the-world that some linguists think desirable.

For application in aphasia therapy, amongst the relations within the semantic field of a word, researchers have singled out a few which they believe to be the most influential. Kogan (cited by Maruszewski 1975, p. 161) believed that name retrieval could be facilitated in amnesic aphasia by 'enacting' the key word in a number of its different semantic relations. The relations he proposed for the word *knife*, for example, were (not necessarily in order of importance): class membership (*tool*), where manufactured (*factory*), where used (*workshop*, *kitchen*), made of what (*steel*), what used for (*cutting*), what kinds (*table-knife*), possible attributes (*sharp*, *blunt*) and similar objects (*scissors*, *razor*). The relations within a semantic field which Goodglass and Baker (1976) have singled out for investigation in aphasia will be described shortly.

At least three direct applications to aphasia have been made of Luria and Vinogradova's conceptualizations of the graded nature of semantic fields. One is in the development over some years of the technique of *deblocking* by Weigl in Berlin. Another is Goodglass and Baker's investigation of aphasic patients' recognition of whether associated words belong in the same semantic field as a key word. A third is an exploration of semantic fields in French using word sorting as the medium.

Weigl's technique of temporary deblocking of the responses which an aphasic patient normally finds blocked makes use of the patient's intact modalities to release the word or sentence in a damaged modality (Weigl 1961). For example, a patient who had difficulty in repeating a word was enabled to do this after he had seen and read aloud the word even though in the interval he had had to struggle with repeating a different word. Weigl (1970a) emphasizes that the nature of deblocking is primarily determined by the factor of meaning, and not any other linguistic factor. Understanding of a word can only be deblocked through an intact ability in 'copying, repeating, naming etc. of the same or a semantically related word lying in the respective semantic field' (p. 341). Observation of what facilitates deblocking in aphasia can therefore be used to study the nature of a semantic field. Weigl's (1970b) diagrammatic version of the structure of a semantic field has two concentric circles with the generic noun related to the key word in the outer circle and the antonymic noun, synonym and semantic proximate noun in the inner circle. A word can be deblocked by prestimulation of the appropriate semantic field either directly by using the key word itself or indirectly by using a word from the field, or perhaps by using both words. With such dual prestimulation the deblocking rate may be increased or there may be a double effect of deblocking with the patient now able to use, for example, the category word as well as the key word. Sometimes indirect deblocking by a related word has an unintended consequence—a 'deviation phenomenon' in which the patient uses the related word for the key word but is convinced that he is correct. Weigl suggests that the deblocking technique can be used to investigate homonyms: it provides a way of studying which meaning or meanings of a homonym predominate. Conflicts can be produced if only one meaning of a homonym is reinforced by prestimulation, and a picture is then shown to the patient of an object showing the other meaning of a homonym. With some patients, however, it is possible to deblock several meanings of a homonym: for example an anomic patient was asked to repeat several words including a homonym *Feder* (pen/feather/spring), and was then able to name pictures of all three of these objects correctly. The word-sound had deblocked all the meanings, though these were contained in different semantic fields.

Goodglass and Baker's (1976) investigation of semantic fields in aphasia began with the assumption that semantic fields have as components specific associative categories. The associative categories they selected were (examples are given for the key word *drum*) superordinate (*instrument*), attribute (*loud*), coordinate (*guitar*), function associate (*beat*), functional context (*band*), clang (*crumb*) and the key word itself. The procedure used was to show the patient a picture of the object and ask him to name it and then, while still looking at the picture and its printed name, to listen to a tape-recorded list of 14 words. Every time the patient recognized a word which he thought might be related to the key word, he pressed a rubber bulb which provided an automatic recording of both the speed with which he reacted and the errors he made. The 14 words included an example of each of the associative categories listed above, together with seven incorrect words. This procedure was repeated in two sessions, for a total of 16 key words, of which 8 were of high frequency in English and 8 were of low frequency. The aphasics' results were compared with other brain-damaged and non-aphasic control subjects'. The results showed that none of the subjects, aphasic or not, paid much attention to clang responses—results compatible with Luria's conclusion that the semantic system is dominant—and this category was excluded from the analysis. The results of the aphasics differed for patients classed as having good comprehension on the Boston Diagnostic Aphasia Examination and those classed as having poor comprehension. On the reaction-time measure the low-comprehension but not the high-comprehension aphasic subjects differed significantly from non-aphasic brain-damaged control subjects. The low-comprehension subjects also showed a different order of difficulty for the various associative categories from the other subjects. Although they reacted about as quickly to the key word itself, they reacted relatively more quickly (in comparison with their average speed) to the coordinate words than did the other groups, identifying them about as easily as they did the superordinate and attribute associations. Reactions were strikingly slower to functional context and function associate words (i.e. words related to the key word by describing an action performed by or on the object or by describing the situation where the object occurs). The error scores essentially corroborated these findings from the reaction-time scores. Goodglass and Baker conclude that low-comprehension aphasic patients, although they know what an object is, no longer know as much about it as they previously did. The semantic field around a concept has become constricted. This conclusion was corroborated by a comparison of the errors made on words which the aphasic subjects had successfully named before they heard the tape-recorded list, and those which they had not named. The low-comprehension subjects (but not the high-comprehension) made significantly more errors in the decision task on those words which they had not been able to name. Further analysis showed that word frequency had not been a significant factor for either of the aphasic groups in their success in responding in the decision task. Impaired naming was equally related to recognition for all of the associative categories. There are two main inferences to be drawn from this experiment. Firstly, naming difficulties in the speech of patients with impaired comprehension can be related to an underlying impairment in semantic knowledge rather than to difficulties at a more peripheral stage. Secondly, when aphasic comprehension difficulties are severe, the impairment in semantic fields amounts to a qualitative distortion, with functional context and function associate words much harder to recognize as being related to a key object when this is pictured under these circumstances. Goodglass and Baker also comment on the fact that superordinates were remarkably easy for all the aphasic subjects to recognize; they suggest that under the circumstances in which the object was presented the superordinate acts almost as a synonym for the object name.

Goodglass and Baker's finding of qualitative differences between groups of aphasics on a measure of semantic comprehension concurs with that of Zurif and his colleagues, who used a different measure of semantic ability, to be described in the section on semantic features. Both of these groups of researchers from Boston identified their groups of patients as being Broca's aphasics (with good comprehension) or Wernicke's aphasics (with poor comprehension). The final experiment to be described here, one undertaken at Lhermitte's unit at the Salpetrière in Paris (Lhermitte, Derouesné and Lecours 1971; Derouesné and Lecours 1972), found that distortions in semantic fields could not be neatly characterized as being of Broca-type or Wernicke-type. The French researchers also preferred not to interpret their results as indicating qualitatively different semantic deficits in the different types of patients they identified, but suggested that amnesic aphasia represents a particularly pure form of a semantic deficit which is all-pervasive, to some degree or other, in aphasia.

They used sorting of printed words in their procedure. Subjects were given two tests. In the first test they were asked to classify twelve words according to whether they were closely related, remotely related or not at all related to a key word. The choice was forced, in that they had to place four words in each of these three categories. There were ten items of this type. All the words to be sorted were nouns or infinitive forms of verbs. An example of a set of such words (translated) is (for the key word *fish*): closely related *ocean, gills, angler, to swim*, remotely related *kitchen, merchandise, smell, to clean*, and unrelated *chair, fantasy, brick, to dye*. For the second test they were given as a key word a homonym which had from two to four meanings. They had to select from seven words as many of these meanings as they could find; the choice in this case was therefore not forced. An example of a key word with four meanings is *division* with the meanings represented by *army, arithmetic, sharing*, and *quarrel*. From prior testing with normal adults it was found that there was an influence of educational level on their abilities, and weightings were therefore given to the results from aphasic subjects to take this into account.

Lhermitte and his colleagues combined the results of both tests to derive information about the status of semantic fields in the aphasic subjects. They therefore were using an interpretation of semantic fields which assumes that homonyms share the same semantic field; they describe the correct words in the homonym test as being 'in the centre of the semantic field', although they represent different senses of the homonym. This identification of a semantic field with the phonological shape of a word rather than primarily with its sense, seems somewhat questionable, in view of Luria's conclusion that semantic relations are dominant.

From the first test they were able to distinguish patients who made errors primarily across the inner boundary between the central and peripheral area of a semantic field, i.e. they made most errors in confusing words which were closely and remotely related to the key words (*hierarchization errors*) but very few errors of including unrelated words or excluding related words. A second group, while still making a number of hierarchization errors, made errors also across the outer boundary of the field. By incorporating the results of the homonym test as well, the researchers distinguished in this latter group a further division: some showed predominant narrowing of the outer boundary of the field in that they failed to include the full number of meanings of the homonyms; others showed predominant widening of the field in that they included, as meanings of homonyms, inappropriate words. The general symptoms of severity of aphasia, as independently classified according to their speech traits, increased from those making hierarchization errors through those making narrowing errors to those making widening errors. Patients whose symptoms could be described as those of a Broca's aphasia without word-finding difficulties scored well on the tests, as did patients with a Wernicke's aphasia dominated by phonemic paraphasias in speech. But patients showing either Broca's aphasia or Wernicke's aphasia characterized by word-finding difficulties in speech produced a high number of either narrowing or widening errors. The small number of amnesic aphasic patients tested, despite their relatively good speech, all displayed grossly abnormal performance on the semantic tests. Like Goodglass and Baker, the French researchers conclude that amnesic aphasia reflects a central semantic deficit and not simply difficulty in finding words for speech. But they interpret this as a relatively pure form of the semantic deficit which is characteristic of aphasia of all types. They also observed that semantic systems are more disturbed in posterior than in anterior lesions in the left hemisphere, and that semantic disturbances do not depend on deterioration of general intelligence, as patients with a score below 38 on the Raven's Progressive Matrices test of intelligence had been excluded.

These studies of aphasia based on the notion of semantic fields corroborate the validity of this notion as representing some aspect of the organization of the mental lexicon. A further interpretation of semantic relationships based on the notion of features is less securely related to psychological correlates.

## Semantic features

Clark's (1970) interpretation of the links amongst associated words is somewhat different from those we have described in the last two sections. It draws on the idea that word meanings are not wholes, but are composed of semantic elements or features—an approach to the analysis of meaning by some linguists which is known as *componential analysis* (Lyons 1969) or *systemic analysis* (Leech 1969).

Clark suggests that the relationships between paradigmatic associations and their stimulus words can be accounted for in terms of four rules, all of which are related to this idea that words can be conceived of in terms of features. One of these rules concerns syntactic rather than semantic features (the *category-preservation* rule which specifies that syntactic class is maintained for noun, verb and adjective), but the other three rules relate primarily to semantic features. The *minimal-contrast* rule specifies that only one feature is to be changed, e.g. from 'boy' which is + Male to 'girl' which is − Male (or as some would prefer to argue, + Female). The *feature-addition-and-deletion* rule leads to responses of superordinate ('fruit' for 'apple' where a specifying feature of kind of fruit has been deleted) or subordinate ('apple' as response to 'fruit' where a specifying feature is added). The third rule, the *marking* rule, draws on the notion that features, conceived of as binary oppositions, have one of these oppositions with a more basic or neutral value (the unmarked feature) with the other having a positive value (the marked value). The rule states that it is more common for a response to a marked term to be an unmarked term, rather than vice versa. For example an association is more likely to go from 'bitch' to 'dog' than from 'dog' to 'bitch', as 'bitch' is a term marked for sex, while 'dog' is unmarked for this feature. We shall return to this question of markedness shortly.

Pilch (1972) makes use of this notion of semantic features in describing aphasic misnamings. He points out that in pairs of words which show *semantic solidarity*, such as 'bite—teeth'. 'rustle—cattle', and 'auburn—hair', the meaning of the second word is contained as a feature of the meaning of the first word. Aphasic patients, when asked to name an item like one of the second words, characteristically substitute the equivalent solidarity word.

Componential analysis of this kind concentrates on that part of associative links which can be described in terms of logical relationships. It can be traced back to philosophical speculation in the seventeenth century that there are certain universal components in meaning which can be identified in all languages. Some modern conceptualizations of these components (called in different theories markers, attributes, sememes, labels or—the term we will use here—features) have drawn on the notion of distinctive features in phonology in imposing on them a binary organization. Examples of these features are ± Animate, ± Human, ± Adult, ± Male, ± Parent. It is immediately obvious that although a large part of the common meaning between two concepts can be explained in these terms (for instance 'woman' and 'ewe' are both ± *Animate*, − *Male*, + *Adult*, but one is + *Human* and the other is − *Human*) such a list of features leaves unaccounted for a large amount of information which distinguishes the two concepts. For this reason Katz and Fodor (1963) contrasted such general features, which they called *markers*, with the features which isolate the meaning of a specific word, which they called *distinguishers*. For the word 'bush' for example, semantic markers would be PLANT and WITH BRANCHES and the distinguisher would be BRANCHES ARISING FROM OR NEAR THE GROUND.

Difficulties arise, however, if all of a word's meaning is thought of as being quantifiable in terms of binary features. Firstly there are taxonomic systems which cannot be satisfactorily defined in terms of binary features (e.g. the meaning relationships amongst *bedroom/hall/kitchen/dining-room* etc.), and scalar systems in which an ordered linear progression is inherent (*inch/foot/yard* etc.). There are also systems, which, although they fall into binary pairs, are not well described in terms of binary opposition. For example with the pair *parent/child*, the intuitive relationships between them cannot be accounted for by classifying child as − *Parent*. To describe someone as − *Parent* implies, not that he or she is a child, but that he or she is an adult who has no children. To account for the interrelationships amongst sets of words like kinship terms, one is also obliged to devise features which are specific to this system, like *linear, second generation* and *collateral*. Any binary system of semantic features therefore proves inadequate.

Lyons (1969) has called into question the conceptualization of semantic features as universal and common to all languages. Furthermore there is a residuum of meaning for each word for which quantification in terms of features is not suitable. This residuum includes the effect of the frequency of that word in the vocabulary, an individual's personal emotive reactions, his encyclopaedic and cultural knowledge about the referent, the perceptual and operative impressions he associates with it—one of which may be described in terms of the visual semantic memory which Warrington has suggested—and so on. Features can be used to describe the quantifiable components of the word's meaning, but more as a convenience in describing logical relationships than as necessarily psychologically valid units. The list of features therefore need not be couched in terms of universals but in terms of what is appropriate to distinguish the usage of an individual word. For instance it is convenient to describe selectional restrictions in sentences in terms of incompatibility of one or more semantic features.

But psychological experimentation does support the validity of making at least two kinds of distinctions in that part of word meaning which can be quantified by semantic features. One is between general or *presupposition* features and specifying or *assertion* features (a distinction not the same as that between Katz's markers and distinguishers). The other is the distinction of polarity between marked and unmarked terms which has already been mentioned. Both of these have been applied in aphasia research.

In making the distinction between presupposition features and assertion features, Miller (1969) drew attention to the fact that negation cancels out only the latter type of feature. For instance if we hear a sentence such as 'That person is not a mother', we would be more likely to assume that the person was a woman who had not given birth to a child, rather than that the person was a man. In other words the presupposition features of − Male, + Adult (and + Human etc.) would be retained, but the assertion feature of + Has-given-birth would be cancelled by negation. As the presupposition features are not cancelled by negation, Millar points out that statements like 'Tom is not a thief' contain a subtle kind of libel; they leave uncancelled the implication of some criminality, even though this does not take the specific form of stealing. If people are asked to sort out words into groups they tend to sort them according to the presupposition features rather than according to the assertion features. The presuppositional structure is

conceived of by Miller as being hierarchical in nature. For example 'being' dominates 'person' which dominates 'man' which dominates 'knight'.

If people, when asked in an experimental task to sort printed words according
to their meaning, are likely to cluster words together according to presupposition
features rather than assertion features, and if they are also more likely to group
together words which share more presuppositions, this offers a method for testing
the integrity of an aphasic patient's knowledge of word meanings. Zurif, Caramazza, Myerson and Galvin (1974) used this technique to examine semantic feature
representations in aphasic and normal language.

Zurif and his colleagues wished to test whether or not aphasic patients would
sort words according to their general presupposition features, their specifying
assertion features or by any other residuum of emotive, encyclopaedic etc. meaning. They selected 12 words to be sorted, all of them concrete nouns of relatively
high frequency. They could be divided into two categories in terms of a very basic
general feature, ± Human (*mother, wife, cook, partner, knight, husband* compared
with *shark, trout, dog, tiger, turtle, crocodile*) which the aphasics at very least might
be expected to recognize. Within the + Human group, words could be classified
in terms of either general presuppositional or assertion specifying features (the
researchers used the term 'residual features' to label the latter, but because we
have used the term residual for the idiosyncratic aspects of meaning which are
not systematically quantifiable in terms of common features, this term will be
avoided here). If the words were to be classed by presuppositional features *wife*
and *mother* would be paired together, as would *husband* and *knight* (with general
features of + or − Male); on the other hand if words were to be classed by their
assertion features, *wife* would be classed with *husband* and perhaps even with
*partner*. The − Human words provided another possible kind of classification, not
only by features but by aspects of the residuum of meaning. They could be classed
according to species membership (presuppositional features) or by ferocity (emotive or encyclopaedic knowledge).

The method which was used was one known as the method of triads. The subject
is presented with three items and asked to indicate which two of these three he
feels go together. If this is repeated over all possible triple combinations of the
words a matrix can be drawn up which shows in each cell the frequency with which
a particular word is grouped with another by the subjects. To acknowledge both
hierarchical and multidimensional models of lexical organization, two alternative
methods of data analysis were used. With a hierarchical clustering analysis, the
pairs of words in the matrix which are most closely related are grouped together
to form a new matrix and this is repeated until all possible groupings have been
made. From this a tree-like structure can be derived which illustrates, in two dimensions, the relationships which the subjects have found amongst the words. The
second method of analysis, multidimensional scaling, allows the relationships to
be presented spatially in several dimensions with varied distances between the
items showing the extent to which each could be positively or negatively loaded
on different factors or dimensions.

The clustering analysis showed that the five non-aphasic control subjects who had been given the task made the +Human/−Human distinction perfectly, and within the animal terms sorted predominantly according to the general features of species membership. With the human terms they sorted partly according to general features but also on their knowledge of referential and social situations. For example *mother*, *wife* and *husband* were closely associated. The five Broca's aphasics showed some similarities to this sorting, in that they made the broad distinction between human and animal, though with one exception: they clustered *dog* with the human group. With the animal terms, however, they sorted not on the basis of presuppositional features but on the emotive residuum of meaning, putting the ferocious animals together. Their sorting of the human terms also suggested that they were influenced by the distance of the terms from their own social experience, hence the classing of *dog* in the human world (as man's best friend?). The results from the five Wernicke's aphasics, however, produced very different clusterings. Even the basic ±Human concept did not appear to have been extracted. Zurif and his colleagues commented that the behaviour of these patients during the task suggested that they were often not sorting on the basis of semantic connectedness but rather on how easily two of the triad could be put into a sentence with the copula *is*, such as 'My mother is a good cook'. The multidimensional scaling analyses, undertaken only with the data from the non-aphasic and Broca's aphasic subjects, were consistent with the findings from the hierarchical analysis. The dimensions which emerged were labelled in terms of humanness, aggressiveness and land-adaptedness (animals) or social distance (humans). The Broca's aphasics' results showed retention of the basic dimensions except for social distance but looser spacing out of items along the dimensions. These patients appeared to be relying more heavily than non-aphasics on extra-linguistic information (such as the fierceness of wild animals) rather than on systematic relations amongst words. With the Wernicke's aphasics, as tested in this metalinguistic task, there appeared to have been a more comprehensive disruption of lexical organization.

In that this experiment showed that normal subjects do not necessarily sort in terms of logical structure, it gives no firm support to the psychological rather than linguistically convenient value of semantic features. It does indicate, however, that there is some degree of semantic impairment even in patients classed as Broca's aphasics, with a more drastic impairment in patients classed as Wernicke's aphasics.

The feature of markedness is more abstract than the features we have been talking about so far. It applies to a basic aspect of organization and can be (and has been) used in phonology and syntax as well as in semantics. There is also a considerable body of evidence that, as a semantic feature, it is influential on language behaviour in children and adults, and that the distinction between marked and unmarked at the semantic level therefore has some psychological reality. At the phonological level, it is presumed that distinctive features have a neutral form and a marked form—for instance voicelessness as in /p/ is assumed to be unmarked, while voicedness as in /b/ is assumed to be marked—and Blumstein's study of whether or not aphasic speech supports this distinction is described in chapter 8. At the syntactic level, similarly, in English the uninflected form of a verb or noun or adjective or the nominative form of the pronoun (*boy, jump, good, they*) can be described as the unmarked form, with any inflected form being marked (*boys, jumped, better, them*). The singular is therefore considered to be unmarked, as is the present tense, while plurality or pastness or adjectival comparison introduces markedness. At the semantic level, as we saw from Clark's example with *dog* and *bitch*, markedness can sometimes be described in terms of a specific feature, in this case sex. But more generally it is now used in a more abstract sense of polarity, which is most easily illustrated by pairs of adjectives, like *old* and *young*. Although these adjectives refer to opposite values on a polar scale, one of them, *old*, also refers to the entire scale in a neutral sense without necessarily implying polarity. For instance we can ask 'How old is that baby?' without in any way infringing the selectional restriction that a baby is necessarily young. Similarly we could also ask how tall a midget was, how wide a narrow strip was, how thick a thin plank was, how deep a shallow pool was and so on. There have been several studies of the way children acquire these polar adjectives (see for example Eilers, Oller and Ellington 1974) which suggest that the two senses of such adjectives are at first undifferentiated, with the marked adjective often being interpreted as having a neutral value. Children asked to show which is *less*, at some stage of language acquisition, point to *more*. With adults, too, studies measuring the time it takes to decide whether or not a statement is true show that it is faster to make decisions about unmarked than marked terms (Clark and Card 1969; Carpenter 1974).

The distinction also appears to hold up when tested against the proving ground of aphasia. Marshall, Newcombe and Marshall (1970) included a comparison of marked and unmarked adjectives in their detailed examination of the types of words which an aphasic patient, who had had a bullet wound in front of the left ear, found difficult to read. The patient's misreadings in a list of marked and unmarked adjectives indicated that his errors tended to preserve the markedness status of the stimulus item: *large* would be misread as *long* rather than *small*, *short* misread as *small* rather than *long*, *little* misread as *short* rather than *big*. A recent experiment (Lesser, in preparation) compared the number of errors made by an unselected group of aphasics on different types of sentences when given a picture choice. Like normal adults used as control subjects in a parallel experiment in which reaction time measures were used, they showed more difficulty with sentences which contained comparative adjectives which were marked ('This bottle has less milk', 'The pencil is shorter than the ruler') than they did with sentences which contained comparative adjectives which were unmarked ('This jug has more water', 'The ruler is longer than the pencil'). Marshall *et al.* (1970, p. 421) have speculated that unmarked adjectives may have a dual representation in the lexicon, one in their neutral dimension-making sense, and one in their polarized sense. If this were to be so, possibly the duality of representation could facilitate retrieval. Alternatively one might speculate that marked terms require a double process of identification—first identification of the particular dimension which is being referred to (height, size, age, etc.) and then an identification of which pole of the dimension is referred to. Although Clark has specifically rejected the proposal that normal subjects' delays in responding to decisions about marked adjectives are due to their first converting them into a negative form of the unmarked (i.e. in changing *short* into *not long*), a few of the subjects who made a large number of errors in the experiment we have just referred to appeared not to be performing at a random level as if they did not understand the sentences, but to be preferring the choice of the picture showing the unmarked term. Whatever speculation may eventually be supported, the abstract feature of markedness, as applied at least to these kinds of adjectives, does seem to have some validity as a proposal about one facet of the mental organization of the lexicon.

The studies outlined in this chapter have mostly supported the hypothesis that the naming difficulties which are common in aphasia are at least in part to be accounted for by central changes in semantic representation, rather than simply by unavailability of intact semantic information. It may be that the aphasic patient's problem is not so much one of difficulty in retrieval from an intact store of words which have maintained their integrity, but is one of changes in the pattern of interrelationships amongst word meanings such that the delimitation of the meaning of a word is less completely clear (if we accept an associationistic semantic-field model) or is one of reconstitution of a word from its features (if we accept a feature model). There are, however, other conceptualizations of the organization of the lexicon, two of which we shall consider in the next chapter. One of these considers words as members of categories; the other attempts to distinguish operational components in the complexes of influences which association studies have shown to be important in the interrelationships amongst words.

# 6

# Semantic relationships in aphasia: categories, complexes and retrieval

The term *semantic field* is used in linguistics more commonly in a different sense from the way we have used it in the last chapter. It is used to denote not the sphere of associated words around any single word, with its physiological implications, but a domain of words which are logically or semantically interconnected. Although this usage is less attuned to the needs of a science which attempts to link language and brain, this kind of interpretation of semantic field has also been applied in research into aphasia. To make it clear that we are referring to a different conceptualization of lexical structure, we shall use the term *semantic category* to describe this interpretation of semantic field.

## Categories

A recent readable account of a linguistic interpretation of semantic categories is one by Lehrer (1974) who has made a special study of cookery and container terms. She describes a semantic category ('field' in her terminology) as 'a group of words closely related in meaning often subsumed under a general term' (p. 1). The categories which have been most studied are ones with relatively well-defined limits and a manageable number of members, such as colour terms and kinship terms, which have served in cross-cultural studies (Berlin and Kay 1969; Greenberg 1966). Some attempts have also been made to describe the logical relationships amongst larger categories within one language such as verbs of motion (Miller 1972). It is from such attempts to characterize these relationships that the notion of semantic features was derived.

Lehrer concludes that most categories are in fact not closed well-defined sets. There are usually peripheral terms which some people would include in a category, but others would exclude. Lexical categories do not seem to be systematically arranged in patterns of oppositions and differences but in a multiplicity of ways. There are frequently gaps in them; for example we have a term for dead bodies which are human, *corpse*, or animal, *carcass*, but not vegetable. Some sets of words are not appropriate for analysis in terms of categorical relationships, because the relationships they show are too diffuse, while the structure in other terms is extremely simple (for example the linear structure in cardinal numbers and alphabet letters).

The concept of categories, however, does seem to capture some realisms about lexical organization. It explains some syntactic regularities, for example, in that the members of the category of *manner-of-speaking* verbs (whispering, shouting, mumbling, etc.) can all be used parenthetically, can all be interpreted as reports of assertion and all have nominal direct objects cognate with the verb. It gives insight into how meanings can become extended: for instance a novel phrase like 'warm war' is readily interpretable because *warm* can be fitted in in its category between *hot* and *cold*. In psychologists' experiments the size of the category of which a word is a member has proved to be a significant variable in the time it takes for someone to decide whether it is a member of that category or not (Wilkins 1971). One possibility is that people may search through the category in making the decision, so that it takes longer to decide whether a canary is a bird than it does to decide whether a collie is a dog (there being more names of birds than of dogs) (Landauer and Meyer 1972).

One observation that is frequently made in aphasiology is that the misnamings made by the aphasic speaker are usually within-category errors rather than wildly off-target. Geschwind (1967) in fact makes this one of the distinctions between classical aphasic anomia and specific anomia, inferring that someone with a specific anomia for colours gives colour names when asked to name a colour not because he is finding an approximation to the word he wishes to name but because the question tells him that it is a colour name of some kind which he is expected to produce. The belief is that he has no perceptual information which could help him to link a colour name with a colour percept. But the extent to which we are willing to interpret aphasic misnamings as being within a category depends on what limits we decide to impose on the category. When (in a real-life example from a patient with a fairly mild degree of fluent aphasia) a patient says 'Half past Monday', this can be interpreted as a confusion of categories in that the category of clock times is confused with the category of days of the week, or as a within-category confusion in that both are measures of the passage of time, but one on a larger scale than the other.

So far only a few semantic categories have been given any special interest in the study of aphasia. These are body parts, colours, alphabet letters, cardinal numbers, geometric shapes, kinship terms, professional roles, room objects, and, as a very large category, 'object names'. In what has been called non-aphasic mis-naming after diffuse brain damage or right-brain-damage, the misnamings noted are often relatable to disease and hospitals: but this has been interpreted in terms of the patient's emotive reactions to his illness rather than in terms of a disturbance in a special category (Weinstein and Keller 1963). Weinstein and Keller considered that the misnamings made by patients who were not aphasic after right-brain-damage were related to disturbances of orientation and data about personal identity, and involved predominantly objects connected with disability. With patients with left-hemisphere lesions, error words were names of objects which were related in function and form to the target object or showed some spatial or temporal contiguity. In a more recent paper Weinstein and Puig-Antich (1974) report on the jargon of two patients with aphasia, suggesting that the use of stereo-types and 'officialese' which they evidenced has its analogue in the *denial* syndromes of people with right-hemisphere damage who refer to their illness with inappropriate terms. However, the sharp separation of non-aphasic misnamings and aphasic misnamings has been questioned. If aphasic misnamings are an intense form of the difficulties which everyone experiences at some time or another, some of the comments which have been made about misnamings after diffuse damage or stress are applicable to aphasia also, and some aphasic misnamings can also be attributed to emotive and personal factors, and related to the psychological distance from the self of the objects to be named.

Semantic categories have been examined in aphasia to test the extent to which, if at all, they can be selectively disturbed. We have already commented that the selective anomia of some patients has been explained in terms of a disconnection of percept from the language system. From the linguistic perspective the question is whether or not selective misnamings of one category can occur within classical anomia, indicating that within the neurological organization of language there are specialized representations of categories, which can therefore be disturbed relatively selectively.

Again we have a polarization of opinions. Some people suggest that aphasia disturbs all semantic processes equally, and that the differences which are found in naming in some categories can be attributed to non-inherent differences like perceptual saliency or frequency. Others believe that the word-finding system in the brain may be subdivided anatomically according to the nature of different word categories. This has its parallel in discussions on asymbolia about whether a general faculty of use of symbols is impaired, or whether specific symbol systems are selectively damaged. From one perspective aphasia can be described as a difficulty in grasping and expressing ideas by means of learned symbols, which permeates through all symbols; and from another, a difficulty with symbols in each individual can be thought of as being primarily specific to certain symbol systems. Leischner and Fradis (1974), for example, describe patients in whom they noted specific asymbolias for mathematical signs, the Morse code alphabet, shorthand writing, chemical formulae, traffic signs, punctuation marks, national emblems and flags, and money. Leischner and Fradis believe such asymbolias to be distinct both from agnosia and from apraxia, in that the asymbolia is consistent however the patient is tested, and through whatever medium: they consider that they are failures in the recognition of the meaning of a direct stimulus rather than in the recognition of the stimulus itself. The asymbolias, according to Leischner and Fradis, form clinically independent syndromes, which may accompany an aphasia but can also occur on their own. Gardner, however (1974a), has pointed out that the difficulty with many descriptions of specific disorders in individual patients is that they do not report in detail how the patient fares with symbolic categories other than the one whose impairment has aroused interest. Gardner therefore examined the capacity of patients diagnosed as having an asymbolia for written materials (i.e. as having alexia) to recognize non-linguistic symbols, and compared this with the abilities of patients diagnosed as aphasic. The categories of symbols he tested were the names of numbers, letters, colours, animals, punctuation marks, domestic objects, mathematical notations, proper nouns (represented by well-known faces), a collection of miscellaneous symbols like the swastika and the dollar sign, a heterogeneous collection of printed words, and of words written in different typographies—eleven categories in all, which were presented for naming, or for multiple-choice recognition, if the patient did not produce the correct name within fifteen seconds. The alexic patients were found to need as much help in naming as were the aphasic patients classed as anomic, and rather more than patients classed as having an anterior syndrome. On the score of recognition, as measured through both naming and multiple-choice of names, the posterior aphasic patients were the worst of all the groups. However, when the order of difficulty for the different categories was plotted, it was virtually the same for anomic aphasics as for all other aphasics. The performance of the alexic patients was qualitatively different: alexic patients made more errors in naming printed words than in naming objects, while anomic patients made more errors in naming objects than words. Gardner concludes that 'the recognition and naming of symbols is impaired across-the-board in aphasic patients, in the same relative order as in non-aphasic subjects' (p. 152). He also observed that alexic patients seem to have a general difficulty in identifying written symbols which is not restricted to verbal symbols. Gardner suggests that it is only those individuals suffering from disconnections between sensory and linguistic areas (Geschwind's explanation of pure alexia) who will show isolated deficits of specific symbolic capacities: with damage to the linguistic areas themselves, and a consequent aphasia, we might expect some general reduction in the capacity to utilize symbols.

We can examine from two perspectives this question of selectivity or generality in impairment in the use of symbols. Disconnection theory implies a complete difficulty in tasks which require the patient to name items in whatever category is disturbed. With aphasic misnamings due to damage to the language system itself, we might in contrast expect qualitative differences within a category reflecting inherent linguistic difficulties: the misnamings should fall into a pattern which suggests that they are not random guesses but are reflecting the inherent organization of language. This is one perspective from which misnamings within a semantic category have been examined. The other perspective focuses not on qualitative differences within categories but in the relationship between impairment in semantic categories and type of aphasia in pursuit of an answer to the question of whether different semantic categories can be functionally distinguished in the neuroanatomical substrate of language. As the first perspective makes finer distinctions within a category, while the second makes broad distinctions across categories, let us consider the second perspective first.

Poeck and his colleagues (Poeck, Hartje, Kerschensteiner and Orgass 1973; Orgass, Poeck and Kerschensteiner 1974; Poeck and Stachowiak 1975) have made a study of the relative impairment of three kinds of categories in aphasia, colour names, body-part names and object names. They examined them through comprehension as well as through naming. For the comprehension test with body parts, given to 45 aphasic patients with different kinds of aphasia (described as amnesic, motor, sensory and global), they asked each patient to point out named parts of the body on a diagram and on their own body. They also gave, for comparison, a test in which they had to point out from their spoken names pictured objects out of a choice of four. Pointing to parts of the body on a diagram or on their own bodies produced similar errors, so these results were combined. Of importance for the question of whether or not categories are separately impaired was the finding that comprehension of object names also followed the same pattern; in fact the correlation between the comprehension of object names and that of body parts was as high as that between the two forms of testing comprehension of body parts. Patients with good understanding of body parts had good understanding of object names, and those with poor comprehension of body parts had poor comprehension of object names. Poeck considers that this result gives no support to the proposal sometimes made that aphasics find it harder to identify parts of a whole because of a general difficulty in analysis. In respect of the human body at least the names of parts seem to be identified in the same way as the names of autonomous whole objects. When aphasic patients make errors in pointing out parts of their body by name, it cannot necessarily be inferred that they have a specific impairment in the sense of the spatial relations of their own bodies (*autotopagnosia*), but the difficulty is more likely to be related to their general difficulty with all names.

Poeck's co-workers also found similar results when they examined the comprehension of colour names. This correlated highly with comprehension of object names and body-part names. When they tested colour names through the patients' abilities in producing names rather than in comprehending them, they also found results which corroborated this conclusion. The ten colours they asked 80 patients to name were yellow, lilac, white, red, blue, brown, grey, orange, green and black. They compared the results with their ability to name twenty pictured common objects (house, cup of coffee, table, door, apple, cigarette, key, banana, tree, chair, handkerchief, walking-stick, watch, sofa, spectacles, comb, telephone, refrigerator, shirt and bottle). Although the different types of patients differed in the nature of the naming errors they made (anomic patients were self-correcting, Wernicke's were not, while Broca's and global aphasics produced phonemic distortions) the numbers of errors made by each group were not significantly different. There was also no difference in the pattern of the naming difficulties; all the groups found the colours slightly more difficult to name than the objects. In each group the majority of individual patients found colours harder to name than objects, although in the Wernicke's group this difference did not reach significance. Poeck considered that in the few examples of patients making more errors with object names than colours, the difference was not great enough to be of diagnostic significance. As colour naming tends to be more difficult than object naming in general, there was no support for the concept of a specific *colour aphasia*. Orgass, Poeck and Kerschensteiner (1974) propose, in fact, that it is highly improbable that there should be specific difficulties with certain semantic categories in aphasia—although, in contrast, it is more likely that different types of aphasics can be distinguished according to their behaviour with different syntactic classes of words. 'In testing the speech-comprehension of aphasic patients for single words, it is not meaningful to classify into sub-tests according to semantic content (objects, colours, parts of the body). It is merely necessary to use words of decreasing frequency, i.e. of increasing degree of difficulty, regardless of whether or not they indicate a unified class of objects' (p. 101, translated).

In line with these observations are the findings of Rochford (1971) that the naming difficulties of aphasics can be distinguished from those of demented patients in that the aphasics' difficulties in body-part naming are equivalent to those they have in object naming, while for demented patients body parts are much easier. Rochford discusses a possible explanation for the discrepancy in the demented patients' performances in terms of a general impairment in visual recognition due to the interacting effects of generalized lesions or a specific impairment in visual perception. In the present context the finding of a highly significant degree of agreement in the aphasics' scores between ability to name parts of the body and eight line drawings of objects gives corroboration to Poeck's position. So does an experiment which used different categories from those which Rochford and Poeck's team had selected: the categories of clothes, household items, foods, living things and (within the syntactic category of verbs) actions. Wiegel-Crump and Koenigsknecht (1973) were interested in the extent to which therapy aimed at improving word-retrieval skills in one semantic category would extend to another category. With four adults who showed an aphasia which was predominantly anomic in nature, they found, for each, those words out of a list of 150 words (30 in each of the above categories) which the patient failed to name. From this list of errors they selected a set of items for which, over 18 therapy sessions, they gave naming drills, using the techniques recommended by Schuell *et al.* (1964) with auditory and visual stimulation. Other items in those categories were not drilled, and from one category, food names, no items at all were drilled. When the patients were re-tested at intervals during the training programme and at the end, they showed a very similar progression of improvement over all the categories, including the food category in which no drill had been given. They also showed improvement in the items within categories which had not been drilled, though the speed of response was significantly faster amongst those items which had been drilled than it was for those items which had not been drilled. The experimenters' conclusion was that in amnesic aphasia there is no reduction in the lexical store itself but an impairment in ability to retrieve information from the lexical store. The generalization from one category of words to another gives no support to the idea that the categories used in this study are differently represented in the brain.

According to Schwartz and Halpern (1973) the ability in aphasia to name parts of the body is related to whether or not the speaker has a hemiplegic paralysis. They report that hemiplegic aphasic patients made significantly more errors with names of body parts than with neutral stimuli. These investigators suggest that the naming of body parts is affected by the patient's emotions relating to his physical impairment rather than to linguistic categories.

In contrast the point of view that selective semantic categories of words can be disproportionately disturbed within the syndrome of aphasia is equally strongly held. Schuell included in her research edition of her test battery for aphasia a subtest for examining names of parts of the body which was eliminated only in the final shortened version. Goodglass and Kaplan (1972, p. 28) allude to the 'frequent selective disturbance of comprehension of names of parts of the body' and include in their aphasia battery a special subtest to examine understanding of this semantic category. They also make provision for the disparate impairment of other semantic categories by including in their other subtests of auditory comprehension six defined semantic categories: letter names, number names, geometric forms, colours, actions and objects.

An experimental study with this test is reported in Goodglass, Klein, Carey and Jones (1966). It examined both comprehension and production of four of these kinds of names but comprehension only for body parts and geometric shapes. The material used for the objects and actions was black and white line drawings. The categories differed, as was expected, in their degree of difficulty due to the number of class members per category and their distinctiveness. But apart from this inherent and expected distinction there were differences amongst the types of aphasia in naming, although their performances in comprehension were essentially parallel. The fluent aphasic patients were markedly deficient in object naming and markedly superior in letter naming, relative to their other categories, although the absolute level of object naming was virtually the same for Broca's and fluent aphasics. In contrast Broca's aphasics tended to find object naming easier than letter naming. The results emphasize the difference made by having to speak a name or having to select a picture or other kind of item to show comprehension of a name. Comprehension, thus measured, did not distinguish amongst types of aphasics, while name production clearly did, and comprehension and production resulted in different overall orders of difficulty. Object names, the easiest to comprehend, were the hardest to name. The objects chosen were conceptually distinct, forming a heterogeneous category—chair, comb, key, glove, hammock and cactus—probably making differential identification of them by name relatively easy; two of them were of relatively low frequency, perhaps contributing to the greater difficulty of naming in a category as wide as object names. Number words and alphabet letters are members of semantic categories of approximately the same size, but the amount of phonological information which distinguishes the members of each category differs for the two categories: more alphabet letters rhyme and are distinguished by minimal contrastive phonological features than is the case with numbers. Consequently we might expect to find that letters were hard to decode and easy to encode, as was found with the fluent aphasics. Goodglass and his colleagues describe their results in the naming task as demonstrating a dissociation between object and letter naming which is related to the site of the brain damage. The difference between the Broca patients, with predominantly anterior lesions, and the fluent patients with posterior temporal and temporo-parietal lesions, indicates, Goodglass suggests, that the word-finding system may be subdivided anatomically according to the psychological character of different word categories, with letter naming related to the structures which are likely to be damaged or isolated in lesions resulting in Broca's aphasia.

Yamadori and Albert (1973) made an even more specific claim based on an individual case. Selective disturbances of semantic categories are more likely to be exposed, they claim, in studies of individuals rather than of groups of aphasics where such selective differences become lost. Yamadori and Albert examined a 54-year-old man, an engineering graduate, who had suffered a depressed left temporo-parietal skull fracture. Six weeks after this accident he was well except for unique defects of language function which the investigators described as *word-category aphasia*. In addition to a generalized anomia, he had a specific and limited loss of the ability to understand the meanings of a set of words relating to body parts and to room objects. Though he could repeat and even spell these words he was unable to attach meaning to them. Yamadori and Albert describe how, when asked to point to a chair, the patient stood up and looked around the room and spelled out the word to himself but finally said, 'I have to double check that word later, I don't know.' When shown a chair, he said, 'Oh yes, you sat down in a chair. Is that what you mean?' Such difficulties were inconsistent, in that he might have difficulty on one occasion with some words within the category of room objects and on other occasions with others. To cope with his difficulties he developed a strategy of self-cuing, so that he learned, when asked to point to a chair, to cue himself in with 'to sit on a chair' and then was able to indicate it. Yamadori and Albert suggest that comprehension of words involves a two-stage mechanism: word-sound perception and word-meaning comprehension, as illustrated by the patient's retained ability to repeat and spell words whose meaning he did not understand. The word-category aphasia moreover indicates, they propose, that categories of word meaning may have a more or less independent neurophysiological existence. A speculation is that semantic categories may develop initially from the self (i.e. with priority for the category of body parts), progress to the immediate environment (the category of room objects) and then to outside objects, and then still further to categories which transcend personal connections, such as colours. The differential neurophysiological basis for the categories would, if this speculation is correct, thus be related to their different relationships to the self and to their development. Yamadori and Albert's patient is unique in that so far no one else has reported any similar observations.

Oxbury, Oxbury and Humphrey (1969), however, propose that there have been a number of instances of a specific colour aphasia, which may or may not be imposed on a more general anomia in aphasia. In colour-naming difficulties which are attributable to disconnection, the patient retains the ability to make verbal to verbal colour associations (i.e. he can answer without difficulty questions such as 'What colour is butter?') although he cannot name colours by sight. But patients can be observed amongst those who have difficulty in naming colours by sight who also cannot make these verbal–verbal associations. The colour-naming deficit seems to be within the language system instead of in access to it from the visual modality. Oxbury proposes that there must be two distinct varieties of colour anomia. As well as the disconnection variety, there is one which is truly an aphasic disorder arising from damage to cortical structures which subserve colour names. In addition to three cases from the literature which exemplify this kind of colour anomia, Oxbury and his colleagues describe a patient they studied themselves, a young jockey who had been thrown from his horse and sustained a severe head injury. He had only mild difficulties in speech and comprehension, apart from a marked nominal aphasia for objects, pictures and colours and severe reading and writing difficulties. When given a verbal–verbal colour association task he described a polar bear as blue, an orange as dark yellow, a pillar box as blue and so on. He found it difficult to learn associations between coloured discs and colour words, performing at about the same level as he did when making associations between coloured discs and unfamiliar words, although he learned easily to make associations between coloured discs and geometrical designs: it seemed that colour words had come to behave for him like rare rather than common words, and that there had been a selective reduction for him in the meaning of this semantic category.

Another patient who makes a candidate for an example of a specific anomia is described by Dennis (1976). This was a 17-year-old girl who had part of the left anterior temporal lobe removed in order to arrest severe epileptic seizures. The verbal deficit she displayed was in body parts. When examined three years after this operation her verbal comprehension was good and her speech well articulated and grammatically well formed, though showing some tendency to perseverative semantic paraphasias. Confrontation naming was fairly good, and verbal–verbal naming was proficient. On naming of body parts, however, she was poor. Repetition was also consistently impaired. Despite the difficulty in naming of body parts, however, she had no problems with a test of body orientation in which the subject has to show on his own body numbered parts on schematic drawings, i.e. on a test which did not require language. Other variants of this test were then used, with combinations of verbal and non-verbal responses and stimuli. When she was asked to give a verbal response, or when the stimulus was verbal (when she heard the name) even though the response was not verbal, her performance was impaired. Only when both response and stimulus were non-verbal was her performance good. This applied to her selection of parts of the body regardless of the side of the body. In discriminating between left and right side her performance was better. Her left–right judgements were as would be predicted for her mental age. For body-part naming, the most difficult condition was when she heard the word and was asked to make a pointing response. She was also tested to see whether or not her naming and comprehension difficulties with body parts was paralleled by difficulties with other parts of wholes, such as bicycle parts and house parts, or by difficulties with other semantic categories. All these other types of nouns proved considerably easier to name. In the naming of body parts all the patient's errors were within-category errors; and when she was given a free word-association task she always gave a body-part response to a body-part word, and never a body-part response to any other kind of word. It therefore seemed that body parts functioned for her as a clear psychological category. Within this category some words were consistently named and understood correctly (*eye*, *ear*, *nose*) while others were almost always wrong (*index finger*, *thigh*). Errors were not random, but implied that not all features had been correctly incorporated. For example *wrist* was called *ankle* and, on another occasion, *knuckle bones*.

Like other questions in aphasia, the question of whether or not there is selectivity of impairment of semantic categories within the language system, as opposed to access to them from one modality, awaits further examination of individual cases.

Dennis's observations that within the category of body parts her patient had no difficulties with some items and many difficulties with others leads us to consider the other aspect of the study of semantic categories in aphasia, the investigation of qualitative differences in impairment within them. With the list of body parts that Dennis mentions, word frequency suggests itself as an influence as the items the patient had difficulty with are ones less frequently labelled. We shall discuss word frequency shortly as one of the many influences which have been put forward as affecting the facility with which words can be retrieved. But there are also theoretical reasons for qualitative differences within some categories which are unique to those categories. One of these categories is colour names. With colour names an order of semantic differentiation can be derived from studies of world languages. Berlin and Kay (1969) observed that all languages have terms for black and white, and that if a language has terms for only three colours, the third colour is always red. Languages with four colour terms have as their fourth term either a term for green or one for yellow, and five-colour-languages have both. The sixth term to be included in a language is blue and the seventh brown. Terms for purple, pink, orange and grey are only included in languages which have at least eight colour terms. If aphasic semantic simplification were to follow lawful rules, one starting point for formulating hypotheses would be this order in which differentiation of colour names has been suggested as occurring.

Poeck and Stachowiak (1975) in the study described earlier found that the aphasic patients made approximately the same number of errors with the words yellow, white, red, blue, brown, green and black, but considerably more errors with lilac and orange: most of the errors with lilac were in calling it blue or combinations of blue, while orange tended to be called yellow. Grey produced the next highest number of errors. Non-brain-damaged control subjects also made most of their errors on lilac and the right-brain-damaged made errors on grey as well as lilac. The colour orange proved the best colour for discriminating between aphasic and non-aphasic. The investigators also commented that the behaviour of types of aphasics differed not in the kind of colours on which they made errors but in the proportion of circumlocutory answers. Amnesic aphasic patients tended to reply in such terms as *mouse grey, sky grey, chocolate* and *dark yellow*.

A qualitative analysis of colour-naming defects in aphasic patients was undertaken also by Wyke and Holgate (1973). They, too, observed that of the eight colours they used in their test (red, orange, yellow, green, blue, brown, black and white), orange was by far the most difficult for the aphasic subjects. They suggest that this may be because, amongst the colour words tested, this word has the lowest frequency of occurrence in the language. (In passing we might note, however, that the arguments about the influence of operativity on naming to be described shortly would predict that a colour which is also a common fruit should be easy to name.) The examination distinguished between naming to sight and naming as completion of a sentence (verbal–verbal naming). The experimenters also distinguished between naming of plastic tokens and of coloured drawings of objects which varied in the strength with which they are normally associated with one colour (e.g. from banana to bird). The semantic resources of the aphasic subjects in naming as many colours as they could with eyes closed were inferior to those of a group of people who had been born blind or become blind during the first year of life. The aphasic patients were found to be slightly better in naming the colours of the tokens than they were in naming black and white line drawings of objects; but they were significantly more impaired in naming the coloured pictures of objects when they had to provide both a colour and object name. Overall, in comparison with a control group of right-brain-damaged subjects, they were significantly impaired in the ability to name colours of tokens, coloured drawings of objects and in the number of colour names they could produce spontaneously in a limited amount of time; but they were not significantly impaired in their ability to complete sentences either with colour names or with object names. The blind subjects, in contrast, although they produced more colour names spontaneously, were impaired on the completion of sentences with colour names.

This study is particularly interesting in that it demonstrates that a group of aphasics with naming difficulties have more difficulties with visual confrontation naming than they do with verbal–verbal naming, the type of performance that is usually attributed to disconnection naming difficulties as distinguishing it qualitatively from aphasic colour misnaming. Wyke and Holgate point out that, when an aphasic subject is asked to complete a sentence with a colour name, the production of the word is assisted by the intermediate contextual and grammatical links. The errors which the patients made were predominantly in colour names which did not have strong associative links with the object which was named in the sentence (orange carrot, yellow butter). A second observation is that the patients found it considerably more difficult to name a coloured object correctly than they did to name either a colour or an object singly: most of the errors they produced could not simply be attributed to the difficulty of having to speak two words as they often provided two words in designating the test object, with one or both incorrect.

Such observations draw attention to the interaction of effects in aphasia: one kind of interaction is that which makes it more difficult to perform a complex task (as in the combination of colour adjective and concrete noun above) than to perform the two separate elements of the task; the other is the interaction of contextual and associative influences on the performance of any task. It is with the study of such interactions, the complexes of influences which operate on semantic retrieval in aphasia, that we continue this review.

## Complexes

When we come to enquire about what it is that makes a word more difficult for an aphasic patient to retrieve accurately than another, or what it is that makes this easy on one occasion but difficult on another, we have to consider a whole set of influences, some of which take us beyond the realm of denotative meaning which we have been attempting to describe so far. The principal factors which have been suggested can be classed broadly under five headings

(1)  Phonological factors, such as pronounceability, length of phoneme, frequency and stress.
(2)  Emotive factors, including connotative meaning.
(3)  Perceptual factors.
(4)  Frequency of the word in the language, or frequency of the use of the object, or age of acquisition.
(5)  Contextual factors and grammatical influences.

It is not proposed to discuss phonological or grammatical factors in any detail in the present chapter, as these will be dealt with in chapters 7 and 8. The present section therefore includes discussions of the factors which affect word retrieval under the headings of frequency, perceptual factors and emotional content. Most of the studies to be described are concerned with one particular aspect of these influences on aphasic word-finding ability; but before we look at these it is useful to consider the findings of one examination which attempted to evaluate the rela-

TABLE 6

*Variables expected to influence confrontation naming*

(based on Corlew 1971)

| *Circumstantial* | *Related to context* |
|---|---|
| *1. Frequency of occurrence of the word in the language | *1. The referent's contextual allocation (i.e. its superordinate or category) |
| 2. Phoneme frequency (composite score reflecting the frequency in the language of the final and initial phoneme) | 2. Its function, purpose or role |
|  | *3. The place it occurs |
|  | 4. Its causes |
| 3. Word length, measured in number of phonemes | 5. What it consists of or includes |
| 4. Word length, measured in number of syllables | 6. The manner of its occurrence |
|  | *7. Its sensory qualities |
| *5. Pronounceability (as rated by control subjects) | 8. Its consequences |
|  | 9. Its actions or potentialities for action |
| *6. Abstractness (as rated by normal subjects) | 10. Its history or development |
|  | 11. Its temporal qualities |
| *7. Frequency of association (the percentage frequency with which the most frequent response was given by normal subjects) | 12. The way it resembles or contrasts with other referents |
|  | 13. An evaluation of the referent |
| *8. Meaningfulness (the number of different associations given) |  |

* Variables found to be significant in Corlew's experiment.

tive importance of a number of factors of many kinds. Corlew (1971) considered 21 classes of variables which might be expected to influence confrontation naming in aphasia. These variables are shown in Table 6.

Fifty-four words (the words used for confrontation naming in five standard aphasia batteries) were first given to normal subjects, so as to obtain predictor values for each word on the variables for which objective counts were not already available. In this way values were obtained for each word on the 21 variables so that the degree to which the aphasics' naming difficulties could be attributed to any of the variables could be calculated. For fluent aphasics, three variables had a significant influence on the time it took to name the object—pronunciability, place and superordinate. When delay in naming was ignored, and the number of totally correct words was examined (i.e. without either phonemic or semantic paraphasia) there were also three significant variables, place, pronunciability and word frequency. With the non-fluent patients, however, different variables were found to be significant in reaction time: association, word frequency, abstractness and superordinate rating values. The number of correct responses (with time ignored) made by the non-fluent was influenced by place and word frequency as it was with the fluent, although the third significant variable was different, the sensory rating. Though the fluent and non-fluent patients did not differ significantly in the total number of errors they made there were therefore indications that they are affected differently by different factors. Corlew suggests that perhaps word frequency contributes more to naming for non-fluent aphasic patients. There was a large number of the possible predictor variables which did not seem to have been of significance in predicting how well or how quickly the patients in either group would respond. For both groups the variable of place had an inverse relationship to the number of items correctly named, i.e. those words for which the normal subjects had made frequent comments about place (such as, for *cactus* that 'it grows in the desert'), proved to result in more errors; words like *girl*, *house* and *dog* were not often connected with a specific location and were easier for the aphasics to name. Corlew suggests that words rated low on place may arouse many associations (they had a high meaningfulness rating), as well as being of higher frequency, and may be easier to name for these reasons. She also suggests that the results of experiments such as hers can be put to practical use by constructing word lists which would be expected to be in order of difficulty for different types of patients, so that these could be used in therapy. It should at least be possible to make better estimates of the variables which need to be taken into account when deciding on what words to use as testing instruments in batteries. Of the five aphasia tests which she had used she found that the naming sections were not equivalent in the number of naming errors which they produced. The Porch Index of Communicative Ability, the Minnesota Test for the Differential Diagnosis of Aphasia and the Language Modalities Test for Aphasia were significantly different in this respect from the Eisenson Examining for Aphasia Test, and the Boston Diagnostic Aphasia Examination. Porch's Index, consisting entirely of high frequency items, was the easiest, and people with mild naming problems often made no errors. The most difficult was the Boston examination, with pictures that could be unrecognized.

Corlew's study confirmed the observation often made that an important factor in word retrieval is frequency.

## Frequency

Since frequency of the word in the language is considered to be of importance in determining the ease with which words can be retrieved in aphasia, it is unfortunate that there is no comprehensive count of the frequency with which words are used in speech. In American English there are at least two counts of frequency in spoken language made by people who have also been interested in aphasic speech (Howes 1966; Jones and Wepman 1966), but the more comprehensive counts which have been used are based on written language collected from a sample of newspapers and magazines. Of these the most used in aphasia research has been the count by Thorndike and Lorge (1944) of 30,000 words, though some studies have used the more recent computerized count by Kučera and Francis (1967). Amongst the studies which have investigated the effect of word frequency on naming in aphasia are those by Rochford and Williams (1965), Halpern (1965), Spreen (1966) and Goodglass, Hyde and Blumstein (1969). One of the first studies of the influence of word frequency on comprehension (in contrast to naming) was by Schuell, Jenkins and Landis (1961), who demonstrated that word frequency was an important factor in the patient's ability to understand words. Siegel (1959) had found that word frequency had to be invoked to account for the unexpected finding that words rated as low for abstraction did not prove to be easier for aphasic patients to read aloud than words rated as high for abstraction. Howes (1964) examined the frequencies of words in the conversational speech of the sample of aphasic men studied by Geschwind and himself. His statistical analysis demonstrated that the shift to words of higher frequency which can be observed in aphasia does not represent a qualitative distortion in the use of words: the shape of the frequency distribution is the same as in normal people's use, with a linear association (when logarithmic transforms are used) between frequency of occurrence of words in an individual's speech and the rank order of the words on frequency counts in the language (see Hörmann 1971 for an account of this phenomenon known as Zipf's law). The potential size of an aphasic speaker's vocabulary therefore is still infinite, even though there is a shift to usage of words of greater frequency in the language. From the fact that the shift in the frequency distribution is proportional to the severity of the aphasia, and therefore presumably to the amount of brain damage, Howes inferred that the neural structures underlying vocabulary may be equipotential within the language areas.

Wepman, Bock, Jones and Van Pelt (1956) examined the question of whether or not the word-finding difficulty of anomic patients was restricted to nouns. They offered two hypotheses. One was that anomia could be due to a suppression of words of low frequency, with nouns being disproportionately diminished as this class includes more words of low frequency. The other was that if anomia was primarily due to a reduction in the availability of nouns *per se*, rather than to this frequency effect, there would still be low-frequency verbs, adjectives and so on. What they found, in their study of one aphasic woman, was that all words of lower frequency were deficient in her speech, and that nouns of high frequency did occur (mostly of the non-specific type of noun like *thing* and *people*). They suggested that the noun-finding difficulty which is the surface characteristic of aphasic speech of this kind in fact obscures a more fundamental effect, the generality of the words retained, which is itself related to the frequency with which words occur in a language.

Rochford and Williams (1962; 1965) undertook a series of studies of effects on aphasic naming. Within the same semantic category (body parts) and with the same visual context (the experimenter's own body) the word-frequency effect was as strong as it was with a heterogeneous set of pictured words. Despite the same semantic and visual conditions a marked effect of frequency obtained. They also examined what happened when aphasic subjects were asked to name composite words which were made up of two words of unequal frequency such as *sun-dial*. They devised a list of composite words in which either both of the component words were common or one of the words was rare, and found that the patients' difficulties in naming were related to the frequency of the first word in the combined pair. Word combinations which were common–common (*penknife*, *lighthouse*) or were common–rare (*wheel-barrow*, *hedgehog*) were easier than words which were rare–common (*padlock*, *spinningwheel*). Homonyms were also tested to see whether their commoner or rarer meaning was named more easily; all the subjects named the commoner object more easily. The effect of frequency also held with pictured verbs as with nouns. Rochford and Williams summarized their findings by saying that high frequency of usage was the main factor responsible for the easy accessibility of words.

Frequency of usage of words correlates significantly with the age at which children acquire those words (Carroll and White 1973) and Rochford and Williams (1962) also tested whether or not aphasic misnamings could be related to the age at which children learned the words. Amongst the picturable words examined were some which were used in their secondary or metaphoric senses: hands of a watch, teeth of a comb, arm of a chair, eye of a needle. Children and aphasic adults were given a series of clues to help them name them if they initially failed. These clues were description of use, sentence completion, a rhyming word and finally the word itself spelled out. There was a close parallel between the number of correct responses given by the aphasic adults to the word and the age at which children had learnt the names. It seems that the names first learned in childhood are the names last lost in aphasia, and Rochford and Williams reported that 'the similarities between the performances of children and dyphasic adults are so close that it almost seems possible to speak of a "naming age" in nominal dysphasia', although children and adults were helped to recall names by different kinds of clues.

Although word frequency can thus be shown to have an important effect on aphasic abilities in naming and comprehending names of objects, there are complicating factors. One is that the error response given to a word may be a rarer word than the one sought: Rochford and Williams comment on an aphasic patient's calling the teeth of a comb *prongs*—a rarer word than the target word required. And indeed not all studies have found infrequent words to present more difficulties than frequent words. For example, Filby, Edwards and Seacat (1963) observed that there was no effect of word frequency when patients were asked to decide which of two words they heard matched a third word. In this case the absence of the frequency effect can perhaps be attributed to the fact that the decision was phonemic rather than semantic. Halpern (1965b) reported also that word frequency was not relevant to the amount of perseveration shown by aphasic patients (perseveration being defined as inappropriate repetition of an earlier response) when they were asked to read or repeat a list of words.

Other possible influences on the triggering off of an inappropriate word can be subsumed under the heading of perceptual factors.


## Perceptual factors

Riegel and Riegel (1961) suggest that it may not be so much the frequency of the word in the language which influences the naming process, as the frequency with which the referent itself has been experienced. In line with this kind of thinking it has been suggested that the retrievability of words in aphasia is related to the sensory impressions which they are capable of arousing. One approach to the examination of this would be to investigate such situations as that described above where a patient faced with a picture he is trying to name produces a word for an object which has a visual resemblance to the object (provided that the misnaming is not due to misrecognition). In terms of a model such as Morton's logogen model the implication is that the visual similarity raises above threshold a word unit which is not entirely appropriate. An alternative and easier way to study the problem is by varying the perceptual factors not in the way the words are presented but in the presumed semantic organization of the words themselves. In other words either naming of a constant list of words can be examined with different modes of presentation, or the words themselves, presented under a constant condition, can be varied for their inherent picturability, operativity (to be described shortly), or capacity for arousing multi-sensory associations.

Most studies in the first category have been concerned with a comparison of naming to pictures and to aurally given definitions or open-ended sentences, though Barton, Maruszewski and Urrea (1969) mention an unpublished study by Vandette in which it was found that aphasics were helped by being able to smell an object as well as see it. In Barton *et al.*'s own study they found that, for the aphasics they examined taken as a group, naming of pictures came midway in difficulty between completing an open-ended sentence and naming in response to a description or definition, although a substantial proportion of the individual patients deviated from this order. If Geschwind is correct in relating the naming process to structures in the parieto-temporo-occipital junction of the left-hemisphere lobes, because this is the supreme association area of the brain where the association areas of the sensory modalities meet, then naming could plausibly be facilitated by increasing the amount of information given to the subject through these modalities. This hypothesis was put to the test by Gardiner and Brookshire (1972). They compared three conditions for naming, one in which the patients were asked to listen to and repeat a name (auditory condition), one in which they were asked to name a picture and to read out a printed name (visual condition) and one in which both kinds of stimuli were used (combined condition). They found that the combined condition produced the best results, with the auditory condition on its own being more successful than the visual condition on its own. Not all the individuals were assisted by multi-sensory presentation, however. Again this could be accounted for in terms of the neurophysiological processes disturbed. A failure in simultaneous synthesis, such as Luria proposes with lesions in the zone Geschwind associates with naming, may mean that increasing the sensory input through two modalities does not improve performance. Alternatively the auditory task can be thought of as tapping chiefly the phonological level of organization. If there was a dissociation between the phonological and semantic levels a combined input would not help.

Bisiach (1966) examined the hypothesis that there are visual perceptive factors in anomia by comparing the naming of realistic coloured figures, outline drawings and drawings defaced by cross-hatching. He found that the percentage of correct answers varied with the clarity of the visual representation but that the impairment on the mutilated drawings could not be accounted for by failure to recognize them. Bisiach deduces that 'Without denying the possibility that the structures responsible for the naming process may themselves be damaged, it is nevertheless apparent that in anomic subjects the language disturbance is at least partly conditioned by factors acting at the level of the mechanisms of interaction between the sensory analyser and the verbal sphere.' Following Bisiach's study, Corlew and Nation (1975) tested whether or not there was any effect on naming of presenting the material as a three-dimensional object or as a reduced-size drawing, using for this test the objects and drawings from the Porch Index of Communicative Ability. They found no significant difference between the two conditions, and cite unpublished studies by Christenson and by Stoler in which the kind of photographs used (cluttered, uncluttered, or reduced size) did not influence naming, nor did the use of objects in a meaningful context or in isolation. In comments on Corlew and Nation's paper Bisiach (1976) defends his claim, and suggests that object identification is not an all-or-none stage between name retrieval and sensory processing, but that sensory processing may directly influence verbal retrieval, or that the identification stage may vary in its efficiency in eliciting naming. Marin and Saffran (1975) describe a fluent aphasic with a naming disorder who performed well in complex perceptual tasks only as long as he was silent or counting aloud. When he talked about what he was doing, he misnamed items and then behaved as if they were what he had wrongly called them. A reverse effect of the interference of poor visual input on naming was therefore found, with poor naming apparently influencing perceptual processes. The authors suggest that such apparently agnosic behaviour may be due to the activation of the left hemisphere by speech, leading to its taking over of a perceptual function normally undertaken by the right hemisphere, and, because of its lack of specialization for such functions, performing it less well—a case of 'pathological verbal dominance'.

The other category of studies examines the influence of sensory factors in the nature of the words themselves on the ease with which an aphasic can produce their names. The earliest formulation of this factor was in terms of the dimension of concreteness and abstraction of words. Head proposed (1926, p. 397) that aphasics had more difficulty in naming abstract items than concrete items. Goldstein developed this theme to emphasize a general impairment in the ability of the damaged brain to adopt an abstract attitude. Siegel (1959), as we have already observed, found inconclusive results when he tested the influence of abstraction on the words which aphasics read aloud. In contrast Halpern (1965a) found that high and medium abstract words presented for reading aloud produced significantly more errors than did words of low abstraction, though there were no differences when the patient heard and repeated the word. A measure of the amount of perseveration produced showed similar results related to the level of abstraction of the word (Halpern 1965b).

In 1971 Paivio suggested that some of the effects that had been attributed with normal subjects to word frequency were in fact related to the imagibility of words, the degree to which what they represented could be pictured. Goodglass, Hyde and Blumstein (1969) tested the extent to which picturability (as well as frequency) influenced the aphasic's ability to retrieve nouns. They hypothesized that the speech of Broca's aphasics would show a higher proportion of picturable nouns than would that of Wernicke's and amnesic aphasics. Nouns were classed as picturable if they referred to objects with a definite visual configuration which would be elicited by most English speakers who heard the name (e.g. *bird*). A word like *animal* was classed as non-picturable because its visual referent is not certain. The hypothesis was supported. In the sample of aphasic speech taken in its entirety, however, there were many more non-picturable words than picturable: the twelve most frequent were *time, year, week, mother, day, work, name, way, wife, father, minute,* and *people*—not the indefinite words which substitute for unavailable picturable nouns, but words common in the small talk which is produced without much effort. Such words, Goodglass and his co-workers suggested, are learned through the contexts of the sentences in which they are heard, rather than by the forming of associations between word and visual referent, as are picturable words. Hence the different proportions of these two classes of words in fluent and non-fluent aphasics reflects the greater facility fluent aphasics have in producing verbal sequences. Rather than being the cause of the difference in the speech patterns of the two kinds of aphasics, the difference in frequency between picturable and non-picturable nouns is therefore an effect.

A second sensory influence suggested on word retrieval in aphasia is related to the kinaesthetic sense rather than to the visual. Gardner (1973) devised four sets of composite pictures illustrating familiar objects and elements which were either *operative* or non-operative and figurative. Operative was defined as manipulatable and discrete, firm to the touch and easily available to several sense modalities. Figurative elements were those which were difficult to grasp and normally recognized by their visual configuration. For instance book, screwdriver and finger were classed as operative, while wall, cloud and hip were classed as figurative. Three levels of word frequency were used for each type of word. Both frequency and operativity proved to have significant effects on the aphasic patients' ability to produce the correct name, though not on their ability to select the correct name from a multiple choice; and operativity appeared to be more influential than frequency. There were no differences in this respect between anterior and posterior aphasic patients. Gardner suggests that operative elements arouse a larger set of associations and acts than do figurative elements. Operative elements might therefore be expected to be relatively more spared in aphasia than elements like colours, alphabet letters and perhaps written words which arouse few if any non-visual associations. Gardner extended his observations (1974b) by comparing the aphasic subjects' results on this test with those of three- and four-year-old children. Children also responded better to words which were more operative and more frequent. Operativity alone, however, cannot be the overriding semantic factor in facilitating retrieval in children and aphasic adults, because aphasic adults find some symbolic categories (numbers and alphabet letters) easier to name than physical objects. These, Gardner suggests, are part of well-developed systems and routines and do not arouse the competing responses which can be aroused by object names.

Beyn and Vlasenko (1974), in one of the few studies to concentrate on the naming of actions (verbs), propose that there are a number of stages in the microgenesis of a name. Using as illustration the action of *to forge* (in the sense of forging iron), they propose that a number of properties and semantic stratifications are aroused when we name the action in a picture. First there are the static elements of the blacksmith, the object which is being made, the hammer, tongs and anvil and the workshop. Then there are the dynamic elements which are superimposed on this picture; the blacksmith wields the hammer, strikes the iron, watches it and so on. It is this dynamic process which constitutes the naming of the action verb. Beyn and Vlasenko propose that the speech process of naming an action is always preceded by a primary reflection of the objects which participate in the action. They therefore suggest that different kinds of misnamings of actions in aphasia, which can be related to types of aphasia, will reveal the different stages in the microgenesis of the word. Apart from misnamings which are phonological in character, or are perseverations of previous namings, most misnamings will reflect either the static stage of word genesis or the dynamic. Static misnamings for *to forge* would be *tongs, blacksmith, anvil*, and a dynamic misnaming would be *chops*. In dynamic misnamings either one element is singled out from the general composition of the action (*piercing* for *sewing*) or an equivalent or more generalized attribute is substituted (*writes* for *draws*). The singling out of a dynamic element sometimes results in a novel word (*bullet-throwing* for *shooting*) which may also contain phonemic errors. Patients with all degrees of severity of fluent aphasia make dynamic-stage misnamings and very few static misnamings; patients with non-fluent aphasia make more dynamic-stage misnamings only when the degree of aphasia is mild; with increasing severity of non-fluent aphasia the number of static paraphasias increases and the number of dynamic paraphasias decreases.

Beyn and Vlasenko propose altogether five stages in the genesis of action-word naming:

(1)  a stage when the static elements are singled out;
(2)  a stage of global formation of the dynamic elements;
(3)  a stage where dynamic elements are differentially singled out;
(4)  a stage where the word becomes structured into its form—the stage at which replacements and neologisms can be formed;
(5)  the final stage where the word becomes realized in its formal shape.

## Emotional content

If naming is assisted by the amount of sensory impact made immediately by the stimulus presented, or by the cumulative sensory impacts which the word meaning itself has acquired, we might expect the emotional content of a word also to affect retrieval. In the first sense in which we examined perceptual influences, in the immediate pressure of emotional content, Jackson's observations that patients who were virtually speechless could produce appropriate words when emotionally stressed would seem to endorse this. However, we are now considering the relatively metalinguistic task of the non-automatic selection of a specific word, and here the role of emotional content is uncertain. Indeed experimental studies with normal subjects (Eysenck 1975), as well as common observation, lead us to infer that the more one wishes to find a word on the tip-of-the tongue the harder it is to find it: it is frequently only when people give up trying that they find that the name they are seeking becomes available. As far as directed motivation is concerned, therefore, it seems that the greater the desire the less is name retrieval facilitated.

A study which is relevant to the question of whether general motivational level bears on naming performance in aphasia is one by Brookshire (1972b). It showed that, if an aphasic patient is given a difficult naming task and then an easy naming task, the second task is less well performed than if it does not follow a difficult task. The converse was also true: if he had been asked to name easy items first, then performance on the difficult items improved. Brookshire comments that 'Although we cannot yet identify the exact processes which produce these effects, it seems reasonable to speculate that placing an aphasic patient in a task where he experiences high proportions of failure may generate emotional responses which are in themselves capable of disrupting the patient's performance' (p. 556). He suggests that these effects can last over a period of time.

But besides the immediate emotional or motivational pressure on word retrieval, there is an affective component in that residuum of word meaning which cannot easily be defined in terms of semantic features. It is this affective component which is described as connotative meaning. Just as denotative meaning has been scaled and words ranked in order of number of associations, picturability and so on, so has connotative meaning been scaled into numbers and rating norms established. The instrument which has been used for this purpose is the measuring technique devised by Osgood known as the Semantic Differential. The Differential consists of a set of bipolar adjective scales on which each subject is asked to rate a certain concept. Starting with 50 different scales, Osgood found that many of them proved redundant and that only three main factors needed to be represented. These factors were identified as Evaluative (i.e. good–bad), Potency (i.e. strong–weak) and Activity (i.e. active–passive). If people are asked to rate a concept or word on seven-point scales representing these factors, a fair degree of agreement is found for many frequent words. The Semantic Differential has found practical applications in advertising and market research as a way of finding out what are people's attitudes towards commercial products.

In their report of a seminar on aphasia, Osgood and Miron (1963) speculated as to whether or not connotative meaning, as measured by the Semantic Differential, should be spared or impaired in aphasia. If connotative meaning is more abstract than denotative meaning, it might be expected to be more vulnerable to brain damage. On the other hand, if it is more primitive and basic a form of meaning, it might be expected to be less vulnerable. Or possibly, if it is part and parcel of the total meaning of a word, it is necessarily impaired to the same degree. If affective meaning is related to the functioning of the limbic and other subcortical systems, however, perhaps it is independent of the cortical systems which subserve language and the denotative organization of meaning.

Doehring and Swisher (1972) put these speculations to the test. They gave 30 Broca's aphasics a version of the Semantic Differential which required them to make a forced choice of a polar adjective for each of 24 words, rather than rating them on scales. They used six pairs of polar adjectives: in addition to the three pairs given above, these were beautiful–ugly, hard–soft and slow–fast. There was near-unanimous agreement from control subjects as to the best adjectives for each of the 24 words. The aphasic subjects proved to be impaired on their judgements in the task, and most particularly in making errors on ratings on the activity factor (active–passive, slow–fast). The number of total errors they made tended to increase with their ratings for severity of aphasia, giving no support to the hypothesis that emotive meaning would be disturbed independently of damage to the language zones of the brain. The errors which the aphasics made tended to be in favouring the positive adjectives and rejecting the negative, suggesting, Doehring and Swisher speculate, that aphasics like to 'look on the bright side'. A problem in drawing conclusions from such an experiment, as the researchers pointed out, is that such a task tests knowledge of denotative meaning as well as of connotative meaning. Although by using Broca's aphasics as subjects an attempt had been made to avoid the major semantic confusions of fluent aphasics, the researchers suggested that the frontal lobes may be involved in the affective meaning systems, and Broca's aphasics with their frontal lesions may therefore show a distinct impairment on connotative meaning for this reason.

A modification of the Semantic Differential has been devised for cross-cultural studies; it uses figural opposites instead of polar scales defined by adjectives (Osgood 1960). It was devised so that the same task could be given to speakers of different languages in order to make multilingual comparisons (amongst Navajos, Mexican Spanish and Japanese). For aphasic subjects it has the advantage that the decisions about the test words are not compounded by difficulties in recognizing the meaning of the adjectival scales. Subjects were asked to select which of each pair of a total of 13 illustrations (like those shown in figure 5) was appropriate for each concept being examined. Mostofsky, Vanden Bossche, Shein-kopf and Noyes (1971) used 12 of these pairs of figures to examine aphasic patients'

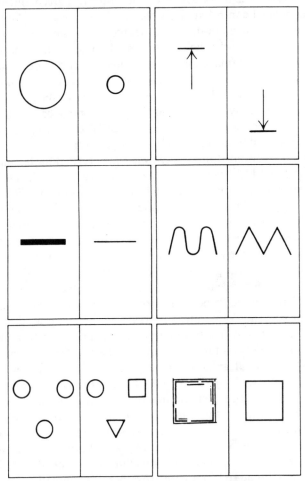

Fig. 5   Six items from a figurative version of the Semantic Differential, illustrating contrasts of large–small, up–down, thick–thin, rounded–angular, homogeneous–heterogeneous, and hazy–clear (based on Osgood 1960)

judgements of the connotative meaning of twenty concepts like *good*, *strong* and *fast*. They also gave the test to non-aphasic right-brain-damaged and to normal people. The results showed that there was the same degree of agreement in the judgements between the aphasic and normal subjects as there was within the normal subjects, indicating a fair degree of affective stability in the aphasics, and suggesting that word-finding difficulty in aphasia does not indicate impairment of connotative meaning. The data, the researchers suggest, 'argue for the existence of residual abstract strengths in a language-disturbed population'.

Although the figurative version of the Semantic Differential avoids some of the reliance of the standard version on knowledge of denotative meaning, one of the hazards is the introduction of a new source of error. Mostofky's right-brain-damaged subjects showed a low degree of within-group agreement, and less agreement with the normal control subjects than did the aphasics. Another study of connotative meaning in brain-damaged people in the same year (Gardner and Denes 1973) reported that the figurative Semantic Differential was so difficult for people with right-brain-damage that some of them refused to do it, protesting that they could not connect the sketchy lines with the meaning of a word: 'Neither of these lines is a woman. I don't see any woman there. What are you trying to pull?' (p. 191). In this study Gardner and Denes compared directly the impairment of connotative and denotative meaning in a group of aphasic subjects. Denotative meaning was examined by asking the patient to select from a choice of two or four pictures the one appropriate for a spoken word; the format for testing connotative meaning using a modified version of the figurative Semantic Differential was similar, with the patient having to select which of a pair of symbolic line configurations was appropriate. The denotation and connotation tasks had ten words in common, and each word was tested against a number of configurations. Some of the words were concrete nouns, some were adjectives appropriate for these nouns, and the others were abstract nouns derived from these adjectives. On the connotation test the aphasic groups scored from an average of 57 per cent correct (global aphasics) to 79 per cent correct (conduction aphasics) and on the denotation test from 52 per cent to 96 per cent correct. There was a significant correlation between denotation and connotation scores, and there appeared to be a regular progression of impairment in both denotative and connotative meaning going from conduction, transcortical motor, and Broca's aphasics, through anomic aphasics to Wernicke's and global aphasics. Unexpectedly scores on concrete common nouns, abstract nouns and adjectives were of about the same difficulty in the connotation test. As the experimenters comment, connotative meaning is complex and probably graded in nature rather than all-or-none as is denotative meaning, and the extent to which the formal task tapped this aspect of meaning was uncertain. That connotative meaning was not related to grammatical class, unlike denotative meaning, supports the notion that it is distinct in nature from denotative meaning, although both were found to be impaired together. If connotation is a more pervasive aspect of meaning it may be both more vulnerable to little brain damage and more spared by greater brain damage.

## Summary

A recent paper by Warrington and McCarthy (1987) will help us to summarize this chapter. It has attempted an integrated account of how semantic information might be categorically coded in the brain. The authors review the kinds of dissociations which have been reported in the comprehension or production of categories of names:

concrete superior to abstract;

abstract superior to concrete;

common nouns and proper nouns superior to action verbs;

action verbs superior to object names;

man-made objects superior to living things;

living things superior to man-made objects;

common objects superior to plants, food and animals;

food, animals and flowers superior to common objects;

body parts superior to foods and animals;

object names superior to body parts;

large outdoor objects superior to indoor objects;

place names superior to names of famous people.

Seven of these are double dissociations, evidence that the difference between the categories is not one of inherent difficulty of one compared with the other. This suggests that the organization of meaning in terms of semantic categories has some neurological validity, though not necessarily to the exclusion of other complementary systems of organization. Simple dichotomies between concrete and abstract or animate and inanimate are not adequate to capture the nature of these dissociations, and Warrington and her colleagues first proposed that the distinction could be cast in terms of the salience of functional or physical attributes of the items to the language user. Applying the principle of minimal pair contrastivity to the analysis, Warrington suggested that object names, for example, tend to be considered in terms of their functional differences: the contrast between shoes and slippers is in their functional use rather than perceptual dissimilarities. Foods, on the other hand, contrast perceptually in terms of their physical attributes, rather than in terms of their functional roles (e.g. the visual contrast between carrot and parsnip). The same applies to other categories of living things, such as flowers.

Warrington's and McCarthy's (1987) fine-grained study of a globally aphasic patient suggested a refinement of this notion. The results of a large number of tests with the names of items, either written or pictured, to which she was asked to point when she heard a word, showed these results:

animals and flowers superior to objects;

large man-made objects superior to manipulable objects;

occupations, vegetables and materials superior to geographical features, colours, kitchen utensils, furniture and parts of the body;

names of famous people superior to common christian names and surnames.

The patient's comprehension for these items was also tested for the effect of rate of presentation in one of the tasks, and it was found that comprehension of object names improved if a five second delay occurred between items compared with when they were presented at two second intervals. Another variable examined was whether making a pointing choice was affected by the type of distractors used, i.e. semantically close or distant distractors. In both reading and listening tasks, semantic similarity was shown to be highly influential on the patient's ability to select from the impaired categories. Over all the set of tests, similar general findings were reported when tasks were repeated, though these were not specific to exact items i.e. it was general category effects which were being discovered, the authors claim, rather than particular difficulties with specific lexical items as such.

Warrington and McCarthy draw several conclusions. The first conclusion is that knowledge is organized in terms of categories. The second is that patients like this have a semantic access deficit in respect of certain categories, rather than degradation of the categories as such, since performance improved if more time was given, and was not item-specific. Furthermore performance tended to deteriorate between the first and second presentation of an item, interpreted as being due to a spreading "refractoriness" in the system, which extended to other members of a category as well as to the specific item. Even the more specific dichotomy earlier proposed of functional/physical was not sufficient to explain the dissociations of categories reported in this paper, and Warrington and McCarthy propose a more elaborate scheme in which categories are distinguished by the relative salience of each of the sense modalities to a category. Visual information, they suggest, for example, may be more important in distinguishing two items within the category of furniture (a chair and a stool), but not so important in distinguishing items in the category of clothing (a shirt and a jacket). Types of visual information (colour, shape, motion, location) also have different saliences according to category. Within the category of vegetables, cauliflower and cabbage are distinguished by colour rather than shape; within the category of flowers, tulip and carnation are likely to be distinguished by shape rather than colour. This characterization of categories in terms of the relative weightings given to sensory and motor attributes can possibly even be extended to apply to the discrepancy between comprehension of names of famous people and common names of people, in that the former have unique and specific referents on which all salient visual and other multiple information sources are focussed.

This challenging proposal of the specificity of categorical knowledge will no doubt provoke considerable research. It is not easy to see how a large lesion resulting in global aphasia could be so selective in its effects on different categories (and it is notable that most, though not all, of the cases reported with category specific deficits have severe aphasia or dementia). The proposal clearly reiterates the need for carefully selected material when semantic abilities are being examined.

To conclude this chapter, it is clear that there are a number of influences on retrieval of word meaning in aphasia. In aphasia itself, and in classical anomia rather than modality-specific anomia, differences in ease of retrieval amongst semantic categories can be at least partially accounted for by these influences rather than by selective damage to certain categories. Prominent amongst these influences are frequency of use of the word and/or its referent, picturability, operativity, concreteness and, in relation to the immediate context of the specific task, the clarity of the perceptual input, the number of sensory media through which the referent is experienced, the emotional content and the carry-over of motivational effects of previous tasks. In addition there is a major influence which we have barely yet touched upon, the influence of the linguistic context in which word retrieval is attempted. All we have said about semantic organization and word retrieval in the last two chapters has been about the sense relationships amongst words out of their syntactic contexts and the relationships between single words and their referents. Yet one of the common methods of facilitating word retrieval in aphasic patients is by cueing them in with a sentence context, particularly one which limits the acceptable choice of words. The ability to name objects or to make conventional word associations may be easier to study experimentally, but may not be of as much moment in revealing the essential nature of an aphasia as the ability to use words appropriately in syntactic constructions or to recognize semantic implication, presupposition and anomaly in sentence contexts. It is principally with these aspects of the language disorder that the next chapter is concerned.

# 7

# Investigations of syntax

The rapport between linguistics and aphasiology blossomed coincidentally with the dominance given to syntax by standard transformational grammar. Since, moreover, one of the most conspicuous characteristics of non-fluent aphasic speech is *agrammatism*, this means that there has been a considerable number of studies of various aspects of aphasic syntax. Grammatical disorders were first reported on in detail in German in 1913 by Pick, a translation of whose book and a summary of whose ideas are now available in the English language (Pick translated by Brown 1973; Spreen 1973). Goodglass and Blumstein (1973), in an introduction to Spreen's summary, comment on the resemblance of Pick's theory of language to current generative grammar: Pick also proposed that a schematic formation of the sentences must precede the choice of words, lexical insertion. Agrammatism, which superficially resembles telegrammese, was therefore first conceived of as a regression from conventional syntax to 'thought' syntax: the equivalent in terms of generative grammar would be that the agrammatic patient utters a phonetic realization of deep structure without its infill of grammatical words and inflections or transformations.

Before the formulation of generative transformational theories another idea of Pick's was adopted by some theorists—the idea that the agrammatic patient's difficulties were in part due to the effort which speech required of him. This interpretation was encouraged by the observation that patients with agrammatic speech were usually those who also had articulation difficulties. It was not even certain to what extent the term *agrammatism* was justified as a comment on grammar rather than on the need to simplify articulatory production. Low (1931) considered, however, that the degree of agrammatism was related to the complexity of the grammar in the speaker's native language. But present-day aphasiologists would not agree with Low's observations that '"typical" cases of agrammatism suitable for detailed study are either rare or rudimentary among English-speaking patients' (p. 556): English, he thought, has a relatively simple grammar while the German language, in which Pick's observations of agrammatism were made, 'has retained the dead weight of a cumbersome grammatical organization which makes the language extremely complex and difficult to handle' (p. 557). Despite the questionableness of some of his observations, Low's proposal is interesting in that he attributed agrammatism not so much to the articulatory effort required of the aphasic speaker but to the grammatical load. One concern of recent linguistic investigations of disorders at the syntactic level has been an examination of the extent to which agrammatism can be explained as a central disruption of syntactic competence which extends to comprehension as well as speech, rather than as economy of effort. Some contemporary aphasiologists accept the interpretation of agrammatism as being primarily related to the need for economy of neuromuscular effort (e.g. Lenneberg 1973); others, who also do not consider agrammatism to be a central loss of competence, have modified the notion of economy of effort to describe it in terms of a memory disorder, an inability to sustain the pre-speech intention long enough to utter it, or of the need to achieve a certain threshold of *saliency* before a word can be uttered. We shall consider these ideas shortly, but some preliminaries are necessary. Firstly, agrammatism is not the only label which has been provided for disturbances of syntax in aphasic language: another label, *paragrammatism*, is used for the speech of fluent aphasics who produce a jumble of phrases using plenty of grammatical words but few complete sentences of complex structure. Out of Goodglass's (1968, p. 179) list of some of the grammatical difficulties which have been noticed in aphasia, it is perhaps the last two which relate to paragrammatism, as well as to agrammatism:

(1) Omission and within-category interchangeability of articles, prepositions and personal pronouns.
(2) Substitution of verb-stem or infinitive for inflected form.
(3) Loss of coordinating and subordinating syntactic constructions.
(4) Loss of speech melody as an indicator of segmentation.
(5) Loss of comprehension of grammatical words and inflections.
(6) Use of incomplete sentences or the mixing of grammatically incompatible sequences.

However paragrammatism has been less well studied than agrammatism, and we will leave discussion of it to the end of this chapter. To impose some kind of structure on the many linguistic studies of aphasia at the syntactic level, let us begin with a brief account of the methods of investigation used, followed by examples of studies which have progressed from the taxonomic interest in parts of speech, through the study of grammatical words and syntactic features expressed through inflections, to the most recent emphasis on structure and sentence types. Then, as a preliminary to the final section on paragrammatism, it will be appropriate to consider those studies which have tested the question of whether syntactic and lexical abilities can be dissociated by aphasia.

## Methods of investigation

Unlike investigations within the semantic level, where it is useful to have a specific stimulus so that there is some certainty about the word the patient is trying to find, investigations at the syntactic level often rely on spontaneous speech to provide data for analysis. Indeed, perhaps because of the difficulties inherent in assessing a patient's abilities in syntactic comprehension, some linguists and psycholinguists make spontaneous speech the sole data for their analysis of grammatical disability. There is a considerable diversity in the systems of analysis of syntax used by various investigators, not only in the linguistic theories on which they have based their analysis but on the compromises with these theories which they have made due to the practical impositions of their applications. We will look briefly at examples of these from American, British, Canadian, Dutch, French, Japanese, and Romanian reports. Most of these investigators make no distinction between spontaneous speech as recorded in interviews and speech which has been elicited through story-picture description. Although a meticulous analysis would perhaps distinguish the two as representing different levels on the metalinguistic-functional scale, for convenience both are assumed to provide the same kind of data for syntactic analysis.

The second method we shall illustrate is the use of set tasks to elicit speech in order to examine syntactic knowledge. These can be distinguished from story-picture description because each task is aimed at examining a specific aspect of syntax. Examples of these tasks are sentence-completion, repetition, spelling, construction of sentences from given words, and tasks where the patient is asked to substitute pronouns for nouns, conjoin sentences or perform other transformations.

The third principal method of investigation of syntactic abilities does not require the patient to speak, and so provides a method of investigation of patients with major difficulties in speech. Like the second method it has the disadvantage of requiring structured material, so that the information which can be extracted depends entirely on what the investigator has included in the task, rather than being open-ended as with spontaneous speech. It is necessarily completely at a formal level. Favourite tasks under this method are picture-choice, judgement of syntactic acceptability, sorting or pairing of words and following of directions (although, as we suggested in chapter 4, tasks which require more than the simplest of gestures may be compounded by factors which are not linguistic). These tasks have mostly been used by investigators interested in testing whether or not patients whose speech is agrammatic show parallel difficulties in tests of syntactic comprehension or knowledge, where speech is not required.

## 1. Spontaneous speech

Goodglass and Blumstein's (1973) collection of papers on studies of syntax in aphasia includes an account by Panse and Shimoyama of an examination of the speech of an agrammatic Japanese speaker. Josephs's introduction to this account describes the authors' approach to linguistic theory as rather impressionistic and non-rigorous. But despite the contrasts between Japanese and the Indo-European languages in which aphasia has been principally studied, Panse and Shimoyama conclude that agrammatic disturbances in Japanese are just like those in German. Though Japanese lacks some of the articles and inflections of German, it has a number of prefixes, infixes and suffixes which express stylistic nuances of meaning. The Japanese agrammatic patient's errors are in omissions of these affixes with some substitutions of one affix for another and some uncertainties related to word order. The authors interpret their observations as indicating that agrammatism is a reflection of a disturbance in memory availability.

Lebrun (1967) has described the spontaneous speech of two patients with 'emissive' aphasia, both speakers of French. One was compared with Jakobson's predictions for *contiguity disorder*. Of his utterances, 93 per cent were made up of strings of less than four words, and there was only one example of his using a subordinate clause. Instead of using intensifiers he would repeat the substantive word; for example instead of 'a very long rest' he would repeat 'rest, rest'. However, neither this patient, nor the other one whose syntactic constructions were more elaborate despite his lack of fluency, supported Jakobson's dichotomy of disorders into ones related to contiguity and ones related to similarity. The agrammatic patient retained the ability to precede a substantive word by an article and to use connectives, and most of his breakdowns occurred between rather than within phrases.

Voinescu (1971) also used Jakobson's theory in the analysis of interviews from 20 Romanian aphasic speakers. The first 100 sentences spoken were analysed according to whether they were simple, complex (including compound) or elliptical. The sentences were further classified according to the number of verb qualifiers and noun attributes they contained, and a ratio was calculated for the proportion of nouns and 'substitutes', the latter category including pronouns, adverbs, adjectives and numerals. Voinescu comments that attempts to describe the utterances in terms of Chomsky's tree-diagrams proved unsuccessful. He observed from his analysis that most of the aphasic speakers showed a reduction in the ability to form attributes and use verb qualifiers, but they formed a far from homogeneous group. They could be classified in terms of syntactic complexity according to the noun/substitute ratio and three other parameters: the elaborateness of the sentences they used (i.e. the proportion of complex sentences to simple or elliptical sentences), the complexity of the internal structure of the clause in terms of the number of qualifiers used, and the absolute number of verb qualifiers. One group was most impaired in the ability to use nouns, though sentence elaboration was close to normal. A second group showed marked reduction of sentence elaboration, but a normal proportion of nouns. A third group showed some impairment of both elaborativeness and availability of nouns, while a final fourth group showed only mild syntactic disturbances (their main disturbances being phonemic or semantic). Irrespective of the group they belonged to, all but one of the aphasic speakers showed some impairment in the use of attributes. Voinescu comments that placement into groups is useful for rehabilitation purposes, indicating the areas of weakness around which therapy should be designed; but it would seem that the ability to use attributes can be retrained only in an advanced stage of rehabilitation.

For the study of the syntactic structures evidenced in the spontaneous speech of five French-speaking conduction aphasics, Marcie (1967) used the following categories:

(a)  elementary structures which could be subclassified according to whether they consisted of nominal phrases only, noun and verb phrase constructions, or negative transformations

(b)  complex structures showing relativization, relativization plus negative transformation, embedding, clauses linked by conjunctions, and sequential clauses where subordination is indicated by proximity.

He reports that the speech of conduction aphasics showed a richness of syntactic structure. The patients' abilities in using tenses and different forms gave a normal profile, with a preponderance of the present and past tense, the affirmative, the first person singular and the third person with an animate subject.

To elicit samples of spontaneous speech from 107 Dutch-speaking aphasics, Wagenaar and his colleagues (1975) used three conversational questions 'What do you usually spend the day doing?', 'How did your speech problems start?' and 'Tell me something about the place you live'. They used 30 measures to analyse the samples, which included such aspects as number of words produced in six minutes, number of complex utterances as a percentage of the total number of utterances, number of deletions and number of substitutions of function words, and number of mistakes in tense as a percentage of the number of utterances. From a factor analysis on these variables, six significant factors emerged as the best distinguishers of different types of aphasia. These factors were labelled by the investigators as fluency, telegraphic speech, grammatical errors, articulation, verbal (i.e. semantic) paraphasias and empty speech. As far as grammatical errors were concerned there was no difference amongst the various kinds of mistakes, and the investigators suggest that simply counting up grammatical errors without distinguishing amongst different types of errors would be an adequate scoring procedure. Semantic paraphasia and substitutions of grammatical words patterned together but were not found to relate closely to either neologisms or to literal perseverations. The investigators also found that classification of patients according to number of words uttered needed to be supplemented by classification by mean length of utterance, so that not all patients with relatively long utterances need be classed as fluent if their rate of utterance was slow, and not all who produced relatively few words need be classed as non-fluent if their mean length of utterance was high. The incidence of grammatical mistakes proved to be quite separate from the incidence of articulatory difficulties in the speech of aphasics. The primary dimension along which the aphasic patients could be characterized was fluency, supporting the previous analyses of aphasia along this dimension, and the investigators found that fine-grained linguistic analysis was not necessary to make this distinction. The linguistic distinctions they had made between content and grammatical words and types of grammatical errors failed to make distinctions between groups, and the time-consuming scoring of sentences for syntactic complexity provided no more classificatory evidence than did the seemingly less valid measure of mean length of utterance. Obtaining classificatory evidence is of course only one aim of the examination of aphasic speakers: the Dutch researchers' findings do not detract from the value of examining an individual aphasic speakers utterances for syntactic complexity so as to obtain evidence of the nature of his individual problems for application in therapy or for studying linguistic breakdown.

The study from Amsterdam just described was mainly concerned with the extent to which different classes of aphasic patients could be distinguished through an analysis of their spontaneous speech. Another major study of free samples of aphasic speech has been initiated at Victoria BC in Canada by Gosse, Wachal and Spreen (1972; Wachal, Spreen and Gosse 1973); this aims to analyse the ways in which aphasic can be distinguished from normal speech. In order to cope with a large number of measures and speakers these investigators have developed a system whereby speech characteristics can be coded for computer processing. Tape-recorded interviews are transcribed so that not only words can be analysed, but so can pause fillers, unrecognizable sounds, neologisms, vocal gestures, part-words which can be related to the surrounding material or phonetically distinct utterances which cannot be identified as being neologisms or word substitutes. The grammatical theories on which these researchers have based their analysis have been derived from Fries and from Jones, Goodman and Wepman's classification of parts of speech. For example a noun can be coded in one of 23 ways, such as common noun which is subject of a phrase, noun possessive determiner which is part of a prepositional object phrase, or unmarked non-final adverbial noun, while there are nine ways of classifying WH- words, such as introducing full or reduced relative clauses. Spreen and Wachal (1973) have reported on some preliminary results of this investigation. Aphasic speakers need more responses and prompts from their interviewers than do normal speakers, and other variables which distinguish them are vocal gestures, mispronounced words, neologisms, pause fillers, and parasyntactic words. These procedures therefore provide a means of quantifying characteristics of aphasic speech which seem to be obvious enough at a superficial level, but whose careful examination should be able to tell us more about the nature and types of aphasia.

Turning now to the USA, let us consider a quantitative analysis of agrammatism based on the recorded interviews which Howes collected for his examination of word frequency. De Villiers (1974) took eight transcripts of at least 5,000 words and examined them according to whether or not inflections or grammatical words were used in contexts where they were required syntactically—for example the definite and indefinite articles and the progressive verb inflection -*ing*. There was a considerable similarity amongst the patients in the rank order of omission of the morphemes. The progressive -*ing* was used most often, followed by plural -*s*, contractible copula (e.g. *is*, *'s*), uncontractible copula (e.g. *were*) the articles *a* and *the*, the regular past, the irregular past and finally the third-person regular -*s*. De Villiers comments that this order is not the same as the order in which these morphemes are acquired by children. But Jakobson's prediction for the relative difficulty of various uses of -*s* was supported. The third-person verb inflection was disrupted more than the possessive, which was disrupted more than the plural. But explanations in terms of the size of the unit which has to be processed (clause, phrase, word) do not provide a complete answer, as the marked difference between copula and inflection forms of the verb shows. Transformational complexity also proved not to account for the rank ordering of difficulty nor did the ranking of the morphemes in terms of 'semantic complexity', which Brown has offered as an account of the order of acquisition in children. De Villiers tried out three other possible explanations: stress, redundancy and frequency. Goodglass (1968) had found that agrammatic patients have more difficulties with non-syllabic endings like -s and -d than they do with the syllabic versions of the same grammatical morphemes -es and -ed and has proposed that the Broca's aphasic's difficulties are related to the saliency of a word. (Saliency is an as yet not clearly defined construct which is related to prosodic stress, phonological prominence and informational and affective content, thus mingling phonological and semantic components with a syntactic measure). But de Villiers's analysis did not find any evidence to support the saliency hypothesis in the eight samples of aphasic speech she studied; there was no evidence that syllabic endings were more intact than non-syllabic. Redundancy did not provide a useful measure of analysis because of the difficulty of establishing a criterion in spontaneous speech, where obligatory contexts for a morpheme can only be recognized through some cue which itself makes the morpheme strictly speaking redundant. The frequency with which the morphemes occurred in normal speech also did not provide a satisfactory explanation for their order of difficulty. The inevitable conclusion is that a number of influences must be invoked to account for the difficulties agrammatic patients have with grammatical morphemes in speech.

A recent British handbook on the grammatical analysis of disordered language (Crystal, Fletcher and Garman 1976) applies to aphasia and to children's language a scheme derived from Quirk's description of English in the general structuralist tradition (Quirk, Greenbaum, Leech and Svartvik 1972). This description tunes in well with Jakobsonian approaches to the analysis of aphasic data because it refers to three levels of sentence structure, the clause (and sentence), the phrase and the word. It also incorporates intonation as an index of grammatical groupings, and is comprehensive enough to cover most of the constructions which the analyst is likely to come across in samples of speech. A child's acquisition of syntactic structures and features from age nine months to four and a half years and more provides the arrangement for an assessment sheet on which the number of examples of each structure that are observed in the patient's speech can be recorded. Though the assessment procedure was originally designed for use with children with disordered language, its use has been extended to aphasic patients, and the rank order of difficulty established for the acquisition of language by children is used as a guideline for the order of difficulty to be expected for aphasic adults. Although its authors make the point that they are not necessarily accepting the theory of aphasic regression to levels of earlier acquisition, they report that they have so far found it useful to base remedial work with aphasic adults on this rank order of difficulty.

## 2. Elicited speech

De Villiers's study described above illustrates one difficulty in using spontaneous speech, and that is that the number of occurrences of examples of what the investigator is trying to assess cannot be controlled, nor can the speaker's intentions always be clearly ascertained. To overcome this difficulty some investigators have used formal materials designed to elicit specific constructions or words of certain syntactic classes, so that the patient's rates of success on various tasks could be compared. One ingenious method used by Noll and Hoops (1967), of asking them to spell words from different categories, will be referred to in a later section. Another is to provide the patient with two, three, or four high-frequency words and to ask him to put them into a sentence: this method is used in the Neurosensory Center Comprehensive Examination for Aphasia (Spreen and Benton 1969) and amongst other studies has been used by Gosnave to examine patients with temporal lobe lesions (in press). Gosnave's findings will be discussed under the section on paragrammatism.

Two other useful methods of eliciting structured samples of speech are to give the patient a lead-in sentence (sometimes referring to a picture or real-life action) so designed that there is a high probability of a normal speaker's producing a certain structure. Another method is to give the sentence to the patient and to ask him to repeat it. Barrett (1961) used the former method, giving a set of pictures to elicit nine sentence constructions and nine grammatical morphemes. He found it most difficult to elicit WH- questions by asking 'Ask me about the colour of the strawberries' or 'Ask me the reason for his being so sleepy', with an appropriate picture, and easiest to elicit a structure like Noun phrase + Link Verb + Adjective by asking 'How are these trees different?' An obvious snag about this method is that the likelihood of a patient's producing a specific construction in response to such questions does not necessarily reflect his ability to produce them in other circumstances, and therefore their general availability for him.

A more reliable approach has been used by Goodglass and Gleason and their colleagues in Boston (Goodglass *et al.* 1972; Gleason *et al.* 1975). They devised what they called a Story Completion Test aimed at eliciting two examples of each of 14 constructions. Prior trials with normal subjects had shown that 86 per cent of the items elicited the expected response in at least 90 per cent of the trials. For example, to elicit a declarative transitive sentence, the story 'Mr Jones wants to hear the news. The radio is off. What happens?' was successful in producing in normal subjects the sentence 'He turns the radio on.' For Broca's aphasics, however, a typical response is 'Father, father, turn on radio.' The easiest constructions for Broca's aphasics proved to be those for which only two elements had to be combined, such as the imperatives 'Sit down', or 'Drink the milk', while those for which three elements must be combined (comparatives, transitive declaratives, embedded sentences, etc.) were harder. An exception was WH- sentences which proved easier than predicted, and Gleason puts this forward as further support for the enhancement of availability when an item is salient, since WH- questions begin with an emphatic stressed word with some informational content, unlike Yes–No questions. The least easily elicited structures of all were the future tense and Adjective + Adjective + Noun constructions. Like de Villiers, Gleason *et al.* report that they could not attribute the fairly consistent order of difficulty they found amongst the agrammatic patients to any one explanation, although length appeared to be an important factor. The investigators reported that although the order of difficulty of constructions was significantly similar amongst the patients, all the patients showed themselves capable of producing at least one response which was very nearly conventional. Of great theoretical importance is the observation that each patient's attempts at the target sentences were not consistent over repetitions of the test a week apart. Sometimes one part of the construction was achieved; sometimes another. They also rarely tried to improve on correct responses, indicating that they were aware of what the target sentence should be. If their best responses were selected out of all their attempts, the list was close to normal. The investigators conclude that Broca's aphasics have a relatively large repertoire of constructions, and their problem lies in immediate access to these rather than loss of them. Though these patients show impaired prosody and absence of unstressed function words, it seems that, at the deepest levels of production of sentence syntax, they are functioning fairly normally: according to these investigators, therefore, agrammatism seems to be a defect at the level of encoding of surface structure, rather than a general impairment across a certain class of linguistic forms. Summarizing these findings on the elicitation of structures in agrammatic patients Goodglass (1976, p. 258) writes: 'The performance of agrammatic patients makes it clear that their difficulty does not lie so much in the conceptualization of relationships between terms as with the recovery of the grammatical forms for their expression.' Other researchers have come to somewhat different conclusions about the nature of agrammatism, as will be described later.

The final method of eliciting syntactic structures from agrammatic speakers we shall mention here is repetition, a technique well known to investigators of children's language. Repetition is of course one task through which conduction aphasia is diagnosed, but one of the earliest modern studies of repetition of sentences by Broca's aphasics is described by Goodglass (1968). The sentence types used were imperatives, present progressive, simple past, simple negative, conditional, Noun + Adjectival clause, and Yes–No and WH- questions. Of these, WH-questions again appeared to be surprisingly easy, as easy as imperatives and easier than simple declaratives. Yes–No questions in contrast proved amongst the most difficult to repeat, together with conditionals and subordinate clauses. Fluent aphasics were more consistent in their difficulties with all types of sentences, but although the Broca's aphasics showed more spread of difficulties with the different types of grammatical constructions, the gap between the two types of aphasics was not as wide as had been expected. It seems that this kind of task does not clearly distinguish fluent from non-fluent.

Bliss (1971; Bliss, Tikofsky and Guilford 1976) has used this technique to test aphasic patients' sensitivity to grammatical violations, and found that they (like normal speakers) have greater difficulty in repeating ungrammatical than grammatical sentences. Clearly, if this is so, they must be drawing on an existing store of syntactic knowledge when they repeat a sentence. In her later published experiment, Bliss gave 20 aphasic adults 32 grammatical and 32 ungrammatical sentences, each of which consisted of five or six syllables. The ungrammatical sentences represented four kinds of violations of grammatical rules: violations of phrase-structure categories, of strict subcategorization, of selectional restrictions and of morphological inflections. Phrase-structure categories, for example, could be violated by inserting a verb in the slot which should be filled by a noun ('The sang helped the boy'). Strict subcategorization could be violated by omitting the object of a transitive verb ('The rich owner surprised'). Selectional restrictions could be violated by putting an indefinite article in front of a mass noun ('A weather is warm'). An example of an incorrect morphological inflection could be 'Mary is hits me'. About half of the patients' repetitions were incorrect, with many more errors on ungrammatical than grammatical sentences. Some of the sentences contained semantic violations (for example 'The sink pushed the cat' or 'Jim around the grass') and it was found that such semantic violations presented less difficulty to the aphasics in repetition than did violations which were classed as syntactic with preserved semantic relations (such as 'Mary has changes them'). The evidence in general, Bliss and her colleagues decided, supported the view that syntactic competence was retained in aphasia, and that repetition errors resulted primarily from a reduced retention span and articulation difficulties; aphasics displayed in this task a greater residual semantic and syntactic knowledge than might be inferred from their spontaneous speech.

## 3. Investigating syntax without speech

Investigators with a different orientation from those of Goodglass and Bliss—that is to say those who predict that the radical disruption of syntax demonstrated in agrammatic speech represents not memory limitations or economy of expression or a specifically encoding disorder related to saliency, but rather a radical disturbance of syntactic knowledge itself—have naturally sought for evidence for this viewpoint from the agrammatic's ability to understand syntactic structures. In this way any difficulty with encoding of articulation can be by-passed. The evidence gathered from studies of syntax which have not required speech has resulted in the hypothesis that Broca and Wernicke aphasias are distinguished because the first represents a central reduction in syntactic knowledge with relative preservation of lexical knowledge, and the second represents a central reduction in lexical knowledge with relative preservation of syntactic knowledge. The issues are by no means resolved, though they are of considerable importance for neurolinguistics as relating to the possibility that lexical and syntactic organization in the brain may be anatomically and functionally at least partially distinct. They deserve a separate section in this chapter, which we shall come to later.

Some investigators, however, have been attracted by the advantages of being able to examine syntactic abilities without requiring the patient to speak, though they have not wished to extend their findings to propose the radical dissociation suggested above. There is a considerable attraction in a method of investigation which can be used with almost all aphasic (and dysarthric) patients, however little speech they have at their command, and we will look at two examples of studies which have used picture-choice or following-directions to test some aspects of syntactic comprehension.

Picture-choice is a clinically attractive method, because, as well as not requiring speech, it requires very little coordination of gesture for the patient, it is self-explanatory without verbal instructions, the pictures can be attractively presented, and the patient is not necessarily made painfully aware of his failures. It has limitations in that the test is restricted to what can be unambiguously illustrated by pictures, and in that it does depend to some extent on visual interpretative abilities. Like all other tests of 'syntactic' comprehension, the extent to which it is compounded by semantic comprehension is unknown. Parisi and Pizzamiglio (1970) used this method in Italian with a set of 80 sentences for each of which two pictures were presented. Each of the two pictures showed a situation for a sentence which differed only in respect of one minimal syntactic contrast from the other sentence illustrated by the second picture. For example one minimal contrast was between direct and indirect object, illustrated by two pictures showing 'The boy shows the cat to the dog' and 'The boy shows the dog to the cat.' Altogether twenty such syntactic contrasts were examined, nine of them being contrasts of prepositions, such as in 'The ball is on the chair' / 'The ball is under the chair', the others including word-order contrasts ('The train bumps the car' / 'The car bumps the train'), and contrasts of tense, plurality, negation and gender. The test therefore resembles some picture tests of syntactic comprehension since developed for children but with the important difference that the choice is between top and bottom pictures only—a necessity in a test for brain-damaged people who may show visual field neglect. Figure 6 shows some of the picture contrasts from an English version of this test (Lesser 1974). In the Italian study, from the results of 60 aphasic adults, a rank order of difficulty of the contrasts was obtained, from which it seemed that the most difficult syntactic contrasts were the indirect/direct object and the passive sentences where word order was critical ('The cat is chased by the dog' / 'The dog is chased by the cat') while the easiest were the prepositional contrasts between *near* and *far from* and between *in* and *outside*. This rank order was much the same whether the patients were Broca's aphasics or Wernicke's aphasics; and the patients classed as Wernicke's aphasics proved to be more impaired. The rank order of the aphasic patients' results was also similar to the order of difficulty established for 144 three- to six-year-old children. It is, of course, a moot point as to the extent to which such a test is a measure of the syntactic level of language. That Wernicke's aphasics found the test harder than Broca's aphasics could be interpreted as indicating that patients failed on items because of semantic disorders as well as syntactic disorders. Nevertheless it does suggest that, overall, aphasic adults have more difficulties with certain aspects of comprehension, particularly with word sequence, than they do with others, notably prepositions.

M. D. Smith (1974a) looked particularly at the comprehension of prepositions in a task in which aphasic men were asked to arrange objects in specified places according to a sentence they were given. The relationships of the objects were described in sentences which used the words *on, under, in, beside, with, and, or, by, from, before, after, over, in front of, behind, off, about, only, upside down* and *next to*. Ten common objects were used—a comb, cup, key, coin, bowl, ribbon, nail, book, ring and pencil; and the sentence spoken by the investigator would be something like 'Put the coin in the bowl'. Altogether 21 sentences were given, and the task was repeated a few days later. In order to distinguish between errors due to miscomprehension of the lexical items rather than the relational words, the scoring

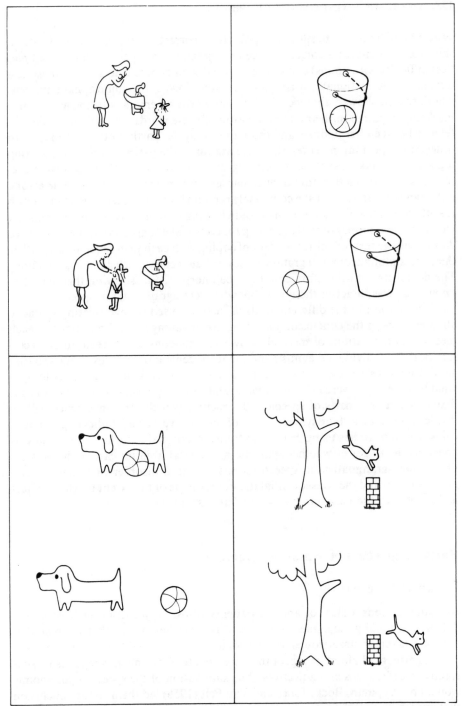

Fig. 6   Four items from an English version of Parisi and Pizzamiglio's Test of Syntactic Comprehension in Aphasia, illustrating 'The mother is washing herself/her', 'The ball is in/out of the bucket', 'The ball is beside/behind the dog', and 'The cat jumps to the wall/from the wall'

system Smith used was to subtract a point for a correct interpretation of a relationship from a point for a correct choice of objects, so that people who scored *plus* (less difficulty with nouns) could be compared with people who scored *minus* (less difficulty with relational words). Smith's study showed that some aphasic patients whose speech showed absence of relational words or errors with them were also markedly impaired in their comprehension of these words: she attributed the difference between her findings and those of Goodglass partly to the fact that word order was important in her test. She also examined the patients' abilities in arranging words to make a sentence describing the situation in which objects were presented, a task which they found much harder, and on which all made some errors, although none performed at a completely random level. In a later experiment Smith (1974b) found that two aphasic men could be taught to order cards into statements with relational terms correctly (e.g. cup on book). She suggests that they may have developed a general cognitive strategy of coping with each item sequentially, rather than the simultaneous integration of several elements which language requires. The demonstration therefore could not be interpreted as showing that syntactic knowledge was intact in these patients who were agrammatic in speech.

This account of the different kinds of methods used in investigating syntactic abilities leads to the conclusion that there are advantages and limitations in each method. Combinations of methods, however time-consuming, seem to be necessary both for individual diagnosis and for advancement of theories about aphasia.

Putting together these results which have used several methods, let us look at what has been discovered about syntactic abilities in aphasia under two headings: firstly as concerns parts of speech and structure (which for convenience will be divided into studies of the syntactic class of substantive words, studies of grammatical words and studies using generative transformational models) and secondly as concerns the issues of whether syntactic and lexical abilities can be dissociated, of whether agrammatism in speech reflects a central disorder of syntactic competence or not and the consequential theoretical issue of the extent to which syntax is disrupted in the paragrammatism of fluent speakers.

## Parts of speech and syntactic structure

### 1. Substantive words

Although there is a class of aphasic patients whose major disorder in speech is difficulty in finding the names of objects, it is nevertheless true that when studies are undertaken of large groups of aphasics it is usually found that nouns are easier to recognize, read aloud or repeat than are the other two main categories of substantive words, verbs and adjectives. An examination of the speech of an anomic woman by Wepman, Bock, Jones and Van Pelt (1956) led them to the conclusion that anomia in speech was not so much a difficulty with nouns as with infrequent words of all the main substantive categories. Siegel (1959) reported that aphasic speakers made more errors in reading out adjectives than in reading out verbs or nouns, though his word list had been selected without regard to frequency. Halpern (1965a), using words of controlled frequency, reported that whether words were read out or repeated from hearing there were more errors with verbs and adjectives than with nouns. Holmes, Marshall and Newcombe (1971) found that a group of men with reading difficulties after left-hemisphere injuries and a residual language impairment could read out nouns with fewer errors than either verbs or adjectives: the same reading lists given to normal subjects, using short tachistoscopic projections, showed that for these subjects nouns were also easiest to recognize, followed by adjectives and then verbs. In a detailed study of one particular patient Marshall and Newcombe (1966) found a clear effect of syntactic class on his reading errors. Out of about a thousand words which could be put unambiguously into one of these substantive classes, this patient read out correctly 45 per cent of the nouns, 16 per cent of the adjectives and only 6 per cent of the verbs. In a recent interpretation of such results Marshall, Newcombe and Holmes (in press) propose that the difficulty of words may relate not so much to the substantive part of speech but to the number of relationships they can enter into with other words. To describe these relationships these reviewers use Reichenbach's term *functions* rather than Fillmore's cases (see chapter 2): but the two notions are similar in essence. Some words can stand on their own, as one-place functions, such as *man*. Other words necessarily implicate two functions, such as *friend* which implies a relationship between two people; while yet others implicate three functions—*gift*, for example, implies object, donor and recipient—or even four, as in *buy*, in which the transfer of money has to be included. Adjectives and verbs can also have different numbers of place functions (e.g. *tall* has 1, *taller* has 2, *tallest* has 3, while *sleep* has 1, *see* has 2 and *send* has 3), but it so happens that verbs and adjectives tend to have more place functions on average than do nouns. The *noun facilitation effect* reported in these studies may therefore be an effect of underlying complexity of number of case relations into which words can enter rather than of syntactic class *per se*. The effect of syntactic class cannot be entirely discounted, however, as some patients read out for a verb its nominalized form, which according to Marshall's criterion would share the same number of place functions. Whitaker and Whitaker (in press) for example describe a patient who would read or repeat verbs as their related nouns, *memory* for *remember*, *reception* for *receive*. (See also the discussion on the lexicalist hypothesis in chapter 5.)

In aphasia research, therefore, interest in parts of speech remains relatively robust. To test whether patients with posterior left-hemisphere lesions would find it easier to classify words in terms of parts of speech than would anterior patients, Gardner and Zurif (1976) gave 36 men a task which included finding the odd-one-out in sets of four words, of which one belonged to a different syntactic class from the others. Their results confirmed the hypothesis that amongst certain groups of aphasics sensitivity to syntactic class remains relatively strong. They found that the overall results with all the aphasics showed a particular difficulty with reading adverbial phrases which included prepositions.

Some studies have not found that nouns presented fewer difficulties than other substantive words. When Noll and Hoops (1967) gave 25 aphasic men 100 words to spell, divided equally amongst nouns, verbs, modifiers (adjectives and adverbs) and 'non-propositional morphemes' including pronouns, prepositions and conjunctions, they reported that there was no selective difficulty amongst the substantive words, but that the non-propositional morphemes were significantly harder. Gardner and Zurif (1975) refer to reports that patients read '2 bee oar knot 2 bee' better than 'to be or not to be', and tested out 38 aphasic patients on a reading task which compared nouns (of different lengths and degree of picturability etc.) with grammatical particles of two or three letters in length and other 'non-nouns'. Long non-nouns (the examples the report gives are *almost* and *replace*) were most difficult, followed by abstract nouns, grammatical particles and short non-nouns. Gardner and Zurif comment that grammatical particles present appreciable difficulties in such a task to all groups of aphasics, including those who use these fluently in speech.

## 2. Grammatical words

Some of the studies which have investigated aphasic understanding of grammatical words have already been mentioned in the section on methods of investigation.

A list of grammatical words includes prepositions, conjunctions and articles (definite and indefinite): some theorists would include pronouns and verb auxiliaries such as the modals *will, may* and so on. A rough-and-ready distinction between substantive and grammatical words is that the former are comparatively free of the context in which they are uttered, while the latter are strongly determined by their context. Several studies of aphasia have confirmed that, taken as a group, grammatical words present more difficulties in comprehension for aphasics, taken as a group, than do substantive words; and if we think of grammatical words as carriers of less information than substantive words this is in line with the other studies which have demonstrated that aphasics have considerably more difficulty with meaningless nonsense words than they do with meaningful words. The aphasic depends, as we all do, on the possibility of connecting what he hears or reads with his pre-existing store of semantic knowledge, and grammatical words have less semantic content to facilitate this than do substantive words. A series of studies undertaken jointly by members of the Academy of Sciences in East Germany and the Academy of Medical Sciences in Romania has been concerned with examining aphasic difficulties with grammatical words (they use the terminology of *operational* or *minor category* words). Kreindler and Mihailescu (1970) analysed the occurrences of grammatical words in the conversational speech of ten Romanian patients, and reported that the aphasics were using the prepositions and conjunctions they did possess much less frequently than normal subjects. There were also distinct individual preferences for some prepositions. On the whole conjunctions were more disturbed than prepositions. Weigl and Mihailescu (1973) gave German-speaking aphasics sets of phrases to read out, repeat and write to dictation. The phrases consisted of either Noun + Preposition + Noun (e.g. in the English translation 'the flower in the vase') or Verb + Conjunction + Verb (e.g. 'he eats and drinks'). The grammatical words were omitted more often than the substantives, prepositions being omitted preponderantly in reading and repetition, conjunctions in writing. Overall, errors restricted to substantive words accounted for no more than 7 per cent of errors in any modality, while errors restricted to grammatical words accounted for up to 54 per cent—a clear demonstration that under these circumstances aphasics find substantive easier than grammatical words. Mihailescu, Weigl and Kreindler (1972) used, in addition to these three-word phrases, the same sets of prepositions and conjunctions in isolation or paired with one other substantive word. The nine patients they studied had predominantly expressive difficulties. The difference in performance between the substantive and grammatical words was more striking when the words were used in phrases than on their own: the percentage of substitutions of grammatical words increased with the complexity of the stimulus (from two-word to three-word) while it decreased in the case of the substantives. After a follow-up study with Romanian aphasic adults which gave similar results, Kreindler, Mihailescu and Weigl (1974) interpret these findings in the following way. A syntactic unit (*syntagm*) confers on words values and functions which differ from those of single words: semantic information becomes more sharply defined, and the number of possible meanings which words in isolation can have becomes delimited by the context. Verbs particularly proved to be read aloud more easily in the three-word syntagms than in isolation. The increase in errors with the length of the item to be read out was largely attributable to misperformances with prepositions and conjunctions, and it may be that words lose their functional identity as the sentence is fragmented. Within these overall findings, it was also possible to distinguish different types of aphasic performance. Some patients' errors, although intermittent, were always of the same type, either semantic or syntactic. Some tried to reproduce the structural and linear order of the syntagm, overlooking the meaning, while others produced only series of un-related words. Kreindler and his colleagues advance this as evidence for the partial dissociation of semantic and syntactic levels of organization, despite their mutual interdependence.

The dependence of grammatical words on their context particularly underlines the disadvantages in studying them as members of a taxonomic category. The study of grammatical words cannot be separated from the study of syntactic structure, in the way that it is possible to consider substantive words in isolation. It is not only that grammatical words form too heterogeneous a category, and that con-junctions and prepositions (and articles and pronouns) present different kinds of difficulties which can be related to their different syntactic roles; in addition gram-matical words like substantive words can be homonyms which perform different roles—in this case different syntactic roles. The word *by* provides a good example. In the sentences 'Vines are cultivated by the river Rhine', 'Vines are cultivated by hand' and 'Vines are cultivated by the peasant farmers', *by* has different mean-ings. It would be quite acceptable to say 'By the river Rhine vines are cultivated by hand by the peasant farmers.' The locative adverbial phrase 'by the river Rhine' and the abverbial phrase of manner 'by hand' are less integral to the structure of the sentence than 'by the peasant farmers' which represents a passivization of the active structure. (For an account of a test of these different uses of *by* by hemidecorticated children see Dennis and Whitaker 1976.) One might hypothesize that an agrammatism which means that sentence structure has become fragmented would impair the use of *by* more when it is a signal of a transformation of the whole structure than when it is part of an adverbial phrase which constitutes an added fragment. In line with this prediction Goodglass, Gleason and Hyde (1970) did find that Broca's aphasics were not particularly impaired on the comprehension of directional prepositions (as tested by asking them to 'Show me the girl *behind* the car' and so on). In fact different diagnostic groups of aphasics were not distinguished by this task (when adjustments were made for overall level of severity of comprehension difficulties). In contrast Wernicke's aphasics were more impaired than Broca's aphasics or anomic patients on a task in which they were required to select prepositions by another criterion. These were prepositions which had a conventionalized grammatical function but no directional significance, for example in phrases like 'waiting *for*' or '*in* Japanese' and 'telling *about*'. The patients were asked which of two prepositions would sound better in such phrases. From the responses of one patient in particular the investigators conclude that response to stylistic factors can be independent of semantic recognition.

However, another recent study by Zurif, Green, Caramazza and Goodenough (1976; Zurif and Caramazza 1976) shows that Broca's aphasics (provided they are categorized as having good comprehension on the Boston test) do make use of sentence structures in a metalinguistic task assessing their grammatical intuitions. Zurif and his colleagues used the method of triads by which they had examined knowledge of lexical meaning (see chapter 5) to test knowledge of syntactic structure. Amongst the sentences they used were 'The ball was hit to John' and 'The ball was hit by John.' The prepositions *to* and *by* differ in their roles in these sentences: in the first case the preposition is part of a directional adverbial phrase, in the second it represents a passivization of the sentence in the more likely interpretation of this ambiguous sentence (in which alternatively 'by John' could be equivalent to 'near John'). A sentence was also used in which *to* was an infinitival complementizer rather than a preposition: 'She likes to eat candy.' The results showed that the Broca's aphasics were able to recognize the strong links both between *to* and *John* and between *by* and *John*, though not between *to* and *eat* and not between articles and their nouns *the* and *ball*. Patients who were nonfluent in speech like the Broca's aphasics, but who in addition showed moderate comprehension difficulties, had difficulties with all the grammatical words. It seemed that the Broca's aphasics retained some sensitivity to grammatical words which express underlying structural distinctions, as between noun-verb relations, but were unsure about the role of articles which are, in these examples, surface structure fillers which carry little semantic content. To explore this latter finding more thoroughly, Goodenough and colleagues (1977) devised an ingenious method of testing whether or not Broca's aphasics were sensitive to the understanding of articles when they were not irrelevant to the meaning of the sentence. They used sentences in situations where an included definite article either hindered or aided the specification of a referent. Subjects were shown an array of three figures, a white circle, a black circle and a black square, and were given instructions which were appropriate ('Press the white one' or 'Press the square one') or instructions which were inappropriate for these circumstances ('Press the black one' or 'Press the round one'). When given such inappropriate instructions most people have to stop and think, and decide that the instruction must refer to the 'black one of the two circles' or the 'round one of the two black figures', and consequently take longer to react to such inappropriate instructions. This was what happened with anomic aphasics. Broca's aphasics, however, showed no difference in their reaction times, indicating insensitivity to the significance of the definite article. It was responded to as if it were an indefinite article (e.g. 'Press *a* black one').

It is clear therefore that grammatical words do not operate as a homogeneous class for Broca's aphasics, and Zurif and his co-workers found further evidence for this in that some patients who were unable to form links between articles and their nouns when pairing words in the triadic comparison procedure found it easier to link a possessive pronoun with its noun in the sentence 'Where are my shoes?' However, this was not always so. In the sentence 'My dog chased their cat' the possessive pronouns were not linked with their nouns. Consequently it could not be concluded that Broca's aphasics were anything more than minimally aware of the semantic distinctions between pronouns and articles, even when their awareness of the significance of prepositions was well retained. Zurif and Caramazza suggest that although they are insensitive to determiners, Broca's aphasics can process adequately those grammatical words which play an important role in encoding semantic relations—specifically noun–verb relations.

Zurif and Caramazza have not yet (at the time of going to press) reported on results of their metalinguistic investigations of syntactic knowledge with Wernicke-type aphasics. Since Broca's aphasics prove to be aware of base syntactic–semantic relationships, there is perhaps no reason to suppose that at this level the two types of aphasia may prove to be distinguished. The major difficulty in examining syntactic comprehension in Wernicke's aphasia is that semantic impairment can cloud the results of syntactic tests, and that the patient with the functional comprehension deficit, which defines Wernicke's aphasia, may perform particularly badly or inappropriately on a metalinguistic task, so that his syntactic knowledge cannot be accessed by this method.

One way in which the integrity of syntactic abilities has been examined in Wernicke's as well as Broca's aphasics is through an examination of the proportion of syntagmatic and paradigmatic responses they give as word associations and their sensitivity to syntactic class in the stimulus words.

With a group of 50 aphasic adults, Sefer and Hendrikson (1966) examined the relationship between part of speech and type of aphasic association, using a list of 40 stimulus words balanced for grammatical classes. The classes they employed were count nouns, mass nouns, adjectives, intransitive verbs, transitive verbs, adverbs and prepositions. When the aphasic adults' results were compared with those of a group of 50 subjects, using as criterion the proportion of paradigmatic responses (the researchers used the term *homogeneous* for these responses which kept the same grammatical class), it was found that the aphasics gave about the same proportion of paradigmatic responses for the various classes as did non-aphasics. In other words, although the aphasics were performing at a reduced level, the general pattern of their behaviour according to grammatical class was that of the normal subjects. Sefer and Hendrikson observed in the aphasics a higher proportion of conventional responses to nouns and adjectives than to prepositions. They found no evidence that the group could be divided into agrammatic and grammatic types of disorders on the basis of their associations, but that both kinds of patients produced syntagmatic and paradigmatic responses; it seemed that the proportion of syntagmatic responses was related to the severity of the aphasia rather than to the kind, and that there was an increase in paradigmatic responses as the patient improved. From these studies it would appear that, although word-association responses can be illuminating about the nature of a semantic disorder, they are not likely to be informative about the quality of a patient's syntactic problems.

Carter (1969) also has taken up this question of whether or not word-association tasks would distinguish aphasic patients with agrammatism (he used Jakobson's term *contiguity disorder*) from patients with *similarity disorder*, the prediction being that those with contiguity disorder would produce very few sequential types of associates. He reported that an unpublished study by Taylor in 1966 with 27 patients had given some partial support to this prediction. Although Taylor had found that syntactic aphasics (classified according to Wepman and Jones's Language Modalities Test for Aphasia) performed better than semantic aphasics overall, and that in general both types of patients were more successful with substantive than with grammatical words, he had concluded that semantic aphasics differed from syntactic aphasics on all the aspects that he had distinguished and that semantic aphasics gave fewer conventional responses than did syntactic aphasics. Carter's own study examined 15 syntactic and 15 semantic aphasics. He measured the time they took to produce an associative response as well as noting the amount of pre-response verbalization and the type of response they made. He found that all three measures did distinguish the two types of patient. Semantic patients talked more before giving responses to conjunctions, prepositions, verbs and auxiliaries. There was a general trend also in both groups for the time taken to respond according to grammatical class to follow the patterns predictable from normal individuals' reaction times. The syntactic aphasics gave a higher percentage of infrequent but listed responses than did the semantic aphasics, for all grammatical classes except verbs, adjectives and conjunctions. Essentially, what distinguished the two groups was not so much the measures of kind of response but the time they took to respond and the amount of pre-response verbalization: it was in these respects that the difficulties of the syntactic patients with grammatical words and verbs became evident. But the difficulties and limitations in using word-association tests as a diagnostic procedure with aphasic adults is indicated by Carter's finding that the most popular response to many of the words, from both syntactic and semantic aphasics, was 'no response'. (See table 7 below.)

TABLE 7

*Effect of the grammatical class of the stimulus words on the ability of 'semantic' and 'syntactic' aphasic adults to give associative responses*

(based on data from Carter 1968)

| Grammatical class | No. of stimulus words given | % of words for which the most popular response was 'no response' | |
| --- | --- | --- | --- |
| | | 'Semantic' aphasic adults | 'Syntactic' aphasic adults |
| Nouns | 27 | 67 | 37 |
| Pronouns | 5 | 80 | 60 |
| Verbs (substantive) | 10 | 80 | 80 |
| Auxiliary verbs | 4 | 100 | 100 |
| Adjectives | 15 | 67 | 33 |
| Adverbs | 15 | 67 | 33 |
| Determiners | 4 | 100 | 100 |
| Prepositions | 6 | 100 | 83 |
| Conjunctions | 4 | 100 | 100 |

## 3. Transformations

Goodglass's studies on the grammar of aphasics (first published in 1968 and reprinted in the collection of studies edited by Goodglass and Blumstein in 1973) report that there was no evidence that any particular grammatical rules were harder for agrammatic aphasics than for fluent aphasics. The hierarchy of difficulty found for a variety of grammatical tasks was substantially the same for all aphasics, and this hierarchy related to a large extent to 'the number of words required in a construction and its frequency of usage'. A number of studies have also examined this hierarchy of difficulty from the perspective of standard transformational grammar, and related it to the number of transformations believed to underlie the surface structure of a sentence.

In the late 1960s the compounding effect of plausibility and pragmatic expectations had not yet been so clearly demonstrated on the way people understand sentences which differ theoretically in the number and kind of transformation that are supposed to have taken place between deep and surface structure. And evidence from aphasia appeared to support the validity of the expectation that sentences in which optional transformations had been applied (passivization, negation) were harder than sentences which contained only the obligatory transformation of the active. Levy and Taylor (1968) reported that, when aphasic patients were asked to read sentences about a boy kicking a girl or vice versa, which were active, passive, negative or negative–passive, and to decide whether or not they were true for a picture they were shown, their comprehension of all but the active sentences was little above chance. The investigators explained this as a failure in aphasics of the transformational decoding process. Doktor and Taylor (1969) also used a generative transformational model to analyse aphasics' comprehension of sentences. They tested the time it took, and the errors made in choosing one of two pictures as appropriate for a sentence—a task very similar to the one used by Parisi and Pizzamiglio, though in this case the sentences were recorded and the reactions were automatically timed. In the grammatical contrasts they used, the investigators distinguished, in the Jakobsonian tradition, amongst contrasts at the word level (The boy/The boys), at the phrase level (The boy is fishing/The boy fished) and at the clause level (The boat pulls the duck/The duck pulls the boat). Doktor and Taylor found that the reaction times for the word-level contrast was not significantly faster than those for the phrase-level contrasts, though both aphasic and normal subjects took longer to react to the clause-level decisions. The researchers suggested that there were three other possible interacting factors in the complexity of the sentences for the patients: the number of transformations in the history of the sentences, the number of clues to deep structure in the surface structure, and the dependence of the decision on whether it is made at a syntactic or lexical level. The number of transformations would predict that a sentence like 'The bear is given the bunny' should be more difficult than 'The boy brings the fish the bird', since not only is it passive but the subject (agent) is deleted, involving in theory an additional transformation. The first sentence did prove to be more difficult, but only with reaction times as the measure: as far as errors were concerned the second seemed more difficult for the aphasics. The surface structure presents some difficulties because the relational preposition *to* has been deleted, leaving two adjacent noun phrases, which it seems the aphasic has difficulty in distinguishing. It may be that in understanding sentences aphasics must pay more attention to surface structure clues to deep structure (such as the inclusion of *to* before an indirect object) than normal subjects need to.

Using a choice of four pictures for a sentence, Shewan and Canter (1971) investigated the relative effects of syntactic complexity, vocabulary and sentence length on the number of errors aphasic patients made in aural comprehension. Length of sentences was increased by adding adjectival and adverbial phrase modifiers ('The girl gives a *large* box to the woman *in the yellow dress*'), and syntactic complexity was increased by passivization or negation in addition to passivization ('Dishes are not washed by queens'). Vocabulary difficulty was related to three levels of frequency of use of words in the language (at the most difficult level: 'The deluge soaked his raiment'). From the results it appeared that it was syntactic complexity which presented the greatest amount of difficulty for the aphasics, rather than vocabulary or length. There appeared to be no qualitative differences between different types of aphasics, but again it was discovered that Wernicke's aphasics fared worst on the test, although it was most influenced by syntactic factors. The discovery that sentence length was not of overriding importance weakens the case sometimes put forward that syntactic disorders are related to limitations of memory. Shewan and Canter had also examined their subjects' memory spans for digits, and reported that the correlation between digit span and length of sentence understood was not significant. They conclude that auditory retention *per se* is not of critical importance in determining the degree of receptive language impairment in aphasia.

Of the studies which have used transformational grammar in the analysis of spontaneous speech of aphasics, two are particularly noteworthy, one because it is one of the few published studies of aphasia in a speaker of an African language, the other because it mapped out in detail a hierarchy of difficulty of syntactic constructions.

The patient examined by Traill (1970) was a speaker of Ndebele, a Bantu language similar to Zulu: he had an 'expressive' aphasia after surgery following a head injury. From the point of view of linguistics and aphasiology Zulu is an interesting language because government by a noun of other sentence constituents is not only made explicit (unlike English) but the explicitness takes the form of making governed forms phonologically similar to the governing noun (*alliterative concord*). As the governing noun changes, so do the prefixes on governed forms (possessives, adjectives, verbs, etc.) Consequently it is inferred that there must be a transformational rule which marks governed forms within the class designation of the governing noun. Traill's analysis of the errors made by this patient suggested that they did not occur at a superficial phonological level but either at a deeper syntactic one or, more commonly, in the lexicon rather than in the syntax. He observed further that, although the patient's speech showed that he was observing the need to make governed forms agree with the governing noun, he was not making them alliterative. Traill comments that although it is tempting to interpret these observations as showing a deficit in competence rather than in a performance mechanism, the patient's comprehension of government appeared to be intact, and thus differed from his speech.

From Meyerson and Goodglass's (1972) transformational grammar analysis of the spontaneous speech of three Broca's aphasics of different stages of severity, they derived the following hierarchy of difficulty:

(a)  the Noun Phrase was better preserved than the Verb Phrase.

(b)  Within the Noun Phrase, the best preserved marker was the plural; if a determiner was used, the best preserved determiner was *the*;
predicate adjectives (*The boy is fat*) were better preserved than adjectives used attributively (*The fat boy*);
words expressing indefinite quantification (*some*) occurred only in the speech of the least impaired.

(c)  Within the Verb Phrase, the *-ing* form was the best-preserved marker; the patients who omitted *be* (and its variants) as an auxiliary verb also omitted it as a main verb;
although prepositional phrases were rare, Verb + Particle was frequently used (*sit down, come out*).

(d)  Adverbials were all retained (*once a week, five years ago*).

(e)  The use of intonation to express emotion appeared to be independent of the ability to use syntax to express ideas.

The most handicapped patient showed no examples of negation expressed other than by including *no* in the sentence, or of comparative constructions, or conjunctions other than *and* between two nouns, or embedded sentences or personal pronouns, or verbs marked for tense. Of theoretical importance for therapy is the demonstration that if a patient's speech showed more complicated structures it necessarily showed also more simple structures. For example if an agrammatic patient used the possessive determiner in front of nouns he could also be expected to use the definite article: if he used verbs he could also be expected to use nouns, and if he used adjectives attributively he also could be expected to use them as predicates.

Although Meyerson and Goodglass describe their analysis as of the 'transformational grammars' of the three agrammatic patients, their conclusions are couched in terms which are appropriate for (general) structural linguistics. Apart perhaps from the concept of competence and performance, which we have discussed in chapter 3, transformational grammar has not proved to be as immediately useful for the analysis of disordered language as might have been hoped (see the discussion in Crystal *et al.* 1976, pp. 33–6). Crystal points out that the salient differentiating features of disordered syntax in speech are precisely those which are not readily describable in terms of transformational grammar. In particular, transformational grammar does not seem to be apt in the examination of comprehension difficulties at the syntactic level. The range of structures from those which present no difficulty to those which require a heuristic approach is so narrow in aphasia that a different theoretical framework for analysis is more useful; for the examination of comprehension which is necessary to throw light on the question of whether agrammatism in speech represents a central or an encoding disorder, the description of language in older structural terms has proved so far to be more practical.

## Dissociation of syntactic and semantic abilities

From some of the studies mentioned so far we have seen that there has been something of a polarization of opinion amongst aphasiologists as to whether or not agrammatism in speech is a surface sign of an impairment of syntactic competence or is a performance limitation restricted to encoding, the character of which can be explained in terms of piecemeal availability, reduced processing capacity, memory limitation or articulatory effort, according to the theoretical orientation of the aphasiologist. Representative of the viewpoint that agrammatism does not imply an underlying loss of syntactic knowledge is Gleason *et al.*'s (1975) discussion of the results of the Story Completion Test. Representative of the viewpoint that the Broca's tacit knowledge of his language is limited in precisely the same manner as his production in speech are the analyses made by Zurif and Caramazza. Caramazza and Zurif (1976) point out that the clinical impression of good comprehension in Broca's aphasia is not incompatible with this limitation in syntactic knowledge. Much of comprehension may depend on heuristics based on sequential regularities and semantic plausibility rather than on decoding of syntactic rules *per se*. When they tested this out with different classes of aphasics, using a picture-choice test to compare sentences which depended to different degrees on syntactic decoding, they found that both Broca's aphasics and conduction aphasics were impaired in ability to use syntactic decoding. For example with a sentence like 'The boy that the girl is chasing is tall' they might choose a picture showing a tall girl rather than a tall boy, or a boy chasing a girl. Such evidence therefore has been used to support a dissociation of semantic and syntactic knowledge in Broca's aphasics: semantic abilities are retained, and syntactic impaired, at the level of tacit knowledge as well as in speech.

The question arises as to whether Wernicke's aphasia reveals the complement of this dissociation, with semantic knowledge impaired but syntactic abilities retained in comprehension as well as in speech. Such a situation would be compatible with the clinical picture of impaired comprehension in Wernicke's aphasia, as functional comprehension depends more on semantic skills than syntactic. But again the evidence is uncertain. Caramazza and Zurif's study found that Wernicke's aphasics were less impaired than the other groups on the picture-choice test, but it is more usual to find that Wernicke's aphasics fare worse than other groups on tests of syntactic comprehension; and Caramazza and Zurif themselves felt that their Wernicke's aphasics must have been only mildly impaired.

One researcher who advances the hypothesis that there is a double dissociation of lexical and syntactic knowledge in Broca's and Wernicke's aphasics is Von Stockert. The method of examination he used, first in a study of two patients (1972) and later in an extended study (Von Stockert and Bader 1976), was sentence arrangement. The basic technique was to cut up a printed sentence either at the boundaries of its constituents ('The girl—from Boston—is pretty') or within the constituents ('The—girl from—Boston is pretty'). It transpired that a Wernicke's aphasic, who was not able to read aloud sentences correctly nor to carry out the instructions they contained, could nevertheless arrange such cut-up sentences into the correct order. A Broca's aphasic, in contrast, despite his ability to read and understand most short commands, performed no better than chance on sentences cut up at their constituent boundaries, although his performance was better on the sentences where the breaks had been made within the constituents and the boundary links retained. Although the Wernicke's aphasic failed to arrange more complicated sentences with embeddings at better than chance level, from his performance on the simpler sentences it was clear that he was able to derive some clues to syntactic structure without (presumably) understanding the lexical items themselves. In a development of this *Sentence Order Test*, or SOT, in German Von Stockert made use of the fact that the definite article in German can be marked for position as subject or object in the sentence. He was thus able to introduce a condition in which a syntactically marked subject was semantically more appropriate as the object, for example, 'The rabbit (marked as subject) shoots the hunter (marked as object).' If this sentence was cut up, its arrangement according to syntactic criteria would produce the semantically anomalous 'The rabbit shoots the hunter', but rearrangement according to semantic criteria would produce the syntactically deviant 'The hunter shoots the rabbit.' (In English an inadequate equivalent would be something along the lines of 'Her gave birth to he'.) Included in the test were grammatically structured nonsense sentences such as (English equivalent) 'The womp yolls the cloppers.' In this study all sentences were cut at constituent boundaries, and only simple declaratives were used. Van Stockert reports that the performance of Wernicke's and Broca's aphasics on the test diverged. Wernicke's aphasics, despite severe reading difficulties, correctly ordered 80 per cent of the normal sentences, and arranged the syntax-versus-semantic sentences usually according to the syntactic criteria without being disturbed by the semantic anomalies this produced. They also succeeded with 75 per cent of the nonsense sentences. On the other hand Broca's aphasics were less successful (75 per cent) with the normal sentences despite superior reading ability, and the errors they made were typically in juxtaposing subject and object and leaving the verb till last. They arranged the majority of the syntax-versus-semantics sentences according to semantic criteria, and when they read them aloud read them as if the syntax was also correct. The arrangement of the nonsense sentences presented major difficulties, and some refused to attempt the task. Von Stockert claims that even global aphasics could be differentiated by the second section of this test according to whether they arrange the sentences by semantic or syntactic criteria.

A study of syntactic comprehension in French patients by Kremin and Goldblum (1975) also used a version of Von Stockert's test, amongst other measures. As when Von Stockert used his first version of the test, they examined a range of different sentence structures and compared those cut at constituent boundaries with those cut within boundaries, as well as including an extra condition where sentences were cut up word by word. They also introduced two further conditions in which sets of three words had to be put together into telegrammatic messages (e.g. Basket—contains—apples) and the patients were asked to classify isolated words according to their syntactic class. From the results they distinguished two kinds of behaviours in some of the patients, which patterned along the lines proposed by Von Stockert. Kremin and Goldblum make further observations: the tests showed up syntactic difficulties in patients without agrammatic features in speech; there was not an exact correspondence between the syntactic/semantic discrepancy in comprehension and the conventional clinical classifications of Broca's and Wernicke's aphasia; and it was only 13 out of 23 aphasics who could be so clearly identified as showing either primarily syntactic or primarily lexical impairment in comprehension. When the general clinical assessments of the two types of patients were examined, it was found that the patients making syntactic errors in comprehension were those with repetition difficulties and those making semantic errors in comprehension were those with naming difficulties in speech.

Further, if qualified, support for Von Stockert's hypothesis can be derived from Gardner, Denes and Zurif's (1975) observations of aphasics' abilities in detecting anomalies in sentences they were given to read or listened to. Like Bliss's repetition task this used sentences which compared sentences which were semantically deviant with those which were syntactically deviant. Both anterior and posterior lobe-damaged patients were better at making accurate semantic judgements than syntactic judgements, and both kinds of patients showed the same relative difficulties with the different kinds of semantic judgements required. But there were qualitative differences between the two kinds of patients on the kinds of syntactic judgements which each found more difficult. For the posterior patients the most difficult syntactic judgement was with incorrect verb forms (He giving the cat milk) with pronoun number and gender proving easy. For the anterior aphasics the hardest decisions were about number and word order, with case decisions (John sat on him/his chair) proving easy. The latter also found the reading version harder than the aural, while the reverse obtained for the posterior patients. Gardner, Denes and Zurif relate their findings to Von Stockert's by suggesting that it is relatively preserved sensitivity to syntax which enables posterior aphasics to deal more effectively than anterior patients with syntactic features such as word order, number and articles.

It is worth reminding ourselves at this point that Luria has contrasted the syntactic comprehension disorders of Broca's (efferent motor) aphasics not only with the lexical comprehension disorders of Wernicke's aphasics but with the difficulties in the comprehension of logico-grammatical relations experienced by semantic aphasics (described by Luria 1975a, p. 47 as a condition in which the 'lexical elements of speech remain relatively unimpaired'). Here also a double dissociation was found. The motor aphasics were unable to judge the correctness of syntactic constructions which reported simple events: the semantic patients were unable to indicate the meaning of such logical relations as *brother's father* or *triangle over a circle*. But each type of patient had no problems with the constructions which the other type found difficult.

Luria recognizes these special difficulties with one kind of syntactic relationship (the integration of a sequence into a whole) in one kind of fluent aphasia; and the extent to which syntactic comprehension is impaired or spared in fluent aphasia is by no means as clearly resolved as the neat dissociation between syntactic and semantic abilities in both speech and comprehension suggested by Von Stockert and others would imply. In the reaction against the dichotomizing of aphasias into receptive and expressive disorders it is tempting to overplay findings which show similar central difficulties in both speech and comprehension, and to divide aphasia up solely along the syntactic-lexical dichotomy. The interaction of levels of language organization should remind us that such an oversimplification is likely in its turn to have to be qualified. And indeed the very existence of *paragrammatism* reminds us that the speech of fluent Wernicke's aphasics reflects some kind of mismanagement at a syntactic level. We end this chapter with a brief account of some analyses of paragrammatism.

## Paragrammatism

Goodglass (1976, p. 238) describes paragrammatism in fluent aphasic patients as involving 'not so much the reduction of grammatical organization as the juxtaposition of unacceptable sequences: confusions of verb tense, errors in pronoun case and gender and incorrect choice of prepositions—the chief defect is paraphasia or the unwitting substitution of ill-chosen words and phrases in the stream of speech.' The central question in paragrammatism is the extent to which these syntactic errors can be attributed to a lexical disorder, and the extent to which they reflect syntactic limitations.

Kinsbourne and Warrington (1963) describe a patient with jargon aphasia who produced words which as individual units were correct and meaningful but did not follow a logical succession. Jargon aphasia in this case appeared to be due to a disturbance in syntagmatic encoding, and grammatical words were also rare in the patient's speech. Kreindler, Calavrezo and Mihailescu (1971) describe another patient with a jargon aphasia which they analysed as being characterized by the utterances no longer representing 'natural logically formed subunits included in a whole, but some agglomerations of disparate verbal ingredients' (pp. 226–7). The patient countered this disintegration of logical structuring by an over-reliance on rhythm and rhyme. Luria (1973) also describes how a patient with semantic aphasia was enabled to write a book ('The Man with the Shattered World') by developing a strategy of using poetical rhythmicized prose. One means of examining the extent to which syntactic relations are preserved in jargon aphasia is that adopted by Caplan, Kellar and Locke (1972). They observed the spontaneous utterances of a patient with neologistic speech and assessed the extent to which these neologisms were correctly inflected for the syntactic role they appeared to be holding in the sentence. Their conclusions were that neologisms were sometimes correctly inflected but sometimes incorrectly inflected and that 'the occurrence of inappropriate inflection of neologisms must indicate that aphasia does not consist of a disorder of "word-finding" alone' (p. 172).

Gosnave (1977) has also reported on grammatical failures in sensory patients with temporal-lobe lesions. He asked them to make up sentences containing two, three or four given words. The majority of errors, however, were in producing semantically anomalous constructions, and they tended to correct any syntactic errors. They also produced longer sentences with more clauses than the instructions required or than the control subjects produced.

The analysis of the speech of sensory aphasics offered by Dubois, Hécaen and their associates (1970) comments on the preservation of syntactic schema. They observed that grammatical words were not affected by word-finding difficulties, as were nouns and verbs, and that neologisms which filled the verb-slot in a sentence were correctly conjugated.

Green (1969b) made the interesting observation that in neologistic jargon aphasia, the neologisms are largely restricted to the predicate of the sentence. Buckingham, Whitaker and Whitaker (1975) have developed this idea in an examination of the stereotyped productions of a fluent aphasic with neologistic jargon speech. Many of his utterances began with a structure characterized by the pattern *I* + *say* + (*you*) + (*that*) + *sentence*. These introductory clauses were intelligible but were followed by neologisms. The authors suggest that introductory clauses such as this may be differentially organized in the brain, perhaps as overlearned stereotypes which are separate from the rest of the syntactic component. But they are represented not as automatized single lexical items like the recurrent automatic utterances of severely aphasic non-fluent patients; rather are they reconstituted as syntactic constructions in themselves, as is evidenced by the fact that modals and negatives can appear sometimes with the verbs in these structures. Although this patient seemed to have virtually no lexical comprehension, it appeared that at the least these aspects of syntax were intact for him.

In their neurolinguistic analysis of jargonaphasia and jargonagraphia Lecours and Rouillon (1976) comment that paragrammatism (they use the synonym *dyssyntaxia*) can usually be traced to substantive word-finding difficulty. Aborted sentences and repetitions of prepositions which result in distorted syntax are in fact secondary to the main phenomenon of word-finding difficulty. Verbal substitutions of one grammatical word for another are frequent, but they too are in the same category of lexical selection difficulties because the grammatical class is observed: pronouns are replaced by an incorrect pronoun not by a different grammatical word. Dyssyntaxia can also result from compounded transformations in which two syntagms become telescoped. The mutual influence of different words on each other in the genesis of dyssyntaxia is more marked in writing than in speech.

On the whole therefore examinations of the syntactic abilities of fluent paragrammatic speakers reflect the inherent difficulties in attempting to isolate syntactic and semantic levels of speech. The majority of studies of comprehension of syntax have found Wernicke's aphasics to be at least as impaired as Broca's aphasics: the exception has been studies with versions of the Sentence Order Test, and even here the capacity of Wernicke's aphasics to order sentences entirely from syntactic information seems to be limited to simple structures. Zurif and Caramazza's studies indicate that in some Broca's aphasics there is also some preservation of comprehension of these simple syntactic relations.

The conclusion must be that speech characteristics are not always reliable indicators of underlying linguistic knowledge—or at least speech characteristics as they are now observed and conventionally classified. Patients with what on the surface appears to be the same quality of non-fluency may show unequal degrees of sensitivity to syntactic constructions and the role of grammatical words. Moreover methods of examination of the comprehension of fluent speakers with Wernicke-type aphasia are not at present adequate for firm conclusions to be drawn about their preservation of syntactic knowledge: these are patients in whom different functional levels of linguistic skills seem to be particularly disparate, and with whom we cannot rely on the results of formal metalinguistic tasks as accurate indices of their abilities.

These studies underline the importance of developing further our means of examining syntactic abilities in comprehension. If we wish to help a non-fluent speaker to re-acquire in speech syntactic strutcures which he is not using spontaneously, it becomes crucial to have some method of exploring the extent to which there has been damage to a central system which includes syntactic comprehension as well as speech.

We shall return to the analysis of agrammatism and paragrammatism (and the question of whether they represent the ends of a continuum rather than a dichotomy) when we look at more recent accounts of cognitive neuropsychological studies of sentence production and comprehension in Chapter 9.

# 8

# Investigations of phonology and prosody

Of all the linguistic levels it is probably phonology which has attracted the most attention in applied work. Perhaps this is because the theory of the phoneme was the first to be fully explored. Perhaps it is because techniques of investigation of phonology had perforce to develop rapidly in the field of children's speech disorders, as deviancy in phonology is the most common and the most obtrusive of the signs of deviant or delayed language acquisition in children. In aphasiology, too, the tradition of interest in phonology is strong, and comprehension at the phonological level has been emphasized nearly as much as has speech at this level: some classifications in fact have attributed the disorders of comprehension in Wernicke's aphasia primarily to difficulties in phonemic decoding.

The earlier studies of aphasia referred to *articulation* rather than to *phonological level*, and it is useful to clarify the difference between the two approaches. The first theories of speech pathology made a distinction between *speech* and *language*, in which disorders of speech were conceived of as being distinct from disorders of language; the organization of sound through articulation was classed as a phenomenon of speech rather than of language, and described in phonetic rather than phonological terms. Linguistic theories in contrast are concerned with language as an integrated process, with speech as one medium of its realization, and with the organization of the sounds of language-speech as one level of this central process. Where earlier theories were unquestioningly prepared to consider articulation as an entirely independent matter of neuromuscular encoding of speech, later theories raise the question of whether, if there is evidence of the disturbance of the phonological level of organization in speech, there should not also be evidence of its disturbance in tests of comprehension as well as speech. Phonology, of all levels, brings most into focus a question we have touched on before, of whether the disorder is one of central linguistic knowledge or one of failure to realize that knowledge adequately through performance in one particular modality. Since phonology is the level closest to surface form, the interface between language and acoustics, it seems inherently more plausible that disorders at the phonological level might be disorders of performance in one modality; and indeed we acknowledge this potential separation of modality performances implicitly by using a different term (graphology) for the visuo-graphic than for the oral-aural media for this level of organization. For this level the case has to be argued whether or not phonemic and graphemic processes are essentially the same; whereas for syntax and semantics the same terms suffice whatever the modality (see figure 7.)

In some interpretations of aphasia, therefore, phonological disorders are seen as simply reflecting peripheral language processes, as disorders of neuromuscular encoding in motor aphasia, or as disorders of the discrimination of speech–sound contrasts in perception in sensory aphasia. In another interpretation, phonological disorders are disruptions in the linguistic system which occur in both Wernicke's

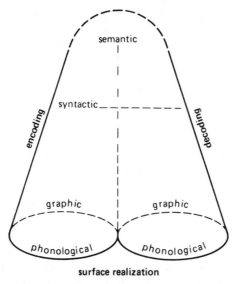

Fig. 7   Schematic representation of the hypothetical relationships between linguistic levels and modalities

and Broca's aphasias, and are part of the language disorder itself. The theories relevant to this level of organization may be categorized under three headings:

(1)   those which emphasize articulation problems in terms of the complicated neuromuscular organization needed for controlled sequences of speech sounds
(2)   linguistic theories in which phonological disorders are considered to be disturbances in encoding which follow lawful linguistic patterns rather than being adequately described in terms of neuromuscular organization
(3)   linguistic theories which consider the breakdown as being a central one of phonological organization, traceable in comprehension as well as in speech.

We shall consider shortly several experimental studies which fall under these three headings, but first there are some thorny matters of terminology to discuss. The penalty for the interest in this level in aphasiology is the number of partially overlapping terms.

There are some disorders in which the first emphasis, on neuromuscular organization, is commonly accepted as appropriate. These are the various kinds of dysarthrias such as those which follow extra-pyramidal, brain stem, cerebellar or lower motor neurone damage. These are due to interruptions at some stage of the linguistic process after the message has been encoded for transmission to the muscles of articulation. They can occur in degenerative neurological diseases such as Parkinsonism, pseudo-bulbar palsy, athetosis or Wilsonian dyskinesis; and in these kinds of disorders the difficulty in speaking is but one example of a general disorder in movement. Movements of the organs of articulation, the mouth, tongue, velum and larynx, may be affected when they are used for purposes other than speech, such as coughing, swallowing or chewing, though it may be that it is in the fine control required for speech that the impairment is first noticed. We must also note that, as no issue is left simple where brain and language are concerned, one line of investigation which is being followed is the exploration of whether patients with these known subcortical lesions and with dysarthria also show some signs of disturbance in other aspects of language, although the lesions are in areas of the brain conventionally described as not being part of the language system. Whitaker (1976) holds that of all the subcortical structures it is only the thalamus which will prove to be concerned with language. Indeed although it may eventually be necessary to modify the conceptualization of dysarthria as relating entirely to neuromuscular control, it seems likely that any central language disorder found in such patients will be of a different nature from that resulting from cortical damage (see Luria 1977).

Even more exposed to question is the dysarthria which frequently occurs after right-hemisphere cortical damage. This is usually reported to be relatively short-lasting. An accumulation of evidence indicates that, in most human brains, the leading control over speech is exercised by the left hemisphere. Since the muscles of articulation are also muscles used for non-speech purposes, and since they are bilaterally innervated, there are advantages in having one dominant system of control for an overlaid function which requires extremely fine and fast coordination. Darley, Aronson and Brown (1975) estimate that control of 14,000 muscles is required in speech. Control is complicated by the fact that messages have to be sent along nerve fibres of different speeds of conduction and of different lengths. Contrarily enough, the nerves involved in voicing for which precision of timing is particularly crucial in many languages, are amongst the longest and the slowest conducting, so that the messages which they transmit must be initiated before those sent along other nerves—a conclusive demonstration that units of speech must be pre-planned. Because of the presumed dominating control of the left hemisphere the dysarthria resulting from right-hemisphere damage usually clears as the left hemisphere replans control to allow for the contralateral dysfunction. When it is the left hemisphere which is damaged, however, there can be a radical disturbance to the articulatory processes even though control from the right hemisphere is intact and is sufficient for the less exacting non-language use of the muscles of articulation. It is this left-hemisphere damage which results in the spectrum of phonological disorders which concern the aphasiologist, as being of a different nature from dysarthria. Nevertheless, it has been claimed that, as with dysarthria, articulation may be the only process which is impaired. If, on clinical testing, aural comprehension, reading and writing are preserved, the patient is considered to have a difficulty specifically in motor programming for speech. Marie in 1906 used the term *anarthrie* to distinguish this disorder from the dysarthrias, as well as from true aphasia, and this term is still used in French studies. Other terms for the same disorder include *phonetic disintegration, cortical dysarthria, verbal apraxia* and *apraxia of speech.* Seventy years after Marie, Darley and his colleagues (1975) endorse the definition of apraxia of speech as a disorder distinct from aphasia, as well as from dysarthria and class it firmly as a motor speech disorder which may occur on its own or as an additional accompaniment to aphasia.

Because this labelling of certain linguistic behaviours as a distinguishable syndrome of apraxia of speech is not universally accepted, it is useful at this point to remind ourselves of the linguistic distinction between *etic* and *emic* descriptions which was discussed in chapter 2 on p. 26, to see if this can help in part to clarify the different descriptions of phonological disorders in speech which have been proposed. Lecours, Dordain and Lhermitte (1970; Lecours and Lhermitte 1976) describe the phonetic level of organization (the 'third articulation' in their terminology) as involving the choice of a number of discrete actions of muscles of the bucco-phonatory apparatus, and their cotemporal integration into phonemes. They further describe the phonemic level (the 'second articulation') as involving the choice of phonemes and their serial integration into more complex segments— morphemes and combinations of morphemes. With this in mind it is possible to make a distinction amongst different kinds of errors at the phonological level which classifications like *apraxia of speech* miss. Patients with a *phonetic disorder* produce distorted sounds, allophonic variants, or sounds which are not part of the inventory of their native language. To transcribe their speech we need not only the phonemic symbols but diacritics to indicate explosive initiation, ingressive air-stream, nasalization, lengthening and so on, together with a description of paralinguistic features such as breathiness. For other speakers with deviancy at the phonological level, however, a phonemic transcription without diacritics suffices. The sounds they produce are well articulated, and are acceptable sounds in the phonemic inventory, but they may be inappropriate for their context, and differ from what is presumed to be their intended realization. For these speakers in particular it is necessary to note prosodic features such as changes of pitch and rhythm as a guide to the speaker's intentions.

As table 8 shows, *apraxia of speech* is a term which can be interpreted with different emphases. Some descriptions emphasize the motor programming nature of the disorder and include phonetic distortions amongst its characteristics (Darley *et al.* 1975), while, according to others, phonemes are well articulated but it is their selection and seriation which presents the difficulties. There are different emphases also in the hypothesized underlying dysfunction: sometimes it is on motor programming *per se*, sometimes on kinaesthetic feedback as essential in the execution of motor plans, sometimes on acoustic feedback. Luria makes the distinction between the first two the key difference between efferent and afferent types of motor aphasia. Another debated distinction is between conduction aphasia as

## TABLE 8

*Disorders at the phonological level in speech*

| | Phonetic (+ phonemic) disorders | | | Phonemic selection and seriation disorders | | Phonemic 'oblivion' |
|---|---|---|---|---|---|---|
| **Hypothetical dysfunction** | Disruption in extra-cortical or peripheral motor apparatus/non-language-specific motor control | Disruption in motor speech programmer (esp. volitional) | Disruption in sensori-motor articulatory apparatus (afferent motor feedback) | Disruption in acoustic-articulatory apparatus (disconnection of Wernicke's and Broca's areas) | Disruption in stability of acoustic verbal traces (temporal lobe damage) | Phonemic system dissociated from semantic? |
| **Label** | DYSARTHRIA | APHEMIA (Broca); PURE ANARTHRIA (Marie); PHONETIC DISINTEGRATION (Alajouanine); EFFERENT MOTOR APHASIA (Luria): APRAXIA OF SPEECH (Darley): LIMITED DISORDER FOLLOWING INFARCT IN BROCA'S AREA (Mohr) | AFFERENT MOTOR APHASIA (Luria); SIMPLE APHASIA WITH SENSORI-MOTOR IMPAIRMENT (Schuell); APRAXIA OF SPEECH (searching for sounds) | CONDUCTION APHASIA (Geschwind): PHONE-MATIC APHASIA (Hécaen); APRAXIA OF SPEECH (attempts at self-correction of words, with well-articulated sounds) | CONDUCTION APHASIA (Warrington, Tsvetkova); ACOUSTIC-AMNESIC APHASIA (Luria) | WERNICKE'S APHASIA (neologisms, fluent phonemic paraphasia without self-correction) |

equivalent to phonematic aphasia, and therefore with an articulatory 'expressive' component (Hécaen 1972), and conduction aphasia as equivalent to acoustic-amnesic aphasia, and therefore conceived of as implicating short-term auditory memory. Goodglass and Kaplan (1972), for example, equate conduction aphasia with afferent motor aphasia, while Tsvetkova (1976) equates it with acoustic-amnesic aphasia. Luria (1976) discusses both types under the heading of conduction aphasia. We might have hoped that the phonetic–phonemic distinction would provide an objective measure through which to make a distinction between these categories of disorders, which could rest on more secure foundations than hypothetical stages of dysfunction in phonological realization. One difficulty is, however, that we cannot in practice make a clear-cut distinction between the phonetic and the phonemic. Errors which may be essentially *phonetic* in nature, in that they are distortions of an intended sound, may result in *phonemic* changes. For example, delayed onset of voicing due to neuromuscular incoordination may result in what to the hearer is indistinguishable from a phonemic contrast (e.g. in English of /v/ to /f/) although in other cases the delay in voicing results only in an allophonic variant (e.g. devoicing of a lateral continuant /l/). If these distortions are consistent we may therefore find changes in the system of phonemes. We have to describe these disorders, therefore, in terms of phonetic and phonemic changes, rather than phonetic only, although other disorders can be described in terms of phonemic changes only.

Phonemic disturbances also occur in the speech of patients with fluent aphasia, and as these phonemic paraphasias occur in a context of apparently effortless speech the question of attribution to difficulties in neuromuscular encoding as such does not arise. Because the Wernicke's aphasic typically does not correct these errors, it is sometimes inferred that they are secondary to a difficulty in perceiving phonemic distinctions of contrast (see Luria's account of acoustic-agnosic aphasia, 1966). The implication is that these patients do not correct their errors because they do not hear them as errors. A different interpretation is that the Wernicke's aphasic has a central impairment at the phonological level which is reflected in both speech and comprehension; the blurring of phonological accuracy in speech is not secondary to auditory perceptual problems but is a prior central difficulty in which the phonological system itself is impaired. Neither of these accounts is entirely satisfactory. On the one hand there can be major reductions in the ability to make phonemic discriminations in hearing in acquired peripheral deafness without any significant effect on speech, so that it seems unlikely that the language disturbances of Wernicke's aphasia can be traced to this source; and on the other hand the impairment at the phonological level in Wernicke's aphasia seems equally unlikely to be a radical disruption at a phonemic level for two reasons. Firstly rules of phoneme distribution in speech seem almost always to be observed in fluent aphasia (for example the cluster /tf/ would not be expected to be produced at the beginning of an English word). Secondly the phonemic inventory does not seem to be reduced, nor the boundaries of phonemic contrasts redrawn, as occurs sometimes in developmental phonological disorders. The phonemic inventory of one's language, once acquired, seems to be remarkably resistant to destruction. Lebrun

(1970) looked for evidence of the 'oblivion of phonemic oppositions' which Jakobson had hypothesized might occur in aphasia and found none. He concluded that confusions in speech between, for example, /l/ and /r/ could be attributed to disturbances in the control mechanisms of the speech apparatus rather than to ignorance of phonological contrasts. Mihailescu and her colleagues (Mihailescu, Voinescu and Fradis 1967; Mihailescu 1970) observed in a statistical analysis of phoneme frequencies in Romanian aphasic speakers that they used all and only the phonemes of the Romanian language, and that the general strategy of using phonemes was similar to that of normal subjects. It is in fact more likely to be in non-fluent aphasics than in fluent aphasics that apparent restrictions of the phonemic inventory can occur. According to Canter (1969), in such cases the restriction can plausibly be related to the degree of precision required for the articulatory gesture; for example fricatives which require precise and selective tongue-tip control may be realized as fricatives where the tongue blade is used instead or as well (e.g. /s/ is realized as /ʃ/). Any restriction is usually not absolute but is related to a specific phonetic context: Sabouraud, Gagnepain and Chatel (1971) point out that the Broca's aphasic may show a restricted range of consonants in initial place in a first syllable (typically restricted to voiceless stops and to /h/) but may use a wider range in the second syllable. Since restriction or disintegration of the phonemic system itself does not seem to be a valid explanation for phonological difficulties in either Broca's or Wernicke's aphasia, and since those of Wernicke's aphasia cannot be accounted for by articulatory problems a further explanation has recently been offered for the phonemic paraphasia of Wernicke's aphasia: and that is that, in this syndrome, there is a dissociation or partial dissociation of phonological and semantic organization.

In this discussion so far we have introduced some of the themes and speculations which have been offered for disorders at the phonological level in aphasia. It is now time to look more closely at the evidence which has been advanced in support of these speculations and different interpretations of the disorders.

## Interpretations in terms of neuromuscular incoordination for speech

### 1.   Phonetic disintegration

Lecours and Lhermitte (1976) have dated the birth of *neurolinguistics* as 1939 when the first major joint study of aphasia by neurologists and a linguist was published, *'The syndrome of phonetic disintegration in aphasia'* by Theophile Alajouanine, André Ombredane and the linguist Marguerite Durand. The syndrome was characterized by slow, slurred speech with difficulty in initiation, frequent phonological errors and distorted intonation. Comprehension was intact or at the most only mildly impaired; repetition showed the same kind of disorder as spontaneous speech, with no marked discrepancies. In those pre-magnetic-tape days, the words repeated by the patients with this syndrome were recorded on Rousselot cylinders for detailed analysis by the linguist. The analysis showed a remarkable constancy in the kind of errors made: they could be classed as examples of assimilation

(/komèse/*commence*→/komèke/), of simplification (/blã/*blanc*→/bã/), of meta-thesis (reversal of phonemes) and of elisions. There was a general trend in the kind of substitutions made; fricatives tended to become stops, voiced consonants to become voiceless, back consonants to be replaced by front ones and nasalized vowels to be replaced by denasalized. But these were trends rather than rules, and there were also examples of changes in the opposite direction; the net result was that there was not an overall reduction in types of phonemes, but rather a confusion of phonemic oppositions. Alajouanine and his colleagues hypothesized that the distortions could be explained in terms of neuromuscular disorders; phonemes whose articulation required more differentiated and more delicate movements were deleted or replaced by those for which grosser movements were adequate. They suggested that the basic problems could be paralytic (resulting in articulatory weakness), dystonic (resulting in excessive force being used) and apraxic (with arti-culatory movements to command more difficult than voluntary ones).

Lecours and Lhermitte (1976) have commented on the inferences made about this syndrome, in particular in one of the patients whom Alajouanine and his col-leagues singled out for a special description because he was bilingual in English and French. He was a commercial agent with an English mother and a French father, who had spoken mainly English at home till the age of six although born and educated in France. At age 63 he suffered an embolic stroke, with initially complete loss of differentiated speech. His reading and comprehension of spoken language were described as normal throughout and his writing showed virtually no deterioration. Hence he seemed to be an example of a *pure anarthria*. He re-covered enough oral expression to reveal semantic and syntactic adequacy but with major articulatory difficulties: speech was laborious and slow, with marked abnor-malities in prosody, and syllabic, explosive, exaggerated movements. Lecours and Lhermitte suggest that the predominating dystonic nature of his speech indicates that articulation difficulties may develop from a paretic stage to a dystonic stage characterized by exaggerated muscular contraction in initiating sounds. In the dys-tonic phase, those phonemes which require relatively intense muscular contraction in normal speech appear to be produced normally (or with an additional intensity which results in allophonic variations but which does not inherently change their character); but those phonemes which require intermediate muscular contractions frequently become transformed into their more intense equivalents as different phonemes (hence fricatives become realized as stops, or, if control for the fricative is eventually achieved after a delay, they become realized as affricates).

This patient illustrates a clear dissociation of the phonological level of organiza-tion in speech from the syntactic, and lexical-semantic levels. He also illustrates a disorder which appears to be limited exclusively or almost exclusively to oral speech. The disorder could not be labelled simply as dysarthria, however. Post-mortem examinations showed that the lesion was unilateral, with Broca's area iso-lated from the left pre-central gyrus and with some destruction of the larynx and mouth areas of the cortex itself in the pre-central gyrus. The disorder was specific-ally in speech, rather than in other uses of the muscles of articulation, and there was no bucco-facial apraxia by the time the patient was examined at six weeks after the stroke. Although the disorder can be described in terms of neuromuscular coding, albeit specifically for speech, there was nevertheless evidence that it related to high levels of coding, because a difference was observed in this bilingual patient between his errors in French and in English. By common agreement from all observers there was a partial dissociation between the two languages: his English phonology, learned earlier, was less abnormal than his French. Lecours and Lhermitte comment that the partial dissociation observed in many aphasic speakers between the more and the less propositional uses of language provides corroborating evidence that even though disorders may appear to be exclusively articulatory in nature, the phonetic disintegration occurs at a relatively high level of cerebral organization.

A quarter of a century after the original observations on the phonetic disintegration syndrome were published, Shankweiler and Harris (1966) undertook a similar careful examination of the errors made by five patients whose difficulties with speech after left-hemisphere stroke were classed as being chiefly of an articulatory nature. This analysis was also based on the patients' repetitions of words, this time tape-recorded. They observed that more errors occurred as initial in the word than medial or final, that more occurred with consonants than with vowels, and that amongst the consonants more errors could be related to attempted affricates and fricatives than to other consonants and more to clusters than to single consonants. Shankweiler and Harris found that many of the errors were apparently unrelated to the target phonemes, and that there was no evidence of particular difficulty with any one group of muscles. They considered that all the evidence pointed to 'a disturbance of coordinated sequencing of several articulators', and that the disorganization is of the process by which phonological units are encoded for production, rather than due to a residual spasticity or weakness.

Lebrun, Buyssens and Henneaux (1973) have also studied two patients as examples of anarthria, using with the advance of technology oscillograms and spectrograms to catch the temporal patterns of their spontaneous speech. The oscillograms revealed that the impression of syllabically spaced speech was misleading: the patients took a longer time in their utterances not because the syllables were spaced out as blocks, but because the entire articulatory process of realization of the phonemes took longer. From the spontaneous speech of one patient they observed that some of the substitutions and insertions of phonemes he had made could be interpreted as anticipations, and that most of these anticipations occurred across word boundaries in connected speech—an observation which the earlier studies could not have made from their method of repetition of single words. Lebrun and colleagues, like the earlier investigators, also comment that there was no evidence for systematic loss or over-use of any phoneme. Indeed they comment on the variability of the errors made; the same word which was articulated correctly at one moment could be mispronounced a few minutes later. It is this variability, they suggest, which aligns anarthria with the phonetic deviations of motor aphasia rather than with those of dysarthria following extra-cortical lesions. Yet these anarthric patients, unlike aphasic patients, retain *inner speech* and linguistic competence, in that comprehension, reading and writing are not impaired, and in that they can pair off words which rhyme, or alliterate, and can tap out the number of syllables in a word which they cannot speak etc. (for a detailed study of the inner speech of one such patient, see Nebes (1975); the term *aphemie* from Broca's original publication is used here instead of anarthria). Consequently Lebrun and colleagues interpret anarthria as a specific linguistic disorder which stands between true aphasia and genuine dysarthria, with its origin in the stage between evocation of the linguistic items and motor actualization.

## 2. Apraxia of speech

The description and analysis of anarthria given by Lebrun and his colleagues bears a close resemblance to Darley's interpretation of what he prefers to label as apraxia of speech (on the grounds that the term anarthria seems to suggest simply a paralysis). The distinction is one of emphasis: anarthria is specified as a condition in which the other language modalities must be 'normal', while for apraxia of speech the requirement is not so strict, in that for its identification speaking performance must be significantly worse than those of the other modalities which need not be normal. The term *apraxia of speech* (or its exact equivalent *verbal apraxia*) is therefore sometimes used to denote the quality of speech in aphasic patients, who undoubtedly have difficulties with other modalities as well, and with writing in particular (hence, for example, Trost's 1970 'descriptive study of verbal apraxia in patients with Broca's aphasia'). Part of the controversy about apraxia of speech has arisen because of this uncertainty of definition. For some people it necessarily is a disorder which, like anarthria, affects only speech, and consequently is outside their definition of aphasia; for others it is a description of certain qualities in speech which can be interpreted as reflecting an underlying central disorder of language. Supporters of the first theory argue that there is a distinct group of patients whose principal disorder is apraxia of speech, that the disorder is exclusively articulatory rather than affecting other language processes, and that they require a specific type of therapy directed at assisting them with articulatory coordination rather than the language therapy required for someone with an aphasic disorder. Supporters of the second theory, in contrast, claim that pure cases of articulatory disorder without any other language disability are unlikely to be met with frequently in clinical practice, and that any categories based on clinical observations and referring to substantial numbers of patients must therefore be describing a disorder in which the articulatory disorder in speech will be accompanied by a disorder in comprehension. An exchange of articles and letters took place in the *Journal of Speech and Hearing Disorders* in 1974/5: Aten, Darley, Deal and Johns on the one hand advocated the separateness of apraxia of speech, and Martin on the other hand advocated the interpretation of the same phenomena as an aphasic disorder at the phonological level. We shall come back to Martin's perspective shortly. For the time being, while we are still considering the interpretations of phonological errors as a deficit in neuromuscular coordination, let us consider Darley's case for apraxia of speech as distinct from aphasia.

Darley (1968) reviewed the descriptions of articulatory disorder which had appeared in the literature (whether under the label of anarthria, aphemia, cortical dysarthria, subcortical motor aphasia or any other term), and concluded that they all support the identification of a distinct syndrome which is separate both from dysarthria (problems due to muscular weakness and incoordination) and from aphasia (problems due to inefficient processing of linguistic units). He makes the overriding justification for separating out this syndrome the fact that a totally different kind of therapy is indicated for patients in whom apraxia of speech is the presenting symptom—direct articulatory therapy rather than 'the general language stimulation appropriate for aphasic patients' (p. 6). The syndrome has thirteen characteristics:

(1)  Absence of significant weakness, paralysis and incoordination of the speech musculature.
(2)  Speaking performance appears worse than performance in listening, reading or writing.
(3)  The most prominent feature of the disorder is the existence of phonemic errors.
(4)  The patient makes effortful groping attempts to produce approximations to the target sounds.
(5)  Errors are inconsistent.
(6)  Imitation of heard words is poor.
(7)  The correctness of the articulation depends on the complexity of the required articulatory positions.
(8)  Longer words are more difficult than shorter.
(9)  There is a discrepancy between automatic and volitional performances.
(10)  The patient is usually aware of his errors.
(11)  Speech prosody is impaired; the pace is slower, with even spacing of syllables (*syllabic*, or *scanning* speech).
(12)  Severe difficulty in initiating words produces an effect like stuttering.
(13)  Some but not all patients also have an associated non-verbal oral apraxia.

A propos of the last item, De Renzi, Pieczuro and Vignolo (1966) concluded from an examination of 134 left-brain-damaged patients that there was a strong association between oral apraxia and phonemic-articulatory disorders of speech, although oral apraxia could occur without any aphasic symptoms and the verbal apraxia could also be more severe than the oral apraxia. Clearly apraxia of speech cannot be explained away entirely as secondary to a general oral apraxia which affects non-verbal gestures such as yawning, whistling and blowing to command.

In support of his claim that apraxia of speech is a specific difficulty in the programming of articulatory movements in volitional speech, Darley and his colleagues have reported a series of experimental studies on apraxia of speech. Johns and Darley (1970) compared the speech of ten apraxic, ten dysarthric and ten normal subjects. They found that initial consonant production in the apraxics was inconsistent, and distinguished their errors from the distortion errors of the dysarthrics as being substitution, repetition and addition (that is to say in this case, aligning apraxia of speech with phonemic selection-and-seriation errors rather than phonetic ones). When the apraxic patients were allowed to make several attempts at a word their performance improved. But the patients' difficulties were not secondary to impairment in the perception of phonemes, as they scored above 90 per cent when asked to listen to words and match them up with ones from a sheet of printed words. From a study in 1972 Deal and Darley again concluded that apraxia of speech is a motor programming disorder; varying the instructions or varying the delay interposed before the patient had to respond, or introducing white noise while the patient was reading aloud or asking the patient to watch himself in a mirror—none of these had an effect on phonemic accuracy. Using a scoring method which weighted errors according to whether they were in a substantive word, or in a word longer than five letters, or occurred early in the sentence, or in a word which had a 'difficult' initial phoneme, the experimenters concluded that word length and grammatical class were important influences. They did not, however, comment further on the implications of the effect of grammatical class other than to suggest that substantive words which carry linguistic or pyschological weight and are essential for communication may impose more stress on the speech system.

Deal (1974) examined in particular Darley's claim that apraxia of speech is characterized by inconsistent rather than consistent errors and can in this way be distinguished from dysarthria. When Deal gave five subjects a hundred-word paragraph to read aloud five times over, he found that as a group they made consistent errors, i.e. that they made errors on the same words at least 60 per cent of the time. This is, however, not to say that the errors themselves were the same.

Some studies have looked at the question of whether apraxia of speech is related to deficits in sensation, or in sensory feedback as is proposed in Luria's interpretation of the syndrome of afferent motor aphasia, with which apraxia of speech is sometimes aligned. Texeira, Defran and Nichols (1974) found that patients whose speech was apraxic performed worse on a test of oral stereognosis than did patients who were dysarthric or aphasic without verbal apraxia. The test consisted of asking patients to identify plastic shapes put into their mouths as being one of four pictured outlines. Rosenbek, Wertz and Darley (1973) also concluded that higher cortical sensory dysfunction frequently accompanies apraxia of speech, when they used a similar test of oral stereognosis together with tests of two-point discrimination on the lip and tongue and of estimation of how wide the mouth was opened. However, although the more severe the apraxia of speech the more severe was the defect in oral sensation, there were some patients with apraxia of speech who performed well on the sensory tests, indicating that a simple account of apraxia of speech in terms of sensory feedback is not adequate.

The researchers point out that as tests of oral stereognosis require the patient to manipulate the shapes with his tongue, some of the difficulty may be motor rather than sensory. However, as apraxia of speech can coexist with good performance on these tests, the disorder as such in apraxia of speech cannot be attributed to sensory deficits, although it would not be surprising if some kinds of phonemic errors in apraxia of speech were enhanced by a major deficit in sensation. Lebrun (1967) has suggested, for example, that more errors are made with the realization of velar consonants than with front consonants, because kinaesthetic feedback from the back of the mouth is inferior to that from the lips and front of mouth. However, these studies have found no support for a division of apraxic disorders in speech into an *efferent motor* type (attributable to problems in motor initiation) and an *afferent motor* type (attributable to difficulties in sensory feedback in the motor process) such as Luria and Canter have proposed. For Darley and his colleagues, apraxia of speech is more homogeneous than heterogeneous.

In summary of this section on the interpretation of phonological disorders in terms of neuromuscular incoordination it appears that:

(1)   the neuromuscular coordinative system is conceived of as being specific to language (and probably under unilateral control), although frequently there are additional complications in motor praxis and sensation which affect non-language skills and which contribute to the severity of the disorder. We cannot at present distinguish whether this specificity to language is more apparent than real because it is the normal motor operations that are put into a different gear for the greater delicacy of control required for speech, or whether it is indeed a kind of language-specific overdrive that is called into play. To test this out we should need to find non-linguistic tasks which are of equivalent complexity to speech, and to search for patients who succeed on these but fail in speech;

(2)   the interpretation of the disorder may be in terms of motor programming or may stress kinaesthetic feedback, but special emphasis is given to serial organization;

(3)   the disorder is conceived of as being specific to the production of speech, and as not implicating any other language modality;

(4)   it is also conceived of as being specific to phonological production in speech, with syntactic and semantic abilities unaffected;

(5)   nevertheless there is some suspicion that higher levels may be involved even in pure cases of anarthria, and that engrams laid down at different ages or which have acquired different degrees of automaticity can be differentially affected. Even though the disorder is one of neuromuscular coordination, the purpose for which that coordination is required is acknowledged to be of considerable influence on the degree to which successful coordination is achieved.

## Interpretations in terms of linguistic encoding

Deal's observations have suggested that there is more to the distinction between dysarthria and apraxia of speech than the identification of errors in the one as being consistent and in the other as being inconsistent; and the emphasis on the linguistic nature of the encoding disorder in apraxia of speech has been particularly on the examination of this claimed inconsistency in apraxia of speech. If the disorder is thought of as primarily one of motor programming which happens to be specifically linguistic, then the description of the errors as being inconsistent is acceptable: the patient is assumed to have an intact 'intention to speak' with the phonological shapes of the words mapped out but not yet realized, and the prime difficulty is in the translation of these shapes into the coordinated pattern of articulatory movements for their phonetic realization. The patient makes hit-or-miss attempts to get it right, tending  on the whole to get nearer to the target as he continues his efforts. If the disorder is a complete breakdown of organization then we should not expect to find linguistic regularities in the kinds of errors made but would predict the inconsistency in errors on which Darley comments. But regularities have been found in the phonemic errors of apraxia of speech. As we have seen these have been interpreted in terms of the complexity of the motor programming required, thus reconciling the finding of consistent regularities with the interpretation of apraxia as a motor disorder. But they can also be interpreted as regularities which reveal linguistic rules, thus making apraxia of speech interpretable as a linguistic disorder. Lebrun (1967) questioned whether the degree of difficulty of different phonemes could be entirely attributed to the motor skills involved. In this section we shall consider this kind of interpretation, but with *apraxia of speech* or the *phonetic disintegration syndrome* considered as a linguistic disorder primarily of encoding, and primarily of the phonological level of organization, though occurring not as an isolated phenomenon but as an accompaniment or integral part of some types of aphasia. We shall leave to a later section the arguments that comprehension as well as speech may be affected in this linguistic disorder and that there are interactions with other levels of linguistic organization.

The two most influential investigators of phonological disorders in aphasia, within a linguistic framework are probably Lecours and Blumstein. Their approaches have been somewhat different in that Blumstein has emphasized comparisons of segmental phonemes against each other in rank order of difficulty (testing out in particular the validity of three linguistic postulates—distinctive features in the abstract framework of generative linguistics, markedness, and Jakobson's regression hypothesis) while Lecours has emphasized the dynamic processes of selection and seriation of phonemes (using an articulatory model of distinctive features). Let us look first at the *rank order* kind of approach.

Blumstein (1973) tape-recorded interviews with 17 aphasic patients who had been diagnosed according to the Boston classification as having Broca's, Wernicke's or conduction aphasia. She used a series of standard questions to elicit conversational speech until she had collected 2,000 word samples from each patient. While this method has the advantage of catching the quality of natural speech, it has the disadvantage that a substantial proportion of the data may have to be discarded as uninterpretable because it bears insufficient phonological resemblance to an inferred target word (a difficulty which does not arise if the data is obtained by asking patients to repeat or read lists of words). Blumstein classed the recognizable errors as being of phoneme substitution, simplification, addition or ones which were influenced by their environment. The relative proportions of these error types were the same for all the types of aphasia; substitution errors were the most frequent, followed by simplifications, with additions being least common. Amongst the substitution errors, regardless of the type of aphasia, those in which the substituted phoneme differed from the target phoneme by one distinctive feature predominated over those where the distance was more than one distinctive feature (but perhaps it should be remembered that some of the discarded data may have included items which were not identifiable because they differed in too many features from the target). The rank order of difficulty of distinctive features was found from those errors which could be classed as of one feature only, and here there was some difference amongst the types of aphasia within a general trend for the features *compact* and *continuant* to be more difficult than the features *grave* and *voice* which in turn were more difficult than the features *nasal* and *strident*. Apart from the relative paucity of errors where the feature of strident was changed, this rank order of difficulty corresponds with that derived from observations of children's acquisition of language, as Jakobson hypothesized; and Blumstein attributes the one discrepancy to the limited distribution of this feature, strident, which serves only to differentiate /tʃ/ and /dʒ/ from /k/ and /g/ or /s/ and /z/ from /θ/ and /ə/. With the substitution errors there was also a tendency for changes from marked to unmarked (e.g. from voiced to voiceless) to predominate over unmarked to marked. With errors classed as simplifications or additions it was observed that most of them occurred in consonant clusters. As for environmental errors Blumstein observed that only a very few resulted in non-English sequences. The majority of environmental errors, whether within a word or across a word boundary ('intra-morphemic and inter-morphemic blends'), occurred when the assimilated and the contaminating phonemes were close together. Blumstein's principal conclusions from her investigation were that phonological errors in aphasic speech can be described according to a system (and are not therefore inconsistent), that the linguistic constructs of distinctive features and markedness can be used in describing this system and that all the types of aphasia she examined showed similar patterns in their errors. This last finding is of considerable relevance to the question of whether phonological errors are essentially difficulties in neuromuscular programming. Two of Blumstein's groups, conduction and Wernicke's aphasics, are conventionally considered not to have articulatory difficulties as such; yet their phonological errors were found to be not qualitatively different on most measures from those of Broca's aphasics with articulatory difficulties. But the transcription of her tapes which Blumstein used in her main analysis appears to have been a broad rather than a narrow phonetic one. It appears to be at this higher level of phonological encoding rather than at the phonetic level that all aphasias show the same quality; a narrow phonetic transcription would presumably have distinguished the Broca's aphasics with laboured speech and impaired articulatory agility from the other two groups.

But Blumstein does make use of a phonetic transcription which includes nasalization and aspiration (allophonic variations in English) to conclude that some errors can be attributed to features which are redundant as well as to those which are used distinctively. She uses redundant features to distinguish the level of formulation at which the disorder has occurred. For example, before /n/ vowels are nasalized (redundantly); some errors where /n/ is omitted (frequently in consonant clusters with /n/) indicate that it is omitted before the vowel has been nasalized (/peit/ for *paint*) while others indicate that it has been omitted after the vowel has been nasalized (/mãdi/ for *Monday*). Blumstein suggests that such observations have implications for linguistic theory in that it appears that redundant features are still represented at the *systematic phonetic level* as well as at the *systematic phonemic level*, i.e. the feature is realized phonetically even though the whole phonemic bundle is not.

Two other studies are pertinent to the description of phonological disorders in terms of rank order difficulties of features. One is Trost's study of apraxia of speech in patients with Broca's aphasia (Trost 1971; Trost and Canter 1974): the other is Hatfield and Walton's (1975) study of the phonological patterns of one patient with Broca's aphasia, undertaken for the purpose of planning therapy.

Trost's main conclusions, from her study of the errors of naming and repetition made by ten Broca's aphasics, were that vowels were produced more accurately than consonants and single consonants more accurately than clusters, that most errors were describable as substitutions, additions or compound errors rather than distortions or omissions, and that the majority of errors were close approximations to the target sounds in that they differed by only one or two distinctive features. Final phonemes appeared to be somewhat easier than initial phonemes (as Luria's inertia-of-excitation hypothesis proposes). Errors of place were the most common (61 per cent) followed by manner (53 per cent), voicing (36 per cent) and oral–nasal (6 per cent). Despite the different method of eliciting speech, like Blumstein but unlike Shankweiler and Harris in their earlier study, Trost comments on the systematic nature of aphasic phonemic errors.

Hatfield and Walton (1975) also sought the rules behind the phonological errors their patient made when asked to repeat syllables (nonsense and real words, though these were not distinguished in the results). They observed a much greater number of errors in the consonants than in the vowels of the repeated syllables, and propose five rules for the consonant errors in this patient; /t/ and /k/ were partly interchangeable, with /t/ tending to be replaced by /k/ before the vowel /o/, and /k/ tending to be replaced by /t/ before /i/ and /u/; syllables ending in a final /t/ were frequently well repeated, and final /t/ was substituted for other consonants; in consonant–vowel–consonant syllables where the consonants differed, the first consonant was often repeated for the second; fricatives and continuants tended to be produced as stops; there was a limited number of examples of inversion of consonants (metathesis). Although it was possible to describe the patient's errors in terms of rules, Hatfield emphasizes that the government by the rules was not sufficiently regular for her to predict whether or not a given phoneme would be correctly or incorrectly repeated in any one instance: the tendency was probabilistic rather than certain.

These three studies have concentrated on the categorical nature of phonemic errors, separating them into those which are environmental (syntagmatic) and those of substitution etc. (paradigmatic). In a major series of studies, Lecours, working at first with Lhermitte in Paris and later on with other colleagues in Montreal, has developed a method for the description of phonological errors in aphasia. The most recent brief accounts in English of his methods are in Lecours (1975) and Lecours and Caplan (1975) with a longer survey in Lecours and Roussilon (1976). Lecours prefers the term *transformations* to the term 'errors', and accepts the implication that the aphasic patient has a model of normal language as his starting point rather than an idiosyncratic 'aphasic system'. The model of language which Lecours has adopted is a hierarchical one of units which combine or are 'articulated' at each level into a higher-order unit, which in turn combines into a higher-order unit, and so on. In the table below, the term *interface* has been substituted for the term *articulation* so as to avoid confusion with the more common use of the latter word in descriptions of speech.

In addition to these main interfaces there can be intermediate ones, as when two phonemes are combined into a cluster which does not yet form a morpheme (e.g. /st/, /bl/) or as when two morphemes are combined but do not yet form a

TABLE 9

*Hierarchical units in language and their interfaces*

(based on Lecours and Lhermitte 1969, with the term 'articulation' replaced by 'interface')

Third interface units:
    Features (anatomically
    related functions, such as
    air expiration movement)
                            Third interface

Second interface units:
    Phonemes
                             Second interface

First interface units:
    Monemes (=Morphemes)
                             First interface

Syntagms: combination of
    morphemes into
    coherent syntactic units

syntagm, as is the case when an inflection is attached to a lexical item (e.g. walk + s). For present purposes we are concerned only with the third interface and its units and with the units of the second interface, i.e. with phonetic and phonemic aspects of language organization.

Lecours uses as a measure of the relationship amongst consonant phonemes the articulatory distance between them in terms of these features: mouth aperture, place of articulation, participation of the vocal cords, participation of the velum, and participation of the mouth muscles which relate to lip and tongue-front co-ordination. The distance between /p/ and /n/, for example, is of three such features (vocal cords, place of articulation and velum), while the distance between /z/ and /ʒ/ is 1 (participation of peri-buccal muscles related to tongue shape). Tables of distance of consonants from each other can therefore be drawn up, as can tables for the distance of vowel phonemes from each other using similar criteria.

If a phoneme is substituted for another one in error, this can be described as a paradigmatic error, or error of selection at the same point in the word. This paradigmatic relationship can be expressed in terms of distance (PD, or paradigmatic distance): for example, the relationship between the intended word *dog* and the paraphasia *dod*, as far as the transformation from /g/ to /d/ is concerned, has a PD of 1 feature (place of articulation). But each phoneme also has a syntagmatic relationship to every other phoneme in the string which forms the morpheme, and this too can be described in terms of the same units of distance. So the initial /d/ in *dog* has a syntagmatic distance (SD) of 1 to the final /g/, and in the paraphasia *dod*, the initial /d/ has an SD to the final /d/ of 0. In a longer word, or longer paraphasia, the SDs amongst all the consonants can be calculated, and the smallest distance is labelled as the MSD (minimal syntagmatic distance)—calculating the distance between consonant phonemes and vowel phonemes does not prove useful in the analysis, and the SD is therefore calculated only amongst the consonants. The MSD is calculated because it is this which appears to expose best the underlying serial links between a paraphasia and the target word on which it is modelled. For example an MSD of 1 in *dog* has become transformed into an MSD of 0 in the paraphasia *dod*. Some measure is also required of the gap over which the MSD operates. In the case of *dog* (or *dod*) it can be called a proximity, or P, of 1 because only one other phoneme intervenes, the vowel /ɒ/ between the two involved phonemes. With a longer word the MSD may have a P with a higher number, for example *abominable* /abɒminabl/ has an MSD of 0 (between the first /b/ and second /b/), but a P of 5 as five phonemes intervene.

Observations of aphasic phonemic paraphasias suggest that they can be described in terms of nine basic rules:

(1)   deletion of a unit figuring only once in the stimulus
(2)   deletion of the first of two identical units in the stimulus
(3)   deletion of the second of two identical units in the stimulus
(4)   addition of a unit which is not in the stimulus
(5)   addition by reduplication of a unit in the stimulus by anticipation
(6)   addition by reduplication of a unit in the stimulus by reiteration
(7)   change of position of a unit in the stimulus by pre-positioning
(8)   change of position of a unit in the stimulus by post-positioning
(9)   change of position of a unit in the stimulus when it is not possible to specify which of pre- or post-positioning has occurred.

(For examples of these transformations in French see Lecours and Lhermitte (1969; 1972.) Paraphasias often can be described in terms of multiples of these rules (e.g. deletion followed by addition or duplication), and up to fourth-order transformations can sometimes be inferred.

Lecours applies this analysis to writing (*literal paragraphia*) as well as to speech. The original data on which he based his system were collected by asking patients to read aloud lists of words; thus the range of effects which could be observed was limited to those occurring within words rather than in connected speech. His system, however, has the advantage of providing a method which can be extended to other levels for the quantification of errors of seriation. It also allows a single transformation to be described in terms of both its syntagmatic and paradigmatic relationships at the same time—an intuitively more acceptable situation than forcing classification into one or other group.

The main conclusions which Lecours reported in 1969 from his analysis of the reading data were that phonemic substitutions were frequent, and that a large proportion of the transformations could be described as sequential errors, with pair creation and pair destruction as the basic phenomena in the generation of these errors. He observed that there is an increased likelihood of syntagmatic errors when phonemes appear in the context of identical or similar phonemes (for cybernetic and physiological accounts of this phenomenon, see Bertaux *et al.* 1968 and Lhermitte *et al.* 1969).

Martin and Rigrodsky (1974) have used a system similar to Lecours's to analyse phonological impairment in aphasic speech. Like Lecours they used a method by which they made sure they knew what was the aphasic speaker's intended utterance, although again there was the disadvantage that connected speech was not used: in their case they asked patients to repeat back meaningful or nonsense words they heard. Unlike Lecours, however, but like Blumstein, the theoretical model they used for the analysis of phonemic contrasts was Chomsky and Halle's (1968), which distinguishes amongst 13 binary features rather than providing a purely articulatory framework. (These features are: vocalic, consonantal, high, back, low, anterior, coronal, round, tense, voice, continuant, nasal, strident.) Martin and Rigrodsky describe the oppositions amongst the consonants and amongst the vowels of English in terms of up to seven of these features at any one time: for example /z/ contrasts in terms of seven features with /k/ (these seven features being high, back, anterior, coronal, voice, continuant, strident). Substitution errors (labelled by these authors as commutation errors) can therefore be described in terms of the number of distinctive features which separate the uttered phoneme from the phoneme appropriate in the intended word. Such a description shows that the majority of substitution errors differ in only one or two distinctive features from the appropriate phoneme. Martin and Rigrodsky also examined the extent to which substitutions could be accounted for in terms of three other possible measures of distinctive feature nearness of phonemes. One measure was of phonemes within the intended word; a second was of phonemes within the paraphasic word; and a third was between the substituting phoneme and the nearest phoneme in the intended word (nearness in this case being in terms of the fewest number of contrasting distinctive features with any other phoneme, rather than nearness in time or referring to the replaced phoneme). They found that the degree of similarity between the phoneme subject to substitution and other phonemes within the intended word did not seem to be a significant factor in instigating substitutions, nor was there a particular pattern of nearness of distinctive features when substituting phonemes in the paraphasic word were compared with other phonemes in the paraphasic word. However, the third measure proved more illuminating. There was a distinct trend for the substituting phoneme in the paraphasic word to resemble a phoneme in the intended word (in addition to the phoneme it directly replaced). In four-fifths of the cases the substituting phoneme resembled a phoneme in the intended word in that the distance was of no more than two features. There was thus a high degree of similarity not only between the substituting phoneme and the phoneme for which it substituted, but also between it and another phoneme in the intended word: such an observation is very much in line with the interpretation of substitution errors in terms not only of selection (paradigmatic) but of seriation for encoding (syntagmatic). But the seriation (and this is the important distinction between this analysis and an analysis in terms of the haphazard programming of apraxia of speech) appears to be systematically related to the realization of the intended word. Martin collected his data by the repetition technique, and consequently postulates that the regularities found in the errors may be reflective of either perceptual problems or memory decay. But he also comments that 'The basic qualitative similarity of performance when error is compared to desired phoneme or the entire stimulus would indicate that there is a basic impairment of a process or processes necessary to phonological production' (p. 343). As he points out this does not preclude the possibility of motor coordination and coarticulation effects occurring as well.

Martin and Rigrodsky did not distinguish amongst classes of aphasia in their analysis. Lecours has mainly collected data from patients with 'pure' phonemic paraphasia, i.e. patients who would be described in some terminologies as having Wernicke's aphasia with phonemic jargon, or as having conduction aphasia. Making generalizations from such findings rests upon the claim, which Blumstein's study supported, that phonemic errors are similar in all types of aphasia, and that they are therefore not closely related to the articulatory nature of the deficits in Broca's aphasia and in apraxia of speech. If they are not, they must be attributable to some prior stage in the encoding process which is vulnerable in all patients who show any kind of phonological disorder in speech. A study by some of Lecours's co-workers (Poncet, Degos, Deloche and Lecours 1972) specifically examined this question, by applying the linguistic distinction between phonetic and phonemic.

They started from the assumption that patients who made phonological errors in speech could be categorized as showing either phonemic (Pm) or phonetic (Pt) transformations (corresponding broadly to patients with Wernicke's aphasia characterized by phonemic jargon, and to patients with Broca's aphasia with articulatory difficulties). They anticipated that Pm and Pt patients would be distinguished on six counts:

(1)  Pm transformations would occur in fluent speech, while Pt transformations would occur in slow laborious speech.

(2)  Pt patients would produce phonetic deviations, while the Pm patients would produce only phonemes conforming to the language stock.

(3)  There would be more errors with Pt patients with structurally difficult words, and a tendency to simplify words by transforming them into conso-

nant–vowel–consonant–vowel–consonant sequences, while Pm patients would often produce difficult series.

(4) Pm transformations would be variable, but Pt constant, through series of repetitions.

(5) Pt transformations would tend to go from voiced to unvoiced whereas there would be no directional preference with Pm transformations.

(6) Sequential errors (metathesis, pair creation, pair destruction) would predominate in Pm transformations but not Pt transformation.

They examined the speech of seven Pm subjects and three Pt subjects obtained by asking them to repeat and read aloud single words. They hypothesized that behind the phonemic errors there was a disorder of programming, while phonetic errors were directly related to a deficit in the execution of motor acts involved in producing phonemic units and series. The results of their analysis gave partial support to the greater constancy of phonetic transformations, and to the greater effect of a dimension which could be called 'structural difficulty' in the latter; but the nature of the structural difficulties was different for both types. Words with repeated phonemes were more difficult for Pm patients, while words with clusters were more difficult for Pt patients. There was a preferential trend in the direction of substitutions in both kinds of patients, whereas it had been predicted only in one. The strongest evidence against the hypothesis that Pt and Pm errors result from different underlying dysfunctions was that there were almost the same proportions of sequential errors in Pt and Pm patients. The investigators came to the conclusion that Pt transformations could be Pm transformations overlaid with articulatory difficulties.

All the analyses described so far rest on the assumption that the aphasic speaker has an intended correct phonemic realization of the word in mind—hence Lecours's use of the term *transformation*. Such an interpretation is fostered by making analyses only of words in spontaneous speech for which the investigator recognizes this target word and discarding other data, or by using as stimuli lists of words to be read out or repeated. But it is also possible that a proportion of the phonemic jargon or neologisms in some patients reflects, not transformations of intended words, but a free spilling-over of speech sounds without any intended words in mind, and without any link with semantic content.

Buckingham and Kertesz (1976) have described three patients with whom neologistic utterances often seemed to result not so much from phonemic distortions of target words but from perseverations and recombinations of various phonemic units which had already been uttered. Howes and Geschwind have suggested that such confabulatory speech may be an outflow of the speech area when brain damage has disconnected it from that part of the language area of the brain which is concerned with semantic sensory-based information. Green (1969b) has also pointed out that many of a patient's neologisms can contain stereotypic phonemic sequences, sometimes uttered singly, sometimes in combination with other elements in meaningless strings. Such observations suggest that neologistic jargon may be essentially of two kinds: in one kind the jargon is the result of a phonemic programming disorder after the stage at which an intended word has been selected (hence the speaker often reveals what the intended word was through a series of approximations and self-corrections), while another kind represents the infilling of speech by a phonemic outflow without intended words having been selected, or during pre-selection gaps which have become prolonged because of the patient's lexical difficulties. In the first kind the target word may often be recognizable by the hearer; in the second kind there are no target words, but the filler neologisms serve to maintain the flow of speech between, or instead of, substantive words, and this speech is an autonomous outflow of phonological units and syntactic filler words and inflections.

Together with Blumstein's observations on the essential homogeneity of phonological errors in the main types of aphasia, these findings suggest that phonological disorders in aphasia can be described in terms of the utilization of a linguistic system rather than principally in terms of neuromuscular difficulties. Taking the argument one step further we will now look at the question of whether the utilization of the linguistic system always pertains exclusively to some high level of selection and seriation programming for speech and writing, or whether it may be a central disorder at the phonological level such that comprehension of phonemic distinctions is impaired as well as production.

## Interpretations in terms of a central linguistic dysfunction

There are four ways of examining this question of the extent to which phonological disorders in speech reflect a specific disorder of encoding or a central dysfunction of language:

(1)  the direct method of testing whether patients with phonemic disorders in speech have corresponding difficulties in making phonemic discriminations in comprehension;
(2)  the examination of the extent to which comprehension disorders in general are attributable to a difficulty in phonemic discrimination;
(3)  the investigation of whether phonological errors conform to independently developed linguistic theories based on models of language competence;
(4)  the investigation of the extent to which a disturbance at the phonological level interacts with disturbances at other linguistic levels.

Let us look at some examples of each of these approaches.

## 1. Comprehension and speech

At the conclusion of their study of the comprehension of patients with either predominantly phonemic or predominantly semantic paraphasias in their speech (without articulatory difficulties) Alajouanine and his colleagues in 1964 proposed 'that there is a sensorimotor auditory phonatory system which underlies the production of phonemic units, that change in this system is one of the factors or is *the* factor responsible for phonemic jargon, and that this system is independent of the system of semantic integration' (p. 19, translated). They had given a group of 19 patients with phonemic jargon but good functional comprehension (i.e. patients who could be called conduction aphasics) a range of auditory tests. Amongst these tests the patients were required to select which one of five pictures matched a word when given pictures whose names were phonemically or semantically similar, to identify distorted words or words which were heard against background noise, and to speak with delayed auditory feedback. The researchers had found that despite their good functional comprehension on standard clinical tests the patients with phonemic jargon were more impaired in phonemic discrimination than were patients whose speech showed semantic paraphasia. Gainotti, Caltagirone and Ibba eleven years later reported a study designed to check on the hypothesis which had been proposed by Alajouanine; they suspected that there might be only a partial correspondence between speech and comprehension in respect of phonemic and of semantic disabilities. The results of their *Verbal Sound and Meaning Discrimination Test* as concerns the relationship between semantic paraphasia and semantic comprehension have been reported on p. 76. Although they found a strong relationship between semantic paraphasias in speech and semantic errors in discrimination, the association of phonemic paraphasias with phonemic errors in discrimination was less convincing—not convincing enough to support the hypothesis of a breakdown of the phonemic level of integration of language. One complication was that sound discrimination errors were related to age, suggesting that there was a non-aphasic effect of presbycusis (impairment in hearing higher frequencies associated with age). The subjects were therefore divided into those under age 60 and those over 60. In the younger group of 54 aphasic subjects, only seven scored below the normal group's cut-off point of one phonemic error: in the older group only eight out of 50 aphasic subjects made more than the non-pathological cut-off of two errors.

Gainotti and his colleagues found that Broca's aphasics could be impaired in phonemic comprehension as well as Wernicke's aphasics, a finding which can be interpreted in two ways: either the syndrome of phonetic disintegration conceals a phonemic disorder similar in quality to that in phonemic jargon, as Poncet *et al.* suggested, or auditory perceptual deficits are universal in aphasia, as Schuell suggested. At all events Gainotti's study does not provide conclusive support for the hypothesis of a separate auditory-phonatory phonological level of language organization which is independent of modality. Unlike the findings at the semantic level, the findings at the phonological level suggest that there may be a substantial proportion of patients who show phonemic jargon in speech who do not have a similar deficit in comprehension—in other words the disorder may be one specific to encoding.

As table 8 indicates, the difficulties conduction patients experience with some tests of comprehension (including repetition) have been interpreted by various investigators as being due to a deficit in short-term memory rather than in phonological decoding as such. Warrington and Shallice (1969) considered that, in at least one case of aphasia which may have been identifiable as conduction aphasia, deficits in repetition were due to reduced span of short-term memory. Tsvetkova

(1976), explicitly identifying conduction aphasia with Luria's syndrome of acoustic-amnesic aphasia rather than afferent motor aphasia, suggests that the basic problem is in the limitation of the amount of material which can be perceived and remembered. Aten, Johns and Darley (1971) report that although apraxia of speech can occur in a relatively pure form without any perceptual impairment, it can sometimes be accompanied by a reduced auditory retention span which impairs the perception of sequences of words which are phonemically similar. However, Strub and Gardner (1974), questioning the extent to which the repetition defect in conduction aphasia is mnestic or linguistic, come to the conclusion that it is better viewed as a linguistic deficit, specifically in the processing, synthesis and ordering of phonemes. Their patient's repetition performance improved when there were longer intervals between stimuli, a result inconsistent with a memory deficit, and he could not repeat even short words if these were nonsense rather than meaningful. Their interpretation of the repetition deficit in conduction aphasia is 'an impairment in proceeding from a phonological analysis to the selection and combination of target phonemes' (p. 253). But both explanations, in terms of memory and in terms such as Strub and Gardner use, admit that adequate phonological analysis in comprehension is potentially retained in patients with phonemic jargon, even if longer processing time is required, an interpretation not incompatible with phonological disorders in speech being restricted to encoding for speech rather than reflecting a central breakdown.

## 2. Comprehension and phonemic discrimination

There is a tradition in speech therapy clinics of attributing language disorders in both children and adults to a failure in auditory processing. Amongst the respected figures whose opinions have been taken to endorse this view are Schuell, for whom difficulty in auditory verbal processing was germane to the unitary phenomenon of aphasia, and Luria, who described an aphasia which is commonly equated with Wernicke's aphasia as being acoustic-agnostic aphasia. Difficulties in auditory verbal processing, primarily at the phonological level, are therefore seen not only as contributing to the slow development of language in some children, but also as accounting for the comprehension disorder in aphasia, both of which views attribute to auditory phonological processing a centrality in the language system. Based on this philosophy many painstaking methods have been developed of retraining in auditory discrimination in aphasia—for example Lane and Moore's (1962) reconditioning of consonant discrimination using hand-drawn spectrographic patterns which were converted into sounds. Experimental evidence has been sought that the pattern of difficulty in phonemic discrimination in comprehension in aphasia is similar to that shown in speech. Consoli (1973) reports that errors of discriminating voicing are less common than errors of discriminating place, and that more difficulties are experienced in discriminating velar consonants than anterior consonants—a similar pattern in comprehension to that reported for speech. Oscar-Berman, Zurif and Blumstein (1975) also made a similar observation through the analyses of error patterns from dichotically presented consonant–vowel syllables: left-brain-damaged subjects (though not all were overtly aphasic) found it slightly easier to recognize the pairs of syllables when the consonants were both voiced or both voiceless, although sharing of other features did not help them. Levinsohn (1969) investigated the disintegration of phonemic abilities in perception and in production in individual aphasic adults and concluded that 'intra-subject responses on perception and production levels tended to be related' (p. 58), in that they substituted the same phonemes in both perception and production tests.

Some studies have reported that aphasic subjects do indeed perceive speech as being distorted. Mostofsky and his colleagues (1973) compared aphasic and normal subjects' judgements of similarity of different versions of a prose passage which had been recorded normally and in four distorted versions (slowed, speeded, reversed and computer-synthesized in a *vocoded* form). From a multidimensional analysis, the researchers reported that the aphasic subjects seemed to perceive speech as more similar to distorted speech than did the normal subjects; but it also seemed that the aphasics' judgements on this task had no relation to either the scores on subtests of auditory comprehension on a clinical battery or to a rating for fluency in speech. In a Japanese study, Sasanuma and colleagues (1973), having confirmed that aphasic subjects were inferior to normal subjects in discriminating the temporal duration of pure tones, tested their ability to make a similar distinction between computer-synthesized pairs of words (*ita/itta*: *oi/ooi*). Although the aphasic subjects showed the same severe perturbation in judgement of duration, nevertheless they recognized the transition between the phoneme boundaries almost as well as the control subjects did, and the results were similar for the consonant contrast *ita/itta* and for the vowel contrast *oi/ooi*. Sasunuma comments that it seems as if the aphasic patients may have had some defect in the auditory system even at a stage preceding speech comprehension, but that some part of their previous linguistic competence, the detection of phoneme boundaries, remained. Carpenter and Rutherford (1971) used edited recorded speech (human rather than synthesized) in a *Discrimination of Acoustic Cues Test* to compare performance on discrimination of perceptual cues with performance on the auditory comprehension subtests of the Boston Test. Of the 15 aphasic patients tested, seven failed both the discrimination test and the clinical test 'thus suggesting that the comprehension disturbance of these individuals may arise from reduced ability to discriminate acoustic cues for speech sounds' p. 2). It was particularly temporal cues (such as distinguish onset of voicing in *hid/hit*) rather than spectral ones (*tail/pail*) which the aphasic subjects found difficult. There were, however, two patients who failed the discrimination test but scored at above the 75 per cent level on the clinical test of comprehension, while three others failed the clinical test but passed the discrimination test. Like Mostofsky's experiment this suggests that poor auditory phonemic discrimination is not the cause of the comprehension disorder in all aphasics, although it leaves open the possibility that it may be in some. In another study, starting from Hécaen's threefold classification of sensory aphasias (predominant defect in reception of verbal signs, predominant defect in verbal comprehension for both written and oral language, attentional disorganization), Goldblum and Albert (1972) found corroboratory evidence from a picture test of phonemic discrimination of a distinction between two of these sensory aphasias. Sensory patients of the first kind, with a receptive deficit like word-deafness, showed discriminatory difficulties primarily when the phonemic distance between words was small, while those with the general comprehension deficit made as many errors when there was a large phonemic distance between words as when there was a small. Overall the aphasic patients were significantly impaired in phonemic discrimination compared with non-aphasic brain-damaged subjects, and within the aphasic group patients with sensory aphasia were significantly more impaired than motor aphasics. The findings could be taken to endorse the association between a deficit in phoneme discrimination and the comprehension disorder in one kind of aphasia (the word-deaf type), while indicating a more complicated breakdown of comprehension in another kind. Goldblum and Albert's test did not include any means of distinguishing true misinterpretations of the stimulus words from random guesses.

Findings such as these, despite the ambiguity of their results, have generally been interpreted as corroborating the importance of auditory perceptual deficits in comprehension difficulties. It is therefore sometimes assumed in therapy that exercises in phonemic discrimination are the key to improvement in comprehension and in language abilities in general. Rees (1973), however, is one of several clinicians who have questioned this assumption both as it relates to children and to adults with disordered language. She reviewed a number of studies and concluded that 'the evidence for an auditory factor at the basis of language disorders is far from conclusive' p. 308). Di Carlo and Taub (1972) found that the impairment noticed in aphasic patients (who had had strokes) when they were given a test of perception of distorted speech, appeared to be related only to age; the hypothesis of a greater difficulty with distorted speech than normal speech due to the aphasic condition itself could not be supported. From the linguistic perspective also the weight of evidence suggests that a model of phonemic perception as the basic stage of a chain of events in language comprehension is too simple. The evidence for what constitutes the basic unit in speech perception is indecisive, perhaps because perception may operate with different units simultaneously, but what is likely is that perception of speech does not normally operate by means of the sequential resolution of discrete phonemes (for reviews of theories of speech perception see Paap 1975 and Darwin 1976).

In particular the concept of Wernicke's aphasia as being secondary to auditory verbal agnosia has been challenged by researchers from Boston and California. Blumstein, Baker and Goodglass (1977) gave Wernicke's aphasics and three other types of aphasics some tests of the ability to make phonological discriminations in comprehension. For the tests they had to listen to pairs of words or of nonsense syllables and to press a button marked *yes* if they were the same, or marked *no* if they were different. The pairs of words in one test differed in one or two distinctive features (voice and place), in another test syllables differed (e.g. *describe/prescribe*), and in a third test the speech sounds were reversed (e.g. *main/name*). The results showed that the Wernicke's aphasics, although diagnosed on the Boston test as having the worst comprehension, were not the most impaired in phoneme discrimination: patients classed as *anterior plus comprehension deficit* and *posterior residual*, despite their better performance on the clinical test of comprehension, made more errors in phonemic discrimination. Moreover all aphasic subjects made fewer errors with real words than in discriminating nonsense words, suggesting that aphasic subjects, like normal subjects, draw on semantic knowledge in making these decisions rather than that they make a decision purely within the phonological level, unless this is the only level possible. For the Wernicke's aphasics place was significantly more difficult to interpret than voice: Blumstein hypothesizes that discrimination of voice, which depends on discrimination of voice-onset time, may be assisted by non-linguistic acoustic processing, a conclusion somewhat at variance with Carpenter and Rutherford's observation that voice discrimination was more difficult for aphasics because it depends on temporally coded distinctions. Rees (1970) cites a study by Rosenthal which came to the same conclusion about aphasic children.

Following an account of Blumstein's study given at a conference in 1973, Naeser (1974) reported the results of an examination of different kinds of aphasic patients on tasks designed to separate out three different kinds of comprehension. Blumstein's study had suggested that there is a dissociation between phonemic discrimination and whatever kind of auditory comprehension the Boston Test measures. Naeser's study goes one step further: it suggests that there is a triple dissociation. The tests she used were one requiring same-different discriminations (similar to Blumstein's), one measuring phonemic discrimination through picture-choice (and hence necessarily requiring the meaning of the words to be understood) and the Token Test, which requires the comprehension of sentences. She found no significant relationship amongst the three kinds of comprehension, and suggested that there may be three qualitatively different kinds of comprehension deficit in aphasia. One, which is picked out particularly by phoneme discrimination, is the element which appears in its most pure form as *word-deafness*, an element of auditory imperception which may be widespread in aphasia but is not sufficient on its own, unless it appears in a very marked form, to result in comprehension difficulties as they are usually recognized. The second is the disorder picked out by picture–word matching tests which examine phonemic discrimination, and where the subject has to link sound and meaning rather than make a decision within the phonological level; it is this which characterizes Wernicke's aphasia, and may be interpreted as an impaired phonemic-semantic association ability (an interpretation that would be in line with Buckingham and Kertesz's proposal that some neologistic jargon may reflect the free running of the phonological system when semantic retrieval difficulties are experienced). The third type of comprehension deficit is shown up most clearly by the Token Test (De Renzi and Vignolo 1962), and may be the syntactic-semantic deficit we discussed in the last chapter which characterizes Broca's aphasia. These suggestions, Naeser emphasizes, are speculative, but they fit in with other observations which have been made of Wernicke's aphasics not being more impaired than other aphasics on tests of phonemic perception, and do indicate that the method by which phonemic perception is tested may be of crucial significance.

But the definition of comprehension disorders is by no means resolved. Many studies have found that tests of phonological comprehension do not separate out types of aphasia. Assal (1974), for example, using a test of phonemic discrimination which required matching words to pictures, reported that patients with Wernicke forms of aphasia were not distinguished from patients with expressive aphasia. He comments particularly on the possibility of poor results amongst patients with anterior lesions. Gainotti's study, again using pictures, found that Wernicke's aphasics did not fare worse than Broca's aphasics on phonemic discrimination. Gardner and Zurif (1976) observe that 'the striking differences found in patterns of expression do not seem to be reflected in patterns of comprehension difficulty, except for certain isolated categories of patients' (p. 186). The picture-choice studies of comprehension by Pizzamiglio and his colleagues (1968) found that their test of phonemic discrimination correlated at ·80 with the clinical rating given for comprehension. When they divided the patients up according to conventional clinical classifications (Pizzamiglio and Parisi 1970) they found no differences amongst the results of Broca's, Wernicke's and anomic aphasics on the test of phonemic discrimination (nor on the other linguistic tests either).

The processes of linguistic comprehension are little understood, despite the attention given to some facets of phonemic perception in speech perception laboratories. To summarize the findings concerning aphasia in this section, we can suggest that:

(a)   distinctions in auditory comprehension as so far examined in tests are not as clearly defined as distinctions in speech;

(b)   the weight of evidence from aphasia indicates that disorders in phonemic perception are not of as much influence in impairment of comprehension as had previously been supposed;

(c)   there is as yet no evidence to suggest that phonemic disorders in speech are paralleled by phonemic disorders in comprehension and no evidence so far to suggest that an interpretation of phonemic and phonetic disorders in speech in terms specifically of encoding processes should be rejected.

## 3. Correspondence with 'central' linguistic models

We have already observed, from Blumstein's (1973) work, that from the linguistic constructs of distinctive features and of markedness predictions can be made about order of difficulty which correspond, at least partially, to what is actually observed in aphasic breakdown. This provides some evidence for the linguistically motivated nature of phonological errors, rather than their neuromuscular nature.

Lebrun, Lenaerts, Goiris and Demol (1969) have described a phonological disorder in terms which indicate that it is not the phoneme but a larger meaningful unit that is the basic unit of speech production. They point out that when patients are helped to pronounce a word by prompting with the initial sound, the incipient movement makes the pronunciation of the whole word possible, indicating that a cerebral programme for the word has been put into gear, rather than its reconstitution sound by sound. An attempt has been made to test whether phonological errors in the reading aloud of one aphasic patient follow the rules postulated by generative phonology (Schnitzer 1971). Schnitzer's aim was to demonstrate that the systematic phonemic representations and the phonological rules proposed in Chomsky and Halle (1968) have psychological reality. Schnitzer suggests that the aphasic patient, a young teacher, who had suffered a subdural haematoma which had left her with a small lesion in the left supramarginal gyrus, made errors in reading which could occur either at the underlying level or through misapplication of transformational rules. An example of an error attributable to the underlying level was a change in vowel tenseness, *radical* read out as /redəkəl/, and of a misapplication of a phonological rule (velar softening, e.g. hard /g/ becoming soft /dʒ/ before certain vowels) was *logicism* read out as /lɒgisəm/ or (in reverse) *allegory* read as /aledʒɒri/. Schnitzer concludes that 'Such evidence clearly demonstrates the psychological existence of the underlying lexical (systematic phonemic) level, in that errors (often of predictable types) made at this level, can, within the framework just noted, account for widespread and seemingly random phonetic-level errors. Such evidence also indirectly validates the phonological rules, since they are needed to derive the observed phonetic forms from the underlying representations' (p. 12). In order to reconcile this conclusion with objections such as those raised by Lebrun to the interpretation of speech production as requiring piecemeal reconstitution of phonological elements, Schnitzer comments that underlying representations and derivations may be used only when one is coining new words or when there is a problem encountered in producing the phonetic form. The majority of words, even with this aphasic woman, may have been stored as units with an easily accessible phonetic representation, which did not require the activation of phonological rules for their production. Other words, later learned, had no easily accessible representation but were subject to various random phonetic errors. The words which were of most interest in Schnitzer's study were those which presumably had no phonetic representation initially for the subject, and which therefore revealed the underlying processes which the subject was obliged to apply (and misapplied) in giving them a phonetic representation.

Reviewing Schnitzer's work Blumstein (1974) comments that the deficits which the patient showed were limited to reading aloud, and do not seem to have occurred in her conversational speech. Blumstein suggests that many of the errors can be explained in terms of reading strategies rather than the relationship between underlying forms and phonetic output—for instance the patient may have hypothesized what the word was from a brief scan, guessed the most likely form of the word (i.e. the underived form), pronounced the word with the stress pattern of this underived form, only to find that there were more letters to be accounted for, and then elided the form so far produced with its revision. Schnitzer (in press, b), however, has pointed out that English spelling resembles underlying forms more closely than it does phonetic forms: the Chomsky–Halle model provides the sort of rules needed for relating underlying representations, which closely parallel standard orthography, to phonetic form in reading aloud.

Again, as frequently in aphasiology, we find ourselves obliged to recall the effect of modality on what it would be simpler to treat as a matter of pure linguistic analysis. Errors in phonological production cannot be unambiguously interpreted as being evidence for a central disturbance of a system of phonological rules, if they are found to occur only in one modality, to which specific qualities apply.

Schnitzer equates the systematic phonemic level with the lexical level, i.e. the phonological shapes which words take. This brings us to the final question to be discussed here.

## 4. Autonomy of linguistic levels

It is a common observation that an overt disorder at the syntactic level is most frequently found in association with a phonetic-phonemic disorder in encoding (in Broca's aphasia) while a phonemic disorder without phonetic distortions is frequently found in association with semantic difficulties (in Wernicke's aphasia). It has also been observed that the phonological encoding difficulties of conduction aphasics are markedly increased when they are asked to repeat a series of grammatical words rather than substantive words ('no ifs, ands or buts'). The alliterative and perseverative behaviour of patients with fluent neologistic jargon is more marked preceding nouns than preceding other parts of speech. All aphasic subjects appear to have more difficulty with nonsense material than with meaningful material. Such observations are consistent with a view that brain damage only partially teases out separate components in language.

One of the most active proponents of this perspective on phonology in aphasia has been Martin with his colleagues in New York. He argues against the concept of isolated impairment at one linguistic level in aphasia, and suggests instead that various processes are operating at reduced levels of efficiency rather than one process being exclusively impaired. Consequently he has raised objections to the term *apraxia of speech* (Martin 1974) because of its implication of an isolated disorder (cf. p. 158 above). He argues against the claim that perception of speech is not impaired in apraxia of speech with the counter-claim that the tests of perception have not been sufficiently sensitive. In a study of the interactions between the phonological and morphological levels in repetition tasks Martin and colleagues (1975) analysed patients' errors when they were asked to repeat a set of monosyllables which consisted of consonant-cluster + vowel + consonant-cluster. In some cases the final cluster was a morphological inflection as in *crossed* /krɒst/. In other cases similar endings were used but not as morphological inflections (*breast*), while in a third condition the final consonant cluster consisted of a combination which is never used as a morphological ending in English (*crisp, plunge*). As predicted there was an increase in errors from the latter kind of words which could only be interpreted as single morphological units, through those with ambiguous endings, to the syllables which could be interpreted as containing two morphemes. It was thus evident that morphological influences had an effect on a phonological task. The kind of errors made also tended to be different between words which could be interpreted as two morphemes and words which could be interpreted only as one: the latter had significantly more substitution errors, while the former had more omission errors, suggesting that these former words were indeed interpreted as being structurally more complex. Martin hypothesizes that substitution errors are more indicative of a basic phonological impairment, while sequencing (including omission) errors are more indicative of interactions between phonological and morphological components.

At the same time that there is a legitimate case for the interaction of linguistic levels, there is also evidence for the potential autonomy of different language operations. Buckingham, Whitaker and Whitaker (in press) have pointed out that knowing what one wants to say and producing the actual word seem to be separate operations. Buckingham and Kertesz's interpretation of neologisms as an overflowing of activity of the phonological system argues for the autonomy of this system in speech. These filler neologisms occur most frequently in slots where nouns would be expected, indicating that although lexical selection may be impaired, phonological output is not.

Further evidence of the separation of phonological and semantic processes in word-finding has been obtained with *tip-of-the-tongue* experiments in aphasia. Since Brown and McNeill's (1966) seminal study showed that, while words themselves may not be retrieved under certain circumstances, some acoustic and orthographic properties of the same words can often be retrieved, this phenomenon has attracted much interest in psycholinguistics (e.g. see Blake 1973). The tip-of-the-tongue condition is a frequent enough phenomenon in aphasia to present the investigator with plenty of opportunities for examination. The problem here is to devise a viable enough method of getting the patient to report what information he has available about the word he cannot produce. At least two studies have been made of this condition in aphasia, first by Barton in 1971 and more recently by Goodglass, Kaplan, Weintraub and Ackerman in 1976. Both used the same technique of presenting patients with pictures to name, and, with any words on which they failed, asking them to identify its initial letter on an alphabet card and to indicate the number of syllables the unavailable word contained on a card marked with dashes separated by slashes. In Goodglass and colleagues' sample of patients, the four groups of aphasics (Broca, Wernicke, conduction and anomic) conveniently turned out to have naming difficulties with approximately the same number of pictures on the list, so that their partial knowledge of the words could be directly compared. The results indicated that the conduction aphasics had much superior information about the words they could not produce than that of Wernicke or anomic aphasics; in fact the latter patients seemed either to be able to produce the word or to have very little information about number of syllables or initial letter, as if word-finding was for them on all-or-none process. The results of the Broca group could not be satisfactorily interpreted due to their variability. Overall, patients were better at identifying the initial letter correctly than they were at pointing out the number of syllables.

A further observation which endorses the possible separation of phonological shape from lexical meaning in anomic aphasia has been made by Diamond, Epstein and Bender (1969). They call it the *paronym defect*. While in the process of trying to find a word patients may actually hear the word they are seeking uttered in a different context, without recognizing it as the target word—indeed they may even repeat the word themselves without recognition. Diamond cites two patients who were seeking the name *tie* for the article of clothing. Although they were able to discuss how they would tie it, they could not name it. One was prompted with 'Can you tie it?' and responded 'Yeah—I can tie it all right—I can tie it—I—I can wear the—the uh—short one—the—like hard for me to tell it—see' (p. 157). Diamond interprets this finding as indicating that words (i.e. the phonologically shaped words) are not the primary units of speech.

Marshall and Newcombe (1973) and Shallice and Warrington (1975) have also identified a dissociation of the phonemic and semantic levels of reading in the dyslexia they have severally called *deep* or *phonemic dyslexia*. In this the patient appears to be able to extract some semantic information from the words he is given to read while being unable to make direct phonemic–graphemic associations. Consequently he can read some words, primarily nouns high in picturability and concreteness, while being unable to respond to function words or more abstract words. A second kind of dyslexia has been described by Marshall and Newcombe as being *surface* or consisting of grapheme–phoneme conversion errors, such as misreading a hard *g* as a soft one and hence *guest* as *just* or vice versa with *barge* misread as *bargain*. Such errors can sometimes lead to the production of neologisms. The existence of (at least) these two types of dyslexia argues for a dual-encoding theory of reading. Marshall and Newcombe propose that there are two complementary routes between visual registration and threshold activation of a word in reading aloud: one goes via a *phonological address*, the other via a *semantic address*. Patients who make grapheme–phoneme conversion errors show that they are relying on the phonological routes, as the semantic route is blocked by the brain damage. Patients with deep dyslexia show that they are relying on the semantic route, with, presumably, the phonological route blocked: hence the semantic imprecisions they make are not corrected by the phonological read-out. In this way a phonological blockage results in semantic errors, a semantic blockage in phonemic errors. The terminology of calling these patients *phonemic dyslexics* becomes somewhat confusing, as, although they are presumed to have a blockage at the phonemic–graphemic level, the kinds of errors they make can be described as semantic (Marshall and Newcombe therefore call this phenomenon *deep* or *syntactico-semantic dyslexia*). Saffran and Marin (1977) studied a secretary who, after a stroke, had great difficulty in reading words which were misspelled but homophonic with their correct spelling (e.g. *phlore*). They concluded that her usual method of reading was holistic rather than phonological. Patients with this deep dyslexia would, therefore, appear to offer a means by which the workings of the semantic system can be interpreted directly through the errors which are exposed in reading without the normal intervention of the graphemic–phonemic process.

Patterson and Marcel (1977) have recently offered evidence which supports the view that the reading difficulties of certain aphasic-dyslexic patients are impaired in use of the phonological–graphemic code in reading. Two such patients were given lists of orthographically regular non-words like *dake* to read out and to repeat. They were able to repeat them fairly well indicating relative preservation of the echoic phonological code for audition-speech, but almost completely unable to read them aloud, indicating a disruption of the phonemic route in reading and a dependence on the semantic route which could not be used with these nonsense words (a similar finding is reported by Schnitzer and Martin 1974 and discussed by Schnitzer 1976). In a second experiment the two patients were given, in a list of words, some non-words which were homophonic with real words, like *flore*, *stane* and *frute*, and asked to indicate which words were real words. With such non-words it has been established (and Patterson and Marcel's experiment also confirmed this) that normal subjects take longer to make decisions than they do with non-words which do not sound like words, indicating that even in this silent task the pronunciation of the non-words has an effect. The aphasic patients examined, however, showed no such effect. From the absence of this effect it could be inferred that there was some lack in the phonological coding abilities of the patients. They were, however, able to perform competently the task of deciding which words were real words and which words were not, indicating the relative preservation of the semantic route.

Japanese dyslexics provide further evidence for a dissociation of phonological and semantic systems in reading. Japanese has three writing systems: two of them are *kana* and are basically syllabic and phonemic in nature, so that the pronunciation of unknown words can be inferred from their writing, as in English. The other is *kanji*, which is basically idiographic, with a symbol representing a semantic concept. There have been several studies of Japanese patients who showed a dissociation in reading abilities between kana and kanji. Marshall and Newcombe cite an early one in 1914 by Asayama. More recent studies by Sasanuma (Sasanuma and Fujimura 1971; 1972; Sasanuma 1974; 1975) and Yamadori (1975) have given detailed accounts of such patients' abilities in both reading and writing.

Schnitzer (1976) summarizes these findings, and others with a blind alexic (for Braille) patient and aphasic deaf-mutes, by saying that two kinds of symptomatology may arise after brain damage (as relevant to phonological organization). In the first case the ability to use a non-articulatory–auditory system may be impaired (as when ideograms or Braille symbols cannot be read) but the patient may be able to use or develop phonological mediation instead. In the second case the system of phonological mediation is disrupted but reading which does not depend on phonological mediation is still possible. In a third case both symptomatologies occur together, as in verbal alexia where the patient can neither read well by Gestalt processes, nor improve his performance by spelling out words aloud. Schnitzer concludes that, though language cannot be described without syntax and semantics, coherent functional linguistic communication can exist in the absence of phonological mediation. 'Language without syntax or semantics is not language. Language without phonology *is* language' (p. 159).

In summary, linguistic investigations of the phonological level in aphasic disorders give a less important role to phonology, particularly in speech perception, than earlier studies have suggested. And although there is enough evidence for a systematic linguistic nature of phonological errors in speech to weaken the case for phonemic disorders being primarily in neuromuscular programming for speech, the case for their being disorders specifically of linguistic *encoding* without consequence for speech perception has not yet been refuted. With perception of language through reading, however, we can get a different picture—an inability to decode at the phonological-graphemic level in reading, but with preservation of phonological abilities in speech. Taken together these observations suggest that not only the phonetic but the phonemic level of language operates at a relatively peripheral part of the language system.

## Prosody

We have so far mentioned only studies of segmental phonology in aphasia, and said nothing about investigations at the suprasegmental level, prosody. Monrad-Krohn suggests that, for aphasia, this may be divided up into rhythm, stress and pitch variation—the latter two being components of intonation. As in linguistics, prosody has played a Cinderella role in aphasic investigations, partly because of this very paucity of theoretical formulations from linguistics, until it began to be considered as of importance in paralinguistic studies of social communication. In aphasia there is some justification for its attracting less initial attention than segmental phonology, as there is evidence that the right hemisphere plays some part in the processing of intonation contours (Blumstein and Cooper 1974), although rhythm is said to be processed by the left hemisphere (Robinson and Solomon 1974). Consequently the extent to which *emic* disorders of prosody are to be expected in aphasia is questionable, although *etic* disorders attributable to articulatory difficulties or grammatical restrictions are the norm in non-fluent aphasia (Mössner and Pilch 1971). Kreindler, Calvarezo and Mihailescu (1971), however, have commented on one case of fluent jargon aphasia as being characterized partly by 'excessive use of the possibilities of rhythmical and esthetical organization of speech' (p. 225). When the patient, a retired schoolmaster, was first interviewed his responses to questions were inappropriate and the characteristics of his speech were a succession of similar sounding and rhyming neologisms and a *hyperrhythmia*, with a progressive increase and decrease in the number of syllables of a complex utterance. A month later, the number of neologisms was much reduced as were the rhyming words, and the element which predominated in the organization of his speech was the rhythmic patterning of phrases. Kreindler suggests that the deterioration in the ability to structure utterances semantically had released the prosodic method of structuring speech with rhythm and rhyme, possibly representing a return to the primary modalities of communication, the paleolanguage.

Two studies support the view that comprehension of at least one *emic* aspect of prosody, stress, is resistant to disturbance in aphasia. Mihailescu and her colleagues in Bucharest (1970) found that the performance of aphasic patients on a test of decoding of correct and wrong word stress was practically the same as that of normal subjects. The subjects were asked to show recognition of the meaning of a multisyllabic word, sometimes correctly stressed, sometimes incorrectly, by showing how it was used and by selecting its referent from amongst a choice of fifteen objects. Although some patients made errors or produced dyspraxic responses, the significant observation was that they made the same kinds of responses however the words were stressed. The patients, like the normal subjects, translated the misstressed words into correctly stressed words, presumably because the incoming stimuli triggered off established neuronal aggregates. Blumstein and Goodglass (1972) studied the phenomenon in a different way, although they too came to the same conclusion that 'although stress perception is a difficult discrimination for both normals and aphasics it is preserved in aphasia' (p. 800). They used meaningful, correctly stressed words, and made use of the fact that stress placement can be used to distinguish noun and verb forms of the same phonemic assembly (e.g. /'transport/trans'port/) and compound nouns from adjective–noun combinations (e.g. /'whitecap/white'cap/). A test was devised in which such contrasts were illustrated with pictures together with two other semantically related items, so that any errors of choice of picture for the recorded word or phrase could be attributed either to incorrect decoding of stress or random factors. Although the aphasics made more errors overall than did a control group of normal subjects, this was accounted for by a higher proportion of random errors; in the comprehension of the distinctions of stress they were not significantly impaired. Both normal and aphasic subjects found it easier to identify nouns than verbs or than the adjective–noun phrases. No differences were found within the aphasic group between Broca's and fluent aphasics.

Patterns of stress play an important role in some aphasic speech as well as in comprehension, though in this case the linguistic analysis is *etic* rather than *emic*. Goodglass (1968) has shown that, when agrammatic patients are asked to repeat short phrases, whether or not the words are stressed may be more important in their success than whether the words are grammatical or substantive. Amongst the phrases given for repetition were /Can Jim 'come?/ (with stress only on the final word) and /'Can't he 'dance?/ (with stress on initial and final words). Despite the greater syntactic complexity of the latter form, it proved easier to repeat. Goodglass suggests that the pattern of stressed word–unstressed word–stressed word is particularly facilitating for aphasics. This would indicate the same facilitation at the word level of rhythmic alternation which has been proposed at the phonetic level, in that alternating patterns of consonant–vowel–consonant–vowel seem to be the easiest to produce. Use has been made of this facilitation by stress patterns as well as by pitch patterns of intonation in the method of Melodic Intonation Therapy which is being experimented with as a releaser for language in global aphasia (for a description of this method see Gardner 1976, pp. 346–7; Sarno's comments in Licht 1975; or Sparks and Holland 1976).

In speech, the preservation of intonation patterns despite semantic unintelligibility in fluent aphasia has frequently been commented on (e.g. Schveiger 1968), and a disturbance of prosody which is not secondary to the articulatory effort required in non-fluent aphasia is considered by Monrad-Krohn (1963) to be rare.

Monrad-Krohn discusses dysprosody in *etic* terms; there are, however, occasional reports of aphasic speakers in whom changes of prosodic and phonetic quality have been so systematic and consistent that they are taken for foreigners. For example, the Norwegian woman who was mistaken for a German (Monrad-Krohn 1947a; Engl and Von Stockert 1976) and other observations do not rule out the possibility that *emic* contrastive aspects of prosody may be impaired. For example in languages where pitch serves as a distinctive feature in phonemic organization, there is reason to believe that this aspect of prosody is under the control of the language dominant hemisphere (Van Lanckner and Fromkin 1973) and is therefore a part of the linguistic system which might be disturbed in aphasia.

Nor is all the evidence in favour of the preservation of *emic* comprehension of intonation in aphasia. Fink (1969) found that aphasic patients had difficulty in judging whether different intonation patterns of a computer-synthesized phrase 'see you soon' were declarative or interrogative. The evidence for a specific aphasic deficit was weakened, however, by the further finding that older non-aphasic subjects showed similar difficulties (compare Di Carlo and Taub's findings at the segmental phonological level). In any case the judgement required here was a metalinguistic judgement about sentence types: when aphasic subjects are asked to judge the emotional tone of meaningless or meaningful sentences and to relate them to moods as illustrated by drawings of faces (anger, happiness and sadness), they seem to be no more impaired than are right-brain-damaged non-aphasic people (Schlanger, Schlanger and Gerstman 1976). Both kinds of brain-damaged people, however, do this task less well than normal people to a significant degree. In this latter study neither a quantitative nor a qualitative difference was found between the aphasic and the non-aphasic brain-damaged subjects, although ideas about the different functions of the left and right cerebral hemispheres would suggest that a more senstive test might show up differences. If the right hemisphere does indeed play a dominating role in emotional processing (Gainotti 1972; Heilman, Scholes and Watson 1976) and in face recognition, a task such as the one given of matching emotional expressions to pictures of faces might well be expected to present difficulties to right-brain-damaged people, quite apart from any linguistic element in the task. Conceivably other components in a task such as the Schlangers used could account for the impairment of their left-brain-damaged subjects.

There is a large body of evidence which implicates the left hemisphere in the timing and sequential organization, on which prosody depends. Bond (1976), for example, demonstrated that aphasic patients were not able to make use of organization of a sequence of non-verbal sounds into a pattern like a tone-group to facilitate recognition, although normal subjects could do so. Nevertheless there are sufficient examples of such patients' using changes of pitch as a means of communication with a limited amount of speech to show that this kind of organization can be spared when other kinds are not (Alajouanine and Lhermitte 1964; Botez, Carp and Mihailescu 1968). Alajouanine and Lhermitte, and also Fry in his comments on their paper in the same book, describe patients whose speech was limited to short stereotypies (e.g. 'one, two') but who used these stereotypies with varied speed and intonation express a range of needs and emotions.

Impairments of prosody after brain damage have been associated as well with damage to the right cerebral hemisphere, which does not produce a frank aphasia in the majority of patients, and there has been the suggestion that this aspect of language in particular may be bilaterally represented in the brain. Prosody, however, has been particularly associated with the expression and comprehension of emotion, and the right hemisphere contribution to the processing of prosody has been mainly interpreted as due to this association (see, for example, Weintraub, Mesulam and Kramer, 1981; Code 1987). Bowers, Coslett, Bauer, Speedie and Heilman (1987) have demonstrated that the problems of right hemisphere damaged patients in deciding whether sentences were spoken in happy, sad, angry or indifferent tones of voice increased if the tone of voice was not congruent with the semantic content of the sentence; it seemed that, in contrast to the left-brain damaged, these patients were distracted by the semantic message. The researchers suggest that this indicates that the left hemisphere (presumably undertaking the processing when the right hemisphere was damaged) is capable of processing emotional prosody, but prefers to attend to the semantic content. When the sentences were given with frequencies between 100 and 5000Hz filtered out, so that the words were unintelligible, the right hemisphere damaged and left hemisphere damaged made equal numbers of errors. Under such conditions the extent to which the prosodic information can still be attributed to the expression of emotion is debatable, and impairment may be due to more peripheral aspects of processing. If this were so, the right hemisphere damaged may be impaired on all tasks which involve the processing of prosody, propositional as well as emotional. Some studies point in this direction. Lonie and Lesser (1983) found that the right hemisphere damaged were significantly impaired on detecting the propositional differences in intonation which distinguish speech acts such as question and apology, in "Sorry?"/"Sorry!". Bryan (1986) followed this with a comprehensive battery of tests of propositional prosody given to left and right brain damaged patients. It comprised tests of the comprehension and production of emphatic stress, the comprehension of speech acts distinguished by intonation and the identification of filtered speech as of a tone language (Chinese) or not. The impairment of prosody demonstrated on all these tests could not be accounted for by poor performance on a measure of discrimination of pitch differences. The 40 right hemisphere damaged patients (none of whom were diagnosed as aphasic by the Western Aphasia Battery) made significantly more errors than the 40 left hemisphere damaged aphasic patients on the identification of the language from which the filtered speech had been derived. It is evident that prosody is an important parameter for study of the effects of brain damage on language, and that its differential impairment according to lateralization is not solely attributable either to its relationship to emotion or to the elementary processing of pitch.

# 9

# Psycholinguistic and sociolinguistic applications of linguistics to aphasia

Over the last decade the two applied fields in linguistics of psycholinguistics and sociolinguistics have begun to make significant contributions to the study of aphasia. Since the application of psycholinguistic models to aphasia originated from cognitive psychologists rather than linguistics, this aspect of aphasiology has become known as a part of cognitive neuropsychology. In contrast, the application to aphasia of sociolinguistics is being developed by linguists rather than sociologists; its main contribution is in clarifying the nature of pragmatics, particularly through the analysis of conversation. This will be discussed in the later part of this chapter.

## Applications of psycholinguistics

### 1. Cross-modality processing of single words

A variety of theories has been proposed as to the nature of the mental lexicon, as was discussed in Chapters 5 and 6, and we shall look here primarily at only one simplified model of lexical processing which has been commonly applied in analysing aphasic disorders (for a review of this and other models, see Harris and Coltheart, 1986, and Ellis and Young, 1988). This is a cross-modality model which employs a system of independent modules to account for the stages of mental processing which intervene between seeing a printed word and reading it aloud, hearing a word and understanding and/or spelling it, and so on. It will be presented here only in a simplified form.

The model assumes a central semantic or cognitive system in which meaning is processed (some models subdivide this into a verbal semantic system and a visual semantic system and/or a higher order conceptual system, but the working model currently being applied to aphasia leaves this question open). Use of this semantic system is either spontaneously initiated or achieved in response to a stimulus, usually through either an auditory word-recognition system or a visual word-recognition system. These word recognition systems are generally thought to include at least two major components: firstly a perceptual analysis and secondly a non-semantic lexicon specific to that input modality. Similarly on the output side, for the production of speech or writing, there are non-semantic lexicons specific to each of these modalities, each accessed prior to a further stage of output phonological or graphemic processing respectively.

This simplified working model therefore consists of four independent lexicons linked to the central semantic system, each with its attendant peripheral input or output processing module. (The assumption is made here of ordered stages of processing, though interactive and cascading models have also been convincingly proposed, as have versions which do not separate input and output lexicons).

The process of repeating a heard word, or reading a word aloud, or writing a word to dictation, does not have to traverse all these hypothesized modules. For each process there are thought to be routes which by-pass the lexicons, but go directly from perceptual input to the output processing (an orthographic-phonological conversion route, for example, used in reading aloud non-words or unfamiliar words, which obviously cannot be represented in a lexicon since they do not already exist as words). Some models also propose that there are routes which go directly from input lexicon to output lexicon, without traversing the semantic system; this would account for the ability (for example) to read words aloud without comprehending meaning even when the ability to read non-words is also lost, a condition in which neither the route via semantics nor the orthographic-phonological conversion route is available.

There are two innovatory aspects about the application of even this simplified model to aphasia. First, it is based on studies of language processing in normal subjects, with later refinements from studies of aphasic (including alexic and agraphic) subjects; it therefore appears to have some psychological validity. Secondly it lends itself directly to a rationale for therapy; patients' disorders can be related to a particular impairment in specific modules and appropriate strategies devised for either strengthening the impaired module and its connections or using strategies which by-pass it (Lesser 1987, in press b). Naming, for example, may be affected by a variety of underlying processing impairments. There may be a disturbance to the semantic component (affecting specific categories or, more commonly, a generalized difficulty in accessing semantics or assembling semantic elements in a degraded semantic system). Another possible difficulty may lie in mapping the meaning onto a complete phonological form in the output lexicon (although some partial information about the phonological form may frequently be achieved—interactive models can account for this more easily than a simple stage model). Further problems may lie in assembling the phonological form once achieved, or in planning the phonetic execution of the phonological form or in actually executing this. For each disturbance it is reasonable to assume that the appropriate treatment must differ (Lesser, in press c). This application of psycholinguistics to aphasia is therefore currently a very rewarding one for speech therapists, and lends itself easily to case studies of patients with naming difficulties either with pictures or with written words, expressed either in speech or spelling. In the simplified form described here it provides a manageable framework for hypothesis-based intervention which can form a routine part of work in the clinic.

The response of patients to therapy aimed at remediating impairments defined by such a model provides one means by which the model can be tested and refined or redrawn. Another means currently being developed is by the use of brain imaging techniques. Petersen, Fox, Posner, Mintun and Raichle (1988) have undertaken a study using PET to examine changes in regional blood flow during lexical processing by 17 normal volunteers. A series of six to ten scans were made of each subject at ten minute intervals while they performed tasks designed to increase in difficulty, so that the effect on blood flow of an easier task could be subtracted from the effect of the next one. The first task compared passive visual fixation on a point with passively looking at or hearing a word. The next task added the requirement to speak the word, and the next one to say a use for the presented word (i.e. production of an associate). The PET scans showed relatively few areas of activation added by each task, so that a clear picture emerged of distinct areas activated by auditory and visual presentation in the passive condition. This is consistent with the proposed division into modalities of input in the cognitive neuropsychological model. The visual tasks did not engage areas thought to be involved in phonological coding, giving no support to an alternative model which claims that reading is mediated through phonology. Sensory specific information appeared to have independent access to semantics and to output modes. Moreover, simple repetition of a heard or seen word did not activate the area concerned with semantic processing. This seminal study therefore provides some objective evidence for the biological validity of some aspects of the cognitive model proposed, in particular for the modular nature of language processing. It does not, however, provide support for the classical localization of language functions. Semantic processing was found to be located (contrary to expectation) in the frontal rather than temporal region of the brain.

## 2. Processing sentences

The processing of single words provides a limited framework for examining aphasia, useful though it is proving in respect of certain aspects of the disorder. Models of grammatical processing have not been able to draw on the same basis of experimental data as have models of lexical processing. The model currently being applied in examining disorders of grammar in aphasia, that proposed by Garrett (1982), has been based, not on experimental data, but on empirical colletions of spontaneous speech errors from normal subjects. Nevertheless there have been some claims made by theoretical linguists that their grammars have psychological validity, and aspects of these grammars have been used as a conceptual framework through which to examine the processing of sentences in aphasia. These are two derivations of the linguistic theories of transformational grammar in their more recent versions i.e. Bresnan's (1978) lexicalist grammar and Chomsky's (1981) government-binding theory. An introduction to these theories can be found in Sells (1985).

Lexicalist grammars allocate to the lexicon functions which earlier transformational grammars had attributed to the syntactic component. The passive form of verbs, for example, is considered to be included within the lexicon, rather than being computed as a syntactic operation in which an active sentence is transformed into a passive one. Bresnan argues this partly on the practical grounds that it is much easier to retrieve items from a lexicon than to compute them by syntactic operations, and that grammars should therefore maximise the lexical component and minimize the syntactic. It is proposed, therefore, that lexical entries for predicative words such as verbs include specifications for their functional structure i.e. the permissible grammatical relations into which they can enter. The active form of a verb, e.g. *eating*, would therefore have a different functional structure from its passive form, *eaten*. The functional structure of a verb is not the same as its semantics (its sense and any semantic entailments), nor even, in Bresnan's exposition, with the thematic roles into which it can enter, such as agent, theme, source, goal. It is, rather, conceived of as a specifically grammatical functional structure; it would, for example, specify two distinct structures for a verb like *give* for which either double objects ("He gives the baby a toy") or to-objects ("He gives a toy to the baby") are acceptable.

Zatorski and Lesser (1981) tested a prediction that follows from Bresnan's claim; that is that anomic but non-agrammatic patients would have problems with to-complements, since these are specified within the lexical component of the grammar, but not with question inversion, since this is speified within the syntactic component. Their study of four patients, using a story completion, story repetition and story re-telling technique, supported by the prediction. In a second experiment looking at comprehension as well as elicited speech (Lesser, 1984), fluent aphasics were shown to be more impaired than agrammatic patients on understanding to-complements of the type "The donkey is inclined to kick" and "The donkey is fun to kick". Although the agrammatic patients made more errors than control subjects on this and other types of sentences (using verbs of directional motion such as "follow", or verbs of aggression such as "hit") their pattern of responses was similar to those of the control subjects, and there was no evidence of exceptional difficulty with the to-complement sentences. Fluent aphasics, in contrast, found these types of sentences particularly difficult to understand, including the ones where the gapped subject of the to-complement was the same as the sentence subject (as in "The donkey is inclined to kick"), although these had produced few errors from the other subject groups. These findings are compatible with the hypothesis that difficulties in lexical retrieval affect grammatical functions as well as semantics.

Comprehension of to-complements of a similar type formed one part of a syntactic comprehension battery used to examine a patient with mild agrammatism, apraxia of speech and anomia, but the linguistic theory to which they were related was a different one, i.e. Chomsky's (1981) government-binding (GB) theory. Hildebrandt, Caplan and Evans (1987) looked in particular at how this man interpreted "empty" categories, which refer to antecedent noun phrases in the sentence, and which GB theory identifies as traces ("t"s). In the sentence about the donkey given above, for example, the gapped subject of "to kick" would be described as a trace which was coreferential with the sentence subject, and labelled as a PRO structure. A PRO structure has the properties of both + anaphor (in that it refers to an antecedent and is bound by the governing category of that antecedent) and + pronominal (in that its antecedent noun phrase occurs outside its governing category); the result of this is that such constructions are limited in occurrence to embedded sentences containing infinitive verbs. Another class of empty Noun Phrases (NPs) represented by traces is that of WH-traces, as in "Who does John like?", where the object "Who" has been moved to the beginning of the sentence, this movement being acknowledged by a trace in the object position. WH-traces are classed as – anaphor and – pronominal. Reflexives, on the other hand, (as in "Patrick told Joe that Eddie had scratched himself") are overt NPs which are classed as + anaphor and – pronominal. This means that the reflexive must be coreferential with an antecedent occurring within the same domain i.e. Eddie in the sentence above, and not Patrick or Joe.

Hildebrandt and her colleagues used a procedure in which the patient, KG, was asked to act out sentences manipulating toy animals or dolls when a sentence was read out to him. Some of the sentences contained empty categoris. Of these KG had particular difficulties with – pronominal ones and sentences which used "seemed" or "appeared" (NP raising). Sentences which were + pronominal and relatively easy, such as "John promised Bill to shave", became more difficult when an extra referential dependency was introduced in the shape of a reflexive ("John promised Bill to shave himself"). Evidently it was not so much the processing of empty categories, or of reflexives or of thematic roles as such which presented difficulties to KG as, rather, a limitation of capacity, such that each complexity added interacting difficulties. The authors' interpretation of the difficulty with the "seem" NP-raising sentences, for example, was that in such sentences the thematic role of the subject cannot be assigned until the final verb has been reached. The problem seemed to lie in the necessity to hold items in a parser, while other processing demands are maintained. This could not be attributed to a memory deficit as such, since KG's span for single words and digits was relatively good, and the authors emphasize that the memory demands "arise *internal* to the parsing operation after a syntactic structure is created" (p. 301).

Caplan and Hildebrandt (1988) have used their technique to make a specific comparison between predictions made about sentence comprehension in government-binding theory and lexical functional grammar. Four of the patients from their studies showed dissociations in the types of sentences which they had difficulty in understanding, which could be accounted for best in terms of government-binding theory. Double dissociations were found between structures with NP–trace and structures with + PRO, and also between structures with + PRO and WH–trace. Caplan and Hildebrandt note, however, that other inferences have to be made in their interpretation of the pattern of comprehension errors i.e. that patients use heuristic strategies to compensate for their difficulties, and that the local processing load on the mental parser for sentences is influential.

A similar proposal of trade-off in difficulties in processing syntax was made by Linebarger, Schwartz and Saffran (1983), but in terms of semantic operations interacting with syntactic. Linebarger and her colleagues found that patients classed as having agrammatic comprehension on picture-choice tests retained in many respects the ability to judge whether sentences were grammatical or not: their comprehension of syntax as such, therefore, appeared to be largely retained, despite their inability to cope with both syntax and semantics on the picture-choice tests. It may be that "agrammatic aphasics are simply less efficient parsers than normal listeners", that "where substantial syntactic analysis is called for, semantic processing may be unusually 'shallow'" and that aphasics are unable to back-up over the sentence ambiguities. This kind of explanation, while maintaining the notion of separate modules for semantic and syntactic processing, suggests how an impairment in one can have an effect on the operation of the other. As Saffran and Schwartz (1988) have pointed out, however, the notion of impaired ability to cope with processing load in parsing needs to be modified. Agrammatic patients' judgements of the plausibility of sentences is not made worse if the sentences are padded out with inessential material (e.g. "As the sun rose, *the worm* in the cool wet grass *swallowed the bird* quickly and went away"); it is impaired, however, if the canonical order of the NP arguments has been changed ("We saw the bird that the worm swallowed" "The bird was swallowed by the worm").

The last decade has seen a flowering of accounts of the nature of agrammatism, not least the proposal that there is no such syndrome (Badecker and Caramazza, 1985) and that individual explanations need to be sought for apparently agrammatic or paragrammatic speech and comprehension. The validity of making a distinction between agrammatism and paragrammatism has been questioned, since they share many cardinal features and have been contrasted primarily by disparity in fluency, which may be a quite separate factor from syntax (Goodglass and Menn, 1985). A study by Bates, Friederici and Wulfeck (1987), comparing aphasic listeners in Italian, German or English and also using the method of asking subjects to act out sentences they heard, found, in fact, that the comprehension of grammatical words and inflections was vulnerable in all types of patients in all the languages. Indeed Broca's aphasics were better able to take advantage of a convergence of grammatical cues (i.e. word order and agreement) than were Wernicke's aphasics; moreover deficits in morphology of this kind occurred also in aging and when non-aphasic subjects were under stress. Nonetheless, Friederici (1988b) prefers to interpret such results as indicating that "the underlying impairment of agrammatics and paragrammatics may well be distinct and (that) the observed similarities are due to processes of a central processing component which serves as a basis for interpretation" (p. 279); off-line tasks (such as matching words to pictures) are influenced by compensatory strategies (and do not distinguish the two types of grammatical disorders), while on-line tasks (such as responding to probes of sensitivity to priming) reveal the underlying processing which distinguishes the types.

The label of agrammatism has been attached to a heterogeneous set of symptoms. Some patients omit main verbs, others nominalize them; some keep inflections despite limited sentence structure, others omit them or produce them incorrectly. A variety of explanations has attempted to capture the generality of this heterogeneous syndrome. As well as the multicomponent theories in terms of processing overload, grammatical impairments have been accounted for as a phonological disorder affecting unstressed words or clitics (Kean, 1979), or as a specific impairment in use of grammatical words in their syntactic though not semantic roles (Zurif 1980) or in their automatic processing (Friederici, 1982, 1988 a). Specific problems in processing word order have been suggested (Saffran, Schwarz and Marin, 1980; Saffran and Schwartz, 1988) and accounted for in terms of difficulty in mapping thematic roles (agent, theme etc) onto syntactic structure (subject, object). It seems, however, that sensitivity to how word order as such reflects thematic roles in simple active and comparative sentences (e.g. "The pencil is longer than the twig") is lost only in the most severely impaired patients. It has also been suggested that some aphasics with grammatical disturbances in speech may have particular difficulty with verbs (McCarthy and Warrington, 1985), and this has been interpreted as due to the fact that all argument structure representations of a verb are activated when it is heard, even those not relevant to the particular sentence (Grodzinksy and Shapiro, 1988). Verbs do not present the same difficulties to all aphasic patients, however: some have been described whose retrieval of verbs is superior to that of nouns (Miceli, Silveri, Nocentini and Caramazza, 1988; Zingeser and Berndt, 1988), and difficulty in naming verbs can be dissociated from difficulty in comprehending them (Miceli et al, 1988).

Indeed the claim discussed in Chapter 7 that agrammatism is necessarily a central disorder of syntax which impairs both comprehension and production has been refuted by a number of studies in which patients classed as agrammatic on the basis of their speech production have performed well on tests of comprehension (Miceli, Mazzucchi, Menn and Goodglass, 1983; Kolk, Van Grunsver and Keyser, 1985). On the other hand the large-scale international study of agrammatism aimed at distinguishing universal and language-specific aspects of grammatical impairment has produced data which show that in the majority (though not all) of the cases comprehension and production do appear to be linked (Obler and Menn, 1988).

How can these varied views be reconciled, other than by proposing idiosyncratic problems in each individual? A preliminary attempt to propose a model, sufficiently complex to incorporate many of these proposals, while being sufficiently manageable to act as a diagnostic framework for therapy, has been made by applying Garrett's (1982) psycholinguistic model of sentence production (Schwartz, 1987; Lesser, 1987). Garrett's model distinguishes five levels of representation in the mental processes underlying sentence production: these representations are, respectively, the message level, the functional level, the positional level, the phonetic level and the articulatory level. The message level is linked to the functional level by a search through the semantic lexicon, in which the action which is to take the form of the verb plays a key role. At the functional level thematic roles, which the verb's argument structure dictates, become specified e.g. who-does-what-to-who, ("put", for example, dictates that a "where" role must be introduced). The functional level is essentially abstract and formless; for example no distinction is yet made between potentially active or passive forms in surface structure. Form and order has to be achieved at the positional level, and this is done on the one hand by retrieval of the appropriate items in the phonological lexicon which correspond to the selected semantic items, and on the other hand by the creation of a syntactic planning frame, or tree structure, into which these items will slot in order like a "scan-copier" (Shattuck-Hufnagel, 1983). The appropriate grammatical inflections are attached to this frame and the phonetic level of representation acts on the output so that the correct form of inflections is used, for example, the syllabic or non-syllabic form of the plural /z/ in "bridges" or "birds". We know this from the evidence of speech errors, since if words are transposed in error, the inflection becomes appropriately realized.

The schema suggests a number of points at which sentence production may breakdown. A problem in verb retrieval could have major consequences; even if the semantic information was available, the argument structure might not be. In turn, even if the argument structures of the verbs were fully available, problems could occur in mapping the thematic roles on to the appropriate NPs which realize the syntactic functions of subject and object. Difficulties could occur in creating a planning frame as such, or in selecting inflections. The sentence might also abort if there were difficulties in mapping the semantic information onto a phonological form (as in some kinds of word-retrieval/naming problems) or in the sequential ordering of the lexical or phonological forms where possibilities of confusion arise through semantic or phonological similarity with other items in the string. This model therefore has potential for accounting for many of the grammatical disturbances which occur in aphasia (as well as in the speech errors of normal subjects, on which it was based).

Sketchy though the model is, implications from it for therapy for grammatical disorders have already been applied. An implication of the model is that processes at and between the message and functional levels are "central" and that the mapping of thematic relations concerns sentence comprehension as well as production. Jones (1986) and Byng (Byng and Coltheart, 1986; Byng, in press) have reported on successful therapy with patients with long-lasting agrammatism; the therapy focussed on restoring the ability to understand and map thematic roles on to syntactic frames. In Byng's study improvement was assessed partly by performance on picture-choice tests of reversible sentences, partly by Saffran, Berndt and Schwartz's (1987) method of analysis of spontaneous or elicited narrative. Amongst other measures this characterizes each utterance (prosodically defined) as sentence, noun phrase, verb phrase, topic/comment etc., counts the lexical content (number of open class words, determiners, verbs, pronouns etc) and specifies the morphological and structural complexity (embeddings, auxiliaries, verb inflections etc). Another method of analysing narrative or other connected speech, which has been used with aphasic adults, is Crystal's (1982) PRISM-G. This interprets the semantic functions, or thematic roles, of clause elements as e.g. Actor, Experiencer, Dynamic Activity, Static Process, Goal, Locative, Temporal. Where the clause elements are word sequences, they are further specified in terms of Scope, Attribute, Definiteness, Possessive, Quantity.

The number and type of deictics are also tallied.

Evaluation of the effectiveness of intervention based on these models is valuable, not only for demonstrating the effectiveness (or not) of therapy, but for the information it can feed back into modification of the models in the light of patients' behaviours. Methods of evaluation which can be applied in working clinics are discussed by Howard (1986) and Pring (1986). But evaluation is dependent on the availability of reliable measures for testing and re-testing performance. Saffran et al's measures of elicited speech provide one means. Complementary ones are in the psycholinguistic batteries being developed by Lecours and his colleagues in Montreal and by Lesser, Coltheart and Kay in England and Australia. The latter, to be published as PALPA (Psycholinguistic Assessments of Language Processing in Aphasia) (Kay, Lesser and Coltheart, in preparation) provides a comprehensive set of materials for examining every stage in the hypothesised cognitive neuropsychological model described above. It includes, for example, measures of semantic judgements, lexical decision, homonym judgement, picture naming, repetition, spelling, letter discrimination, reading of words differing in length or regularity of spelling, phonemic discrimination and comprehension of reversible or gapped sentences. The measures are controlled for variables which are expected to influence results, such as word frequency and imageability. It is hoped that the availability of measures such as these will make the interpretation of patients' language abilities against a model which provides hypotheses for remediation a routine practice in speech therapy clinics.

## Applications of sociolinguistics

In this section we move to an examinaton of how aphasia has been studied in respect of the use of language in functional communication, or pragmatics i.e. the relationship between the language user and the world around him or her. This particularly includes the social aspects of language, and is therefore of interest to the branch of linguistics known as sociolinguistics.

The interest of sociolinguists in aphasia, however, is relatively recent. It has focussed so far principally on such matters as code-switching in bilingual speakers (Perecman, 1984), and on the analysis of conversation. As usual there are converging streams in the study of aphasia, and before we look at how the clinical and sociolinguistic streams are beginning to mingle, in the same way as the clinical and psycholinguistic streams have already mingled so perceptively, let us consider separately both the pre-sociolinguistic clinical approach and the non-clinical sociolinguistic approach to the examination of communication.

## 1. Clinical measures of "functional communication"

Many aphasia therapists have attempted to devise measures of functional communication which avoid the pitfalls of formal tests, and which can be used to test and re-test what is after all the prime aim of therapy, the patient's success in using natural language and effective communication. We have already referred to the earliest one of these to be published with reliability and validation data, Taylor's (later Taylor Sarno's) Functional Communication Profile (1953, 1965). This rates the patient on 45 language-related activities (grouped under the headings of "movement", "speaking", "understanding", "reading" and "other"). Examples of these are "indicating floor to elevator operator", "saying own name", "understanding television", "reading street signs" and "handling money". Information on these activities can be obtained from a semi-structured interview, supplemented by information given by other carers.

This early attempt to scan functional communication has been followed by other clinical explorations, some of them as broad in scope, others looking more closely at selected aspects of conversation, such as patients' comprehension or production of the speech act of requesting. The term "speech act" draws attention to the fact that the grammatical form of a sentence frequently does not correspond to the speaker's intention—the illocutionary force of the utterance. For example intended questions are often couched as grammatical statements ("I wonder if...") and intended requests are typically grammatically couched as questions ("Could you please...?"; Shouldn't you be...?"; "Must you keep on...?"). (For a list of other speech acts, grouped under the headings of ritualizing, informing, feeling and controlling, which the aphasia therapist should be aware of in interactions in patients, see Davis and Wilcox, 1985, p. 138).

Studies undertaken in the late 1970s suggest that most aphasic patients retain sensitivity to the illocutionary force of utterances. Wilcox, Davis and Leonard (1978) made videotapes of 40 situations, each taking about half a minute, in which a person responded either appropriately or inappropriately to an indirect request. The grammatical form was a question using a modal in either affirmative or negative form ("Can you ...", "Can't you ..."), although in both cases the request was positive. Ten aphasic patients who scored as having good comprehension on the BDAE performed well in judging which videotape illustrated the appropriate reply (the performing of the action) or the inappropriate (saying "yes"). Even the eight aphasic patients who scored low on BDAE comprehension performed at 86% correct on this task. A second experiment, in which the indirect request was *not* to perform an action, although the grammatical form did not include a negative ("Must you ...?", "Should you ...?"), presented more difficulty to the patients, in that they were less certain that the response of ceasing the activity was the appropriate one. It is notable that this condition requires comprehension of the grammatical words, as well as of the intent of the utterance, whereas in the first experiment the intent of the speaker can be understood equally well if the modals are not processed.

Speech acts of this kind have been incorporated into two structured assessments of functional communication in aphasia, Communicative Abilities in Daily Living (CADL) (Holland, 1980) and the Edinburgh Functional Communication Profile (Skinner, Wirz, Thompson and Davidson, 1984) (although the latter's stated prime intention is as an observation schedule of communication in the elderly, rather than specifically in aphasia). Of the 68 items in CADL, 21 assess the patient's ability to produce the speech acts of explaining, requesting, reporting, negotiating, advising and correcting misinformation. Other items test the ability to use social conventions and non-verbal communication in the context of a relatively natural situation (albeit in a structured framework in the clinic). Ten of the test items require role playing with pictures and "props" (e.g. "Let's pretend this is a doctor's office") and other items are presented as more formal tasks (e.g. generating divergent alternatives, choosing an appropriate picture for a metaphor). The patient's responses are scored on a 3-point scale in terms of effective communication, regardless of how this is achieved. For example a written or gestured response to "How old are you?" would achieve the maximum score of 2, if the correct information was given, while communicating any age would score as 1, and an inappropriate repetition of the patient's name to this question would score 0.

CADL requires some play-acting from the tester as well as the patient, not only admitted, as in the role-playing activities, but unadmitted, as when the tester (having earlier left his or her jacket on a chair) asks, apparently naturally when about to terminate the session, "Do you know what I did with my jacket?". This method of structuring a naturalistic situation so that a response from the patient can be predicted was used by Prinz (1980) in order to elicit requesting strategies from aphasic patients. In his structured interview, the content of the exchange is immaterial to ten items which are incorporated incidentally. The investigator, for example, asks the patient to sign his name, but does not give him a pencil; when this is supplied after the patient's request, the pencil is blunt; on the patient's further request, a pen is supplied and the patient is asked to sign his name where the X is on the paper, but there are three Xs so that a further request is required. Too much of this might reduce the patient's confidence in the efficiency of the clinician—particularly when an item is incorporated in which the clinician returns from fetching a drink with a large bandage around his neck—but nevertheless this research assessment illustrates the principle that the communication of aphasic patients needs to be examined in naturalistic settings as well as in structured.

Prinz's study showed that even a globally aphasic patient was able to use requesting acts appropriately, and this type of measure may have potential in distinguishing aphasia from dementia. Bayles and Slauson (described in Bayles and Kaszniak, 1987) are using a similar technique in a study of Alzheimer disease patients with differing degrees of dementia. The structured conversational interaction tasks used in their assessment comprise greetings and closing behaviours, as well as reactions to incorrect information, to incomplete information, to a compliment and to a gift.

The Edinburgh Functional Communication Profile, like Taylor's FCP, offers an observation schedule for a semi-naturalistic conversation rather than an itemised interview, although it does not attempt to be as comprehensive as either FCP or CADL. Six language functions are to be noted from the recorded conversation between the patient and the clinician (although, as with the FCP, other carers may need to be asked to supply supplementary information). The language functions to be rated are those of greeting, acknowledging, responding, requesting, propositional communication and verbal problem-solving. Like CADL this assessment therefore uses the terminology of "speech acts" in a somewhat loose way. "Requesting" is examined, for example, not from the linguistic perspective of comparison of grammatical form and speaker's intent, but according to whether and how the patient attracts attention, and whether the request is for an object, an action or information. "Verbal problem solving" appears to be used to assess the ability to produce narrative or procedural discourse, since the patient is asked questions such as "How did you manage to get here today?" and "How would you manage if you needed to ask for help?" The patient's behaviour under each of the twelve sub-headings used is rated for five modalities: speech, gesture, facial expression, vocal productions (other than speech) and writing, each being rated on a 10-point scale. A revised edition of the EFCP is due for publication in 1989 (Skinner, personal communication), which will supplement an analysis schedule similar to the present profile with two other sections: a structured interview designed to help elicit communication particularly with patients who have not produced enough spontaneous communication for the first analysis, and an interaction analysis of particular relevance to the severely linguistically disordered who use several modalities.

Two assessments which are based on a clearer exposition of pragmatics within linguistic theory are those of Prutting and Kirchner (1987) and Penn (1985), the latter being an adaptation of an earlier version of the former. Prutting and Kirchner's Pragmatic Protocol lists 30 aspects of communicative behaviour which can be rated as being appropriate or inappropriate from observation of a 15 minute spontaneous conversation between the patient and a familiar partner. Five of these aspects concern prosody and intelligibility, and seven non-verbal communication. The 18 "verbal aspects" are categorized as concerned with speech acts, topic use, turn-taking, lexical selection and stylistic variation. Though designed originally for use with children, the Protocol has been used to describe the communicative interactions of brain-damaged adults. Prutting and Kirchner describe the results of eleven adults with left-hemisphere damage, the range of whose ratings on the Protocol was from 63 to 93 (out of 100). As a group they were rated as inappropriate in respect of fluency (45%), variety of speech acts (45%), pause time (64%) and quantity (82%). A comparison group of adults with right brain damage received individual ratings varying from 60 to 100; as a group they showed a similar degree of inappropriateness in communication as did the left-brain damaged, though of a different character i.e. quantity (50%), adjacency in turn-taking (50%), contingency in turn-taking (i.e. taking up the other partner's topic appropriately), prosody (50%) and eye-gaze (60%). This is an important demonstration of the value of distinguishing between pragmatic and other aspects of communication, and of the fact that right-brain damaged people who are not classed as aphasic may nevertheless have as great an impairment in functional communication.

Penn's (1985) own version of a similar protocol, the Profile of Communicative Appropriateness (PCA), was devised particularly for aphasic adults and has been used to study types of aphasic communication in more detail. The PCA uses a 5-point scale for degrees of appropriacy, and considers six groups of communicative behaviours: response to interlocutor (e.g. clarification request), control of semantic content (e.g. topic shift), cohesion (e.g. use of indirect speech acts) and non-verbal communication (in which Penn includes prosody, as well as kinesics and proxemics). Fourteen aphasic patients with different ratings for severity on the BDAE were rated on the PCA and the results "suggested that communicative competence is often well retained in aphasia and that difficulties pattern those of normals, occurring however with greater frequency" (p. 22). The results did not reflect the types of aphasia other than a broad relationship with degree of severity.

A survey of other comprehensive clinical assessments of pragmatics in aphasia is provided by Davis and Wilcox (1985).

## 2. Sociolinguistic influences on assessing aphasia

Some of the clinical assessments, as is evident from the account above, have begun to draw on some aspects of sociolinguistic theory, though using the terminology and ideas with a degree of fluidity. The detailed examination of conversation by sociolinguists, however, has been continuing since the devising of these clinical measures, and a complementary approach to these clinical assessments is one which examines in detail a natural conversation in which the patient is participating (Lesser and Milroy, 1987). This follows the example of sociolinguists in exploring nonprescriptively the varieties of normal language through various means of observing and analysing language in natural settings, such as joining the language user's social network by being introduced as a "friend of a friend", whose tape recorder will quickly become unobtrusive (Milroy, 1987).

Sociolinguistics has demonstrated the importance, not only of social networks in resisting or developing phonological and syntactic changes and communicative styles, but also in a broader context the influences on language of social class, age, gender and ethnicity. Also influential are the circumstances in which the language data are collected, formal interview or casual eavesdropping, and the relationship between the speaker and the enquiring linguist. Clinical settings lend themselves more easily to the formal approach, with its unequal relationship between therapist and patient (often complicated by differences in age and sex), with consequent limitations in facilitating the collection of samples of natural language. Most of the clinical assessments of functional communication described above have made no distinction between data collected in structured conversations between the therapist and the patient, or collected between members of a family at home. The author of CADL, Holland (1982), however, recognised this distinction in attempting also to examine functional communication by getting observers to follow a patient around for two hours at home and while shopping, etc., tallying the patient's communicative behaviours according to a schedule. The categories tallied were somewhat broad in terms of current sociolinguistic practice (e.g. answers questions, teases, interrupts, responds to phonemic cues, gestures to maintain conversation, talks on 'phone), but the intention was the laudible one of obtaining truly naturalistic data in a variety of situations. The study distinguished four patterns of communicative behaviour in the patients in terms of degrees of effective communication, and noted strategies used by them which have potential usefulness in planning therapy (such as using circumlocutions or spelling aloud).

Formal tests of language are near the polar extreme of methods of data collection of language, although they may have the advantage for the therapist of being comprehensive and economical of time. It is easy to forget that 'being tested' is an unfamiliar activity to most adults in the age group in which aphasia most commonly occurs. Lesser (1979) reported on the difficulty experienced by the relatives of aphasic patients, who were being used as normal controls, in constructing three-word descriptions of shapes in a production version of a modified Token Test, and commented on the effects of a test situation on people naive to testing. A standard of what is normal, based on people who have actually volunteered to be tested, should be treated with caution.

Another problem with tests requiring convergent responses is that they do not distinguish between pathological and vernacular responses. Milroy (1987) cites examples of speech recorded from patients ("He writing the homework". "She my best friend") which could be cited as examples of agrammatism in the speech community in which they were recorded, but which would be perfectly acceptable responses in Black English. One important message from sociolinguistics, therefore, is that "normal" spoken language varies widely from different communities and different speakers and different circumstances.

Spoken language is also quite distinct from written language, and is typically characterised by ambiguity, incompleteness and repetition. It is primarily a social activity, and requries a different analysis from either that appropriate to written language or to the abstract grammars of theoretical linguists.

## 3. Analysis of conversation

Conversation has been studied both in terms of its structure and how meaning is conveyed. The structure of conversation is founded on turn-taking, in which one speaker has the floor at a time, swift transitions are common and there is very little overlapping. Ellis and Beattie (1986) summarise studies which have examined the turn-taking component of conversation: participants predict possible completion points, and a current speaker selects the next speaker, who assumes the floor when a transition-relevance place occurs. The latter may be signalled by changes in intonation, eye-gaze or kinesics; the last syllable may be prolonged, the final pitch change exaggerated, there may be a gesture of relaxation (Wardhaugh, 1985). Such an analysis emphasises the dependency of turn-taking on signals of facial expression and prosody and implies that the non-aphasic right-brain-damaged might perhaps experience some difficulty with this aspect of conversation, although even the severely aphasic left-brain-damaged may not. If pauses are filled (by "well", "er" "ah" etc.), the speaker may continue to hold the floor while cognitive processing is taking place, and this is a normal behaviour which aphasic patients may need to be encouraged to cultivate, when they need more time for cognitive processing.

The structure of conversation is also characterised by repairs (generally self-initiated) and clarifications: the first depends on the ability to monitor oneself, the latter on the ability to monitor the listener's reactions. These are aspects of conversation in which some aphasics may be deficient, e.g. when paraphasias are produced without correction. Listeners generally tolerate a substantial degree of ambiguity without seeking clarification, on the presumption that the ambiguity will eventually be resolved, and errors are rarely corrected or remarked upon. In these aspects also clinical interactions between aphasic patient and therapist are unusual, and an implicit permission to make such corrections may be required and acted on with discretion.

With this development of the analysis of conversational structure, the extent to which aphasic difficulties in word-retrieval and grammar affect the structure of the conversations in which they participate is now beginning to be studied. Lubinski, Duchan and Weitzner-Lin (1980) studied the conversations of an aphasic woman with her husband and with her therapist in order to examine the repair of breakdowns due to search for words, mispronunciations, semantic paraphasias and inability to follow a topic shift. It is notable that two hundred and fifty repairs were used in response to only 23 breakdowns. In contrast to "normal" conversation, repairs were often initiated by the partner, and took the form of hints, guesses, WH questions, corrections, rejections, repetitions and reinforcements. Different types of repair pattern emerged e.g. hint-guess-resolution, correction-limitation, selfcuing-reinforcement. Repairs between an aphasic speaker and partner have also been studied by De Bleser and Weisman (1986). These researchers made videotapes of three model dialogues, all of which were concerned with dyadic negotiations. One situation was domestic: a wife wished to make vegetable soup, but her husband wanted to go out to eat. The two others were public situations: a shopper wanted a refund of money, but the sales assistant refused it as there was no sales slip; a traveller was in conflict with a customs officer in refusing to pay the necessary duty. These dialogues were watched by pairs of couples who did not know each other, and who were then asked to re-enact them twice, each playing both roles; in two couples the partner was a non-fluent aphasic. The interactions were analysed in terms of content units (e.g. introduction and continuation of a topic), conflict units relating to the negotiation (e.g. proposal of possible solutions) and language units (repairs, modelling, repetition etc). The non-aphasic partners adjusted their speech to maintain the co-operative nature of the conversation, typically using indirect repairs such as checking the partner's intention, rather than direct repairs such as corrections. These kinds of analyses differ significantly from the clinical assessments of functional communication described above, in that they examine the partner's communication as much as the patient's. They are therefore likely to lead more productively to inferences about how communication can be assisted, than would analyses which focus only on the patient. Some practical advice on how to transcribe and analyse conversations is given by Hopper, Koch and Mandelbaum (1986).

When we come to consider meaning in conversation, we need to remember that some sections of conversation are ritual chunks "so banal that they must have some other function than communication" (Wardhaugh, 1985, p.47). They may be a use of language in reinforcing solidarity (in which even abusiveness can play a part), or an avoidance of the embarrassment of silence. Routines such as greetings require a specific response, and we have noted how this has been used in the clinical assessments of functional communication. Much of conversation, however, is concerned with a more overt transmission of meaning, through selection, development and changes of topics. Topics have to be appropriate and developed by consensus, although a speaker can use devices to drop the topic or restructure it ("That reminds me...") or return to it ("As I was saying..."). Conversation works on cooperative principles and it is assumed that each speaker's contribution will be relevant, provide a suitable amount of information, be believable (unless signals are given that the speaker is using sarcasm, metaphor etc) and be matched to the listener's characteristics. As well as having openings and closings, topics are expected to have coherence, i.e. each contribution within the topic needs to make sense in respect of what has gone before.

Associated with coherence, but conceptually quite distinct from it, is cohesion— the use of devices by which parts of a topic are linked with each other e.g. by lexical substitutions, lexical repetition, conjunctions ("but..."), ellipsis and anaphoric pronouns. Texts can be cohesive but not coherent, or coherent but not cohesive (Newman, Lovett and Dennis, 1986), and the analysis of aphasic discourse requires both dimensions to be considered. Anaphora in particular (referring backwards to another linguistic entity which has the same identity) may need to be examined carefully in aphasia due to its necessary dependence on short term memory. Topics can be expanded through illustration, generalization, digression and return, and be linked through equivalence ("similarly"), alternation ("on the other hand"), causation ("because") and summarization ("so"). The extent to which these are deficient in aphasia has yet to be studied in detail.

Extended topics may take the form of narratives or description of procedures. Narratives represent past experience as a sequence of events which is followed temporally in the re-telling. Procedural discourse is similar in that a prescribed sequence must be followed, but in this case the account is of a repeatable activity or procedure, such as how to make a sandwich; it is therefore goal-oriented rather than person- or event-oriented. Ulatowska and her colleagues (Ulatowska, Doyel, Freedman-Stern, Macaluso-Haynes and North, 1983) have studied both procedural and narrative discourse in aphasia, and came to the conclusion that aphasics with moderate impairment retain the ability to produce well-structured discourse, although this is reduced in amount and complexity when compared with normal controls. The reduction of language in respect of discourse structure in these studies was in the decrease of optional steps in procedures and a smaller number of introductions; errors were made in the use of connectors and reference.

Despite errors at the sentential level, and some errors of fact in retelling the stories, aphasics' narratives also included all necessary structures, such as settings, complicating actions and resolutions, although including fewer episodes and optional codas, abstracts and evaluations.

The relative preservation of discourse and conversational structures in aphasia suggests that, even if the ability to construct and understand semantically and syntactically well-formed sentences is impaired, alternative communicative strategies can be used. Green (1984) has discussed the relevance of discourse analysis to therapy for aphasia, in particular in respect of training the patients' communication partners. She has stressed the need to incorporate components of normal conversation into treatment (Green, 1982) by maintaining the need to communicate, incorporating contextual settings, working with numerous speech acts and maintaining the need to communicate, incorporating contextual settings, working with numerous speech acts and maintaining linguistic realism. This has been good practice in some clinics for many years, particularly where, for example, use of occupational therapy settings has been available, or truly interactive group therapy has been used. But Green's papers provide salutary reminders that the blossoming of the application of linguistic theory to components of language up to the sentence level must not distract the therapist from using these applications in the service of communication rather than simply in their own right.

The evaluation of the effectiveness of intervention in respect of functional communication is yet to be satisfactorily achieved. One well-known programme of therapy, Promoting Aphasics' Communicative Efficiency (PACE) (Davis and Wilcox, 1984), which encourages a naturalistic interaction in the clinic in which the patient supplies "new" information to the therapist, is structured in such a way that quantification of responses is possible, and hence lends itself to evaluation of effectiveness. The means for examining whether intervention assists in a truly natural communicating situation, however, depends on the development and application of the descriptive techniques of conversational analysis from sociolinguistics described above.

The last decade has, therefore, seen heartening developments from the application of linguistics to aphasia. Further advances will occur in computational linguistics and in psychobiology, but already psycholinguistic models and sociolinguistic methodology have brought more systematic and scientific approaches to the understanding of the nature of language behaviour in aphasia and, no less significantly, to the art of aphasia therapy.

# References

## Abbreviations

| | |
|---|---|
| Am. J. Psych. | American Journal of Psychology |
| BJDC | British Journal of Disorders of Communication |
| B. J. Psych. | British Journal of Psychology |
| Int. J. Ment. Health | International Journal of Mental Health |
| J. Ch. Lang. | Journal of Child Language |
| J. Com. Dis. | Journal of Communication Disorders |
| J. Exp. Psych. | Journal of Experimental Psychology |
| J. Math. Psych. | Journal of Mathematical Psychology |
| JSHD | Journal of Speech and Hearing Disorders |
| JSHR | Journal of Speech and Hearing Research |
| JVLVB | Journal of Verbal Learning and Verbal Behavior |
| Q. J. Exp. Psych. | Quarterly Journal of Experimental Psychology |

AARONSON, D. 1974: Stimulus factors and listening strategies in auditory memory: a theoretical analysis. *Cognitive Psychology* **6**, 105-32.

ALAJOUANINE, T. and LHERMITTE, F. 1964: Non-verbal communication in aphasia. In A.V.S. De Reuck and M. O'Connor (eds), *Disorders of Language*. London: Churchill.

ALAJOUANINE, T., LHERMITTE, F., LEDOUX, RENAUD, D. amd VIGNOLO, L.A. 1964: Les composants phonémiques et sémantiques de la jargon aphasie. *Revue Neurologique* **110**, 5-20.

ALEXANDER, M.P., NAESER, M. and PALUMBO, C.L. 1987: Correlations of subcortical CT lesion sites and aphasia profiles. *Brain,* **110**, 961-991.

ALBERT, M.L. 1972a: Note: Auditory sequencing and left cerebral dominance for language. *Neuropsychologia* **10**, 245-8.

—1972b: Aspects de la compréhension auditive du language après lésion cérébrale. *Langages,* **25**, 37-51.

—1976: Short-term memory and aphasia. *Brain and Language* **3**, 28-33.

ALBERT, M. and BEAR, D. 1974: Time to understand. *Brain* **97**, 373-84.

ARBIB, M.A., CAPLAN, D. and MARSHALL, J.C. 1982: *Neural Models of Language Processes*, New York: Academic.

ASSAL, G. 1974: Note: Troubles de la reception auditive du langage lors de lésion du cortex cérébral. *Neuropsychologia 12,* 399-406.

ATEN, J.L., DARLEY, F.L., DEAL, S.L. and JOHNS, D. 1975: Comment on A.D. Martin's 'Some objections to the term "apraxia of speech"'. *JSHD* 40, 416-20.

ATEN, J.L., JOHNS, D. and DARLEY, F.L. 1971: Auditory perception of sequenced words in apraxia of speech. *JSHR* 14, 131-43.

AU, R., ALBERT, M.L. and OBLER, L.K. 1988: The relation of aphasia to dementia. *Aphasiology,* **2**, 161-73.

BACH, E. 1975: Order in base structure. In C.N. Li (ed.), *Word Order and Word Order Change*. Austin: University of Texas Press.

BADECKER, B. and CARAMAZZA, A. 1985: On consideration of method and theory governing the use of clinical categories in neurolinguistics and cognitive neuropsychology: the case against agrammatism. *Cognition,* **20,** 97-125.

BARRETT, R. 1961: *Some grammatical characteristics of aphasic speech*. PhD thesis, University of Michigan.

BARTON, M. 1971: Recall of generic properties of words in aphasic patients. *Cortex* **7,** 73-82.

BARTON, M., MARUSZEWSKI, M. and URREA, D. 1969: Variation of stimulus context and its effect on word-finding ability in aphasics. *Cortex* **5,** 351-65.

BASSO, A., DE RENZI, E., FAGLIONI, P., SCOTTI, G. and SPINNLER, H. 1973: Neuropsychological evidence for the existence of cerebral areas critical to the performance of intelligence tasks. *Brain* **96,** 715-28.

BASSO, A., FAGLIONI, P. and SPINNLER, H. 1976: Non-verbal colour impairment of aphasics. *Neuropsychologia* **14,** 183-93.

BASSO, A., CAPITANI, E. and MORASCHINI, S. 1982: Sex differences in recovery from aphasia. *Cortex,* **18,** 469-75.

BATES, E., FRIEDERICI, A. and WULFECK, B. 1987: Comprehension in aphasia: a cross-linguistic study. *Brain and Language*, **32,** 19-67.

BAY, E., 1966; The classification of disorders of speech. *Cortex* **3,** 26-31.

—1969: The Lordat case and its import on the theory of aphasia. *Cortex* **5,** 302-8.

BAYLES, K.A. and KASZNIAK, A.W. 1987: *Communication and Cognition in Normal Aging and Dementia*. London: Taylor and Francis.

BEAUMONT, J.G. 1974: Handedness and hemisphere function. In S.J. Dimond and J.G. Beaumont (eds.), *Hemipshere Function in the Human Brain*. London: Elek.

BEILIN, H. 1975: *Studies in the Cognitive Basis of Language Development*. New York: Academic.

BENDER, H.B. and FELDMAN, M. 1972: The so-called visual agnosias. *Brain* **95,** 173-86.

BENSON, D.F. 1967: Fluency in aphasia: correlation with radioactive scan localization. *Cortex* **3,** 373-94.

BENSON, D.F., CUMMINGS, J.L. and TSAI, S.Y. 1982: Angular gyrus syndrome simulating Alzheimer's disease. *Arch. Neurol.* **39,** 616-20.

BERLIN, B. and KAY, P. 1969: *Basic Color Terms: their Universality and Evolution*. Berkeley: University of California Press.

BERTAUX, D., LECOURS, A.R. and LHERMITTE, F. 1968: *Analogy between sequential errors in aphasia and the behaviour of a cybernetic system (SARF)* . Proceedings of IFAC Symposium on Technological and Biological Problems of Control, Yerevan.

BEVER, T.G. 1970: The cognitive basis for linguistic structures. In J.R. Hayes (ed.), *Cognition and the Development of Language*. New York: Wiley.

BEYN, E.S. and VLASENKO, I.T. 1974: Verbal paraphasias of aphasic patients in the course of naming actions. *BJDC* **9,** 24-34.

BISIACH, E. 1966: Perceptual factors in the pathogenesis of anomia. *Cortex* **2,** 90-95.

—1970: Characteristics of visual stimuli and naming performance in aphasic adults: comments on the paper by Corlew and Nation. *Cortex* **12,** 74-5.

BISHOP, D.V.M. 1988: Language development after focal brain damage. In D.V.M. Bishop and K. Mogford (eds.) *Language Development in Exceptional Circumstances*. Churchill Livingstone: Edinburgh.

BLAKE, M. 1973: Prediction of recognition when recall fails: exploring the feeling-of-knowing phenomenon. *JVLVB* **12,** 311-19.

BLISS, L.S. 1971: *Sentence repetition, evaluation and revision of behavior of aphasics as a function of grammaticality*. PhD thesis, University of Michigan.

BLISS, L.S., TIKOFSKY, R.S. and GUILDFORD, A.M. 1976: Aphasics' sentence repetition behavior as a function of grammaticality. *Cortex* **12,** 113-21.

BLOOM, L. 1974: Talking, understanding and thinking. In R.L. Schiefelbusch and L.L. Lloyd (eds.), *Language Perspectives, Acquisition, Retardation, Intervention*. Baltimore: University Park Press.

BLUMSTEIN, S. 1973: *A Phonological Investigation of Aphasic Speech*. Janua Linguarum Series Minor **153**. The Hague: Mouton.

—1974: Review of 'Generative Phonology—Evidence from Aphasia' by M. Schnitzer. *Cortex* **10**, 206.

BLUMSTEIN, S., BAKER, E. and GOODGLASS, H. 1977: Phonological factors in auditory comprehension in aphasia. *Neuropsychologia* **15**, 19-30.

BLUMSTEIN, S. and COOPER, W.E. 1974: Hemispheric processing of intonation contours. *Cortex* **10**, 146-58.

BLUMSTEIN, S. and GOODGLASS, H. 1972: The perception of stress as a semantic cue in aphasia. *JSHR* **15**, 800-806.

BOND, Z.S. 1976: On the specification of input units in speech perception. *Brain and Language* **3**, 72-87.

BOSSHARDT, H.G. and HÖRMANN, H. 1975: Temporal precision of coding as a basic factor of laterality effects in the retention of verbal auditory stimuli. *Acta Psychologica* **39**, 1-12.

BOTEZ, M.I., CARP, N. and MIHAILESCU, L. 1968: Prosody as a means of communication in aphasia. *Revue Roumaine de Neurologie* **5**, 197-202.

BOWER, G.H. and MINAIRE, H. 1974: On interfering with item versus order information in serial recall. *Am. J. Psych.* **87**, 557-64.

BOWERS, D., COSLETT, H.B., BAUER R.M., SPEEDIE, L.J. and HEILMAN, K.M. 1987: Comprehension of emotional prosody following unilateral hemispheric lesions: processing defect versus distraction defect. *Neuropsychologia* **25**, 317-28.

BRAIN, R. 1964: Statement of the problem. In A.V.S. De Reuck and M. O'Connor (eds.) *Disorders of Language*. London: Churchill.

—1975: *Speech Disorders: Aphasia, Apraxia and Agnosia*. London: Butterworths.

BRESNAN, J. 1978: A realistic transformational grammar. In M. Halle, J. Bresnan and G.A. Miller (eds.) *Linguistic Theory and Psychological Reality*. Cambridge, Mass.: MIT.

BROADBENT, D.E. 1974: Division of function and integration of behavior. In F.O. Schmitt and F.G. Worden (eds.), *The Neurosciences: third study program*. Cambridge, Mass.: MIT.

BROCA, P. 1865: Sur la siège de la faculté du langage articulé. reprinted in H. Hécaen and J. Dubois 1969, *La Naissance de la Neuropsychologie de Langage (1825-1865)*. Paris: Flammarion

BROOKSHIRE, R.H. 1972a: Visual and auditory sequencing by aphasic subjects. *J. Com. Dis.* **5**, 259-69.

—1972b: Effects of task difficulty on naming performance of aphasic subjects. *JSHR* **15**, 551-8.

BROWN, J.W. 1975a: The problem of repetition: a study of 'conduction' aphasia and the 'isolation' syndrome. *Cortez* **11**, 37-52.

—1975b: The neural organization of language: aphasia and neuropsychiatry. In S. Arieti (ed.), *American Handbook of Psychiatry, Vol. 4*. New York, Basic Books.

—1976: The neural organization of language: aphasia and lateralization. *Brain and Language* **3**, 482-94.

—1977: *Mind, Brain and Consciousness*. New York: Academic.

BROWN, R. and McNEILL, D. 1966: The 'tip-of-the-tongue' phenomenon. *JVLVB* **5**, 325-37.

BRYAN, K. 1986: Prosody and other language deficits after right cerebral hemisphere damage. Unpublished Ph.D. dissertation: University of Newcastle upon Tyne.

BUCKINGHAM, H.W., AVAKIAN-WHITAKER, H. and WHITAKER, H.A. 1975: Linguistic structures in stereotyped aphasic speech. *Linguistics* **154/5**, 5-13.

BUCKINGHAM, H.W. and KERTESZ, A. 1976: *Neologistic Jargon Aphasia*. Amsterdam: Swets and Zeitlinger.

BUCKINGHAM, H.W., WHITAKER, H.A. and WHITAKER, H. 1978: Alliteration and assonance in neologistic jargon aphasia. *Cortex* **14**, 365-80.

BYNG, S. in press: Sentence processing deficits: theory and therapy. *Cognitive Neuropsychology.*

BYNG, S. and COLTHEART, M. 1986: Aphasia therapy research: methodological considerations and illustrative results. In E. Hjelmquist and L.G. Nelsson (eds.) *Communication and Handicap: Aspects of Psychological Compensation and Technical Aids.* Amsterdam: Elsevier.

BYRNE, J.M. and GATES, R.D. 1987: Single-case study of left cerebral hemispherectomy: development in the first five years of life. *J. Clin. Exp. Neuropsychol.,* **9,** 423-34.

CANTER, G.J. 1969: *The influence of primary and secondary verbal apraxia on output disturbances in aphasic syndromes.* Paper presented at ASHA Convention, Chicago.

CAPLAN, D., KELLER, L. and LOCKE, S. 1976: Inflection of neologisms in aphasia. *Brain* **95,** 169-72.

CAPLAN, D. and HILDEBRANDT, N. 1988: Specific defects in syntactic comprehension. *Aphasiology* **2,** 255-8.

CAPPA, S.F. and VIGNOLO, L.A. 1988: Sex differences in the site of brain lesions underlying global aphasia. *Aphasiology,* **2,** 258-64.

CARAMAZZA, A. and ZURIF, E.B. 1976: Dissociation of algorithmic and heuristic processes in language comprehension. *Brain and Language* **3,** 572-82.

—1978: *The Acquisition and Breakdown of Language: Parallels and Divergencies.* Baltimore: Johns Hopkins.

CARMON, A. and NACHSHON, I. 1971: Effect of unilateral brain damage on the perception of temporal order. *Cortex* **7,** 410-18.

CARPENTER, P.A. 1974: On the comprehension, storage and retrieval of comparative sentences. *JVLVB* **13,** 401-11.

CARPENTER, R.L. and RUTHERFORD, D.R. 1971: *Acoustic cue discrimination in adult aphasia.* Paper presented at ASHA Convention.

CARROLL, J.B. and WHITE, M.N. 1973: Age of acquisition norms for 220 picturable nouns. *JVLVB* **12,** 563-76.

CARTER, J.F. 1969: *A linguistic feature study of aphasic responses to a free word association task.* PhD thesis, University of Maryland.

CHAPMAN, R.S. and MILLER, J.F. 1975: Word order in early two and three word utterances: does production precede comprehension? *JSHR* 18, 335-71.

CHOMSKY, C. 1969: *The Acquisition of Syntax in Children from 5 to 10.* Cambridge, Mass.: MIT.

CHOMSKY, N. 1957: *Syntactic Structures.* The Hague: Mouton.

—1965: *Aspects of the Theory of Syntax.* Cambridge, Mass.: MIT.

—1981: *Lectures on Government and Binding.* Dordrecht: Foris.

CHOMSKY, N. and HALLE, M. *The Sound Pattern of English.* New York: Harper and Row.

CHRISTENSEN, A.L. 1974: *Luria's Neuropsychological Investigation.* Copenhagen: Munksgaard Int. Pub.

CLARK, H. 1970: Word associations and linguistic theory. In J. Lyons (ed.), *New Horizons in Linguistics.* Harmondsworth: Penguin.

CLARK, H.H. and CARD, S.K. 1969: The role of semantics in remembering comparative sentences. *J. Exp. Psych.* **82,** 545-53.

CLARK, R., HUTCHINSON, S. and VAN BUREN, P. 1974: Comprehension production in language acquisition. *J. Linguistics* **10,** 39-54.

CODE, C. 1987: *Language, Aphasia and the Right Hemisphere.* Chichester: Wiley.

COHEN, G. 1973: Hemispheric differences in serial and parallel processing. *J. Exp. Psych.* **97,** 349-56.

COLLINS, A.M. and QUILLIAN, M.R. 1969: Retrieval time from semantic memory. *JVLVB* **8,** 240-47.

CONRAD, K. 1954: New problems of aphasia. *Brain* **77,** 491-509.

CONSOLI, S. 1973: Performances d'un groupe d'aphasiques à un test de discrimination phonémique. *J. de Psychologie Normale et Pathologique* **70,** 325-48.

COOPER, J.A. and FLOWERS, C.R. 1987: Children with a history of acquired aphasia: residual language and academic impairments. *JSHD,* **52,** 251-62.

CORKIN, S. 1974: Serial ordering deficits in inferior readers. *Neuropsychologia* **12,** 347-54.

CORLEW, M.M. 1971: *Word variables and confrontation naming in aphasic patients.* PhD thesis, Cape Western Reserve University.

CORLEW, M.M. and NATION, J.E. 1975: Characteristics of visual stimuli and naming performance in aphasic adults. *Cortex* **11,** 186-91.

CRYSTAL, D. 1969: *Prosodic Systems and Intonation in English.* London: Cambridge University Press.

—1971: *Linguistics.* Harmondsworth: Penguin.

—1975: *The English Tone of Voice.* London: Edward Arnold.

—1982: *Profiling Linguistic Disability* London: Edward Arnold.

—1988: Linguistic levels in aphasia. In F.C. Rose, R. Whurr and M.A. Wyke (eds.), *Aphasia.* London: Whurr.

CRYSTAL, D., FLETCHER, P. and GARMAN, M. 1976: *The Grammatical Analysis of Language Disability.* London: Edward Arnold.

DAMASIO, A. 1981: The nature of aphasia: signs and syndromes. In M.T. Sarno (ed.) *Acquired Aphasia.* New York: Academic.

DARLEY, F.L., 1968: *Apraxia of speech: 107 years of terminological confusion.* Paper presented to ASHA Convention.

DARLEY, F.L., ARONSON, A.E. and BROWN, J.R. 1975: *Motor Speech Disorders.* Philadelphia: Saunders.

DARWIN, C.J. 1986: The perception of speech. In E.C. Carterette and M.P. Friedman (eds.), *Handbook of Perception, Vol 7 Language and Speech.* New York: Academic.

DAVIS, G.A. and WILLCOX, M.J. 1985: *Adult Aphasia Rehabilitation: Applied Pragmatics.* San Diego: College Hill.

DE AJURIAGUERRA, J. and TISSOT, R. 1975: Some aspects of language in various forms of senile dementia. In E. Lenneberg and E. Lenneberg (eds.), *Foundations of Language Development, Vol. 1.* New York: Academic.

DEAL, J.L. 1974: Consistency and adaptation in apraxia of speech. *J. Com. Dis.* **7,** 135-40.

DEAL, J.L. and DARLEY, F.L. 1972: The influence of linguistic and situational variables on phonemic accuracy in apraxia of speech. *JSHR* **15,** 639-653.

DE BLESER, R. and WEISMAN, H. 1986: The communicative impact of non-fluent aphasia on the dialog behavior of linguistically unimpaired partners. In F. Lowenthal and F. Vandamme (eds.) *Pragmatics and Education.* New York: Plenum.

DEESE, J. 1965: *The Structure of Associations in Language and Thought.* Baltimore: Johns Hopkins.

—1970: *Psycholinguistics.* Boston: Allyn and Bacon.

DENNIS, M. 1976: Dissociated naming and locating of body parts after anterior temporal lobe resection: an experimental case study. *Brain and Language* **3,** 147-63.

DENNIS, M. and WHITAKER, H.H. 1976: Language acquisition following hemidecortication. *Brain and Language* **3,** 404-33.

DE RENZI, E. and FAGLIONI, P. 1965: The comparative efficiency of intelligence and vigilance tests in detecting hemispheric cerebral damage. *Cortex* **1,** 410-33.

DE RENZI, E. PIECZURO, A. and VIGNOLO, L.A. 1966: Oral apraxia and aphasia. *Cortex* **2,** 50-73.

DE RENZI, E. and VIGNOLO, L.A. 1962: The Token Test; a sensitive test to detect receptive disturbances in aphasia. *Brain* **85,** 665-78.

DEROUESNÉ, J. and LECOURS, A.R. 1972: Two tests for the study of semantic deficits in aphasia. *Int. J. Ment. Health* **1,** 14-24.

DETTERMAN, D.K. and BROWN, J. (in press): Order information in short term memory. *J. Exp. Psych.*

DE VILLIERS, J. 1974: Quantitative aspects of agrammatism in aphasia. *Cortex* **10,** 36-54.

DIAMOND, S.P., EPSTEIN, J. and BENDER, M.B. 1969: The paronym defect and verbal abstraction. *Cortex* **5,** 152-63.

DI CARLO, L.M. and TAUB, H.A. 1972: The influence of compression and expansion on the intelligibility of speech by young and aged aphasic (demonstrated c.v.a.) individuals. *J. Com. Dis.* **5,** 299-306.

DILLER, L. and WEINBERG, J. 1972: Differential aspects of attention in brain-damaged persons. *Perceptual and Motor Skills* **35,** 71-81.

DOEHRING, D.G. and SWISHER, L.P. 1972: Disturbances of connotative meaning in aphasia. *J. Com. Dis.* 5, 251-8.

DOKTOR, M. and TAYLOR, O.L. 1969: *A generative transformational analysis of syntactic comprehension in adult aphasics.* Paper presented to ASHA Convention.

DUBOIS, J., HÉCAEN, H., CUNIN, S., DAUMAS, M., LERVILLE-ANGER, B., and MARCIE, P. 1970: Analyse linguistique d'énoncés d'aphasiques sensoriels. *J. de Psychologie Normale et Pathologique* **2,** 185-206.

DUFFY, R.J., DUFFY, JR. and PEARSON, K.L. 1975: Pantomime recognition in aphasics. *JSHR* **18,** 115-32.

DUFFY, R.J. and ULRICH, S.R. 1976: A comparison of impairments in verbal comprehension, speech, reading and writing in adult aphasics. *JSHD* **41,** 110-19.

EFRON, R. 1963: Temporal perception, aphasia and déjà-vu. *Brain* **86,** 403-23.

EILERS, R.E., OLLER, D.K. and ELLINGTON, J. 1974: The acquisition of word meaning for dimensional adjectives: the long and short of it. *J. Ch. Lang,* **1,** 195-204.

EISENSON, J. 1954: *Examinining for Aphasia* New York: Appleton-Century-Crofts.

ELLIS, A.W. 1987: Intimations of modularity, or, the modelarity of mind: doing cognitive neuropsychology without syndromes. In M. Coltheart, G. Sartori and R. Job (eds.) *The Cognitive Neuropsychology of Language.* London: Lawrence Erlbaum.

ELLIS, A. and BEATTIE, G. 1986: *The Psychology of Language and Communication,* London: Weidenfeld and Nicolson.

ELLIS, A.W. and YOUNG, A.W.: 1988 *Human Cognitive Neuropsychology,* London: Lawrence Erlbaum.

ENGL, E.M. and VON STOCKERT, T.R. 1976: 'Ausländischer Akzent' bei Aphasie: eine Fallbeschreibung. In G. Peuser (ed.), *Interdisziplinäre Aspekte der Aphasieforschung.* Cologne: Rhineland.

EYSENCK, M.W. 1975: 'I remember you, you're . . .' *New Behaviour 2,* 222-3.

FILBY, Y., EDWARD, A.E. and SEACAT, G.F. 1963: Word length, frequency and similarity in the discrimination behavior of aphasics. *JSHR* **6,** 255-61.

FILLMORE, C.J. 1968: The case for case. In E. Bach and R.T. Harms (eds.), *Universals in Linguistic Theory,* New York: Holt, Rinehart and Winston.

FINK, R. 1969: *Experiments in the perception of intonation by aphasic and normal speakers of English.* PhD thesis, University of Rochester.

FLORES D'ARCAIS, G.B. in press: Automatic and controlled processes in language comprehension: evidence from psycholinguistics for cognitive neuropsyhcology. In G. Denes, C. Semenza, P. Bisiacchi and E. Andreewsky (eds.) *Perspectives in Cognitive Neuropsychology.* London, Lawrence Erlbaum.

FODOR, J.A., BEVER, T.G. and GARRETT, M.F. 1974: *The Psychology of Language.* New York: McGraw-Hill.

FORREST, D. 1977: The first experiments on word association. *Bulletin of the British Psychological Society* **30,** 40-42.

FOX, P.W. 1970: Patterns of stability and change in behaviours of free associations. *JVLVB* **9,** 30-36.

FRASER, C., BELLUGI, U. and BROWN, R. 1963: Control of grammar in imitation, comprehension and production. *JVLVB* **2,** 121-35.

FRIEDERICI, A.D. 1988a: Autonomy and automaticity: function words during sentence construction. In G. Denes, C. Semenza, P. Bisiacchi and E. Andreewski (eds.), *Perspectives in Cognitive Neuropsychology.* London: Lawrence Erlbaum.

—1988 b: Agrammatic comprehension: picture of a computational mismatch. *Aphasiology,* **2,** 279-84.

FREUD, S. 1891: *On Aphasia* (translated by E. Stengel 1953). London: Imago.

GAINOTTI, G. 1972: Studies on the functional organization of the minor hemisphere. *Int. J. Ment. Health* **3**, 78-82.

—1976: The relationship between semantic impairment in comprehension and naming in aphasic patients. *BJDC* **11**, 57-61.

GAINOTTI, G., CALTAGIRONE, C. and IBBA, A. 1975: Semantic and phonemic aspects of auditory language comprehension in aphasia. *Linguistics* **154/5**, 15-29.

GAINOTTI, G. and LEMME, M.A. 1976: Comprehension of symbolic gestures in aphasia. *Brain and Language* **3**, 451-60.

GARDINER, B.J. and BROOKSHIRE, R.H. 1972: Effects of unisensory and multisensory presentation of stimuli upon naming by aphasic subjects. *Language and Speech* **15**, 342-27.

GARDNER, H. 1973: The contribution of operativity to naming capacity in aphasic patients. *Neuropsychologia* **11**, 213-20.

—1974a: The naming and recognition of written symbols in aphasic and alexic patients. *J. Com. Dis.* **7**, 141-153.

—1974b: The naming of objects and symbols by children and aphasic patients. *J. Psycholinguistic Research* **3**, 133-49.

—1976: *The Shattered Mind: the Person after Brain Damage*. New York: Vintage Books.

GARDNER, H., ALBERT, M.L. and WEINTRAUB, S. 1975: Comprehending a word: the influence of speed and redundancy on auditory comprehension in aphasia. *Cortex* **11**, 155-62.

GARDNER, H. and DENES, G. 1973: Connotative judgements by aphasic patients on a pictorial adaptation of the semantic differential. *Cortex* **9**, 183-96.

GARDNER, H., DENES, G. and ZURIF, E. 1975: Critical reading at the sentence level in aphasia. *Cortex* **11**, 60-72.

GARDNER, H., LING, P.K., FLAMM, L. and SILVERMAN, J. 1975: Comprehension and appreciation of humorous material following brain damage. *Brain* **98**, 399-412.

GARDNER, H., and ZURIF, E. 1975: 'Bee' but not 'be': oral reading of single words in aphasia and alexia. *Neuropsychologia* **13**, 181-90.

—1976: Critical reading of words and phrases in aphasia. *Brain and Language* **3**, 173-90.

GARRETT, M. 1982: Production of speech: observations from normal pathological use. In A.W. Ellis (ed.) *Normality and Pathology in Cognitive Functions*. New York: Academic.

GELB, A. and GOLDSTEIN, E. 1924: Über Farbennamen Amnesie. *Psycholigische Forschung* **6**, 127-86. Reprinted in A. Gurwitsch, E.M.G. Haudek and W.E. Haudek (eds.), *Kurt Goldstein: selected papers*, 1971. The Hague: Nijhoff.

GESCHWIND, N. 1965: Disconnexion syndromes in animals and man. *Brain* **88**, 237-94, 585-644.

—1967: The varieties of naming errors. *Cortex* **3**, 96-112.

—1974: *Selected Papers on Language and the Brain (Boston Studies in Philosophy of Science 16)* Dordrecht: D. Reidel.

GESCHWIND, N. and KAPLAN, E. 1962: A human cerebral deconnection syndrome. *Neurology* **12**, 675-85.

GLEASON, J.B., GOODGLASS, H., GREEN, E., ACKERMAN, N. and HYDE, M.R. 1975: The retrieval of syntax in Broca's aphasia. *Brain and Language* **2**, 241-71.

GOLDBLUM, M.C. and ALBERT, M.L. 1972: Phonemic discrimination in sensory aphasia. *Int. J. Ment. Health* **1**, 25-29.

GOLDSTEIN, K. 1948: *Language and Language Disturbance*. New York: Grune and Stratton.

GOLDSTEIN, M.V. 1974: Auditory agnosia for speech (pure word deafness); a historical review with current implications. *Brain and Langiage* **1**, 195-204.

GOODENOUGH, C., ZURIF, E. and WEINTRAUB, S. 1977: Aphasics' attention to grammatical morphemes *Language and Speech* **20**, 11-19.

GOODGLASS, H. 1968: Studies in the grammar of aphasics. In S. Rosenberg and J. Koplin (eds.), *Developments in Applied Psycholinguistics* New York: MacMillan.

—1976: Agrammatism. In H. Whitaker and H.A. Whitaker (eds.), *Studies in Neuro-linguistics, Vol. 1*. New York: Academic.

GOODGLASS, H. and BAKER, E. 1976: Semantic field, naming and auditory comprehension in aphasia. *Brain and Language* 3, 359-74.

GOODGLASS, H. and BLUMSTEIN, S. 1973: *Psycholinguistics and Aphasia*: Baltimore: Johns Hopkins.

GOODGLASS, H. and GESCHWIND, S. 1976: Language disorders (aphasia). In E.C. Carterette and M.P. Friedman (eds.), *Handbook of Perception, Vol. 7 Speech and Language*. New York: Academic.

GOODGLASS, H., GLEASON, J.B. BERNHOLTZ, N.A. and HYDE, M.R. 1972: Some linguistic structures in the speech of a Broca's aphasic. *Cortex* 8, 191-212.

GOODGLASS, G., GLEASON, J.B. and HYDE, M.R. 1970: Some dimensions of auditory language comprehension in aphasia. *JSHR* 13, 595-606.

GOODGLASS, H., HYDE, M.R. and BLUMSTEIN, S. 1969: Frequency, picturability and availability of nouns in aphasia. *Cortex* 5, 104-19.

GOODGLASS, H. and KAPLAN, E. 1963: Disturbance of gesture and pantomime in aphasia. *Brain* 86, 703-20.

—1972, 1983: *The Assessment of Aphasia and Related Disorders*. Philadelphia: Lea and Febiger.

GOODGLASS, H.M., KAPLAN, E., WEINTRAUB, S. and ACKERMAN, N. 1976: The 'tip-of-the-tongue' phenomenon in aphasia. *Cortex* 12, 145-53.

GOODGLASS, H.M., KLEIN, B., CAREY, P. and JONES, K. 1966: Specific semantic word categories in aphasia. *Cortex* 2, 74-89.

GOODGLASS, H. and MENN, L. 1985: Is agrammatism a unitary phenomenon? In M.L. Kean (ed.) *Agrammatism*. New York: Academic.

GOODGLASS, H., QUADFASEL, F.A. and TIMBERLAKE, W.H. 1964: Phrase length and the type of severity of aphasia. *Cortex* 1, 133-52.

GORDON, H.W. 1970: Hemispheric asymmetries in the perception of musical chords. *Cortex* 6, 387-98.

GOSNAVE, G. (1977): Sentence production test in sensory aphasic patients. In S. Rosenberg (ed.), *Sentence Production: Developments in Research and Theory*. New York: Halsted.

GOSSE, A., WACHAL, R.S. and SPREEN, O. 1972: *Linguistic Analysis of Free Speech Samples: Manual of Instructions for Transcription, Pre-editing and Coding*. University of Victoria, BC.

GREEN, E. 1969a Psycholinguistic approaches to aphasia. *Linguistics* 53, 30-50.

—1969b: Phonological and grammatical aspects of jargon in an aphasic patient: a case study. *Language and Speech* 12, 103-18.

—1970: On the contribution of studies in aphasia to psycholinguistics. *Cortex* 6, 216-35.

GREEN, G. 1982: Assessment and treatment of the adult with severe aphasia: aiming for functional generalisation. *Aust. J. Hum. Comm. Dis.*, 10, 11-23.

—1984: Communication in aphasia therapy: some of the procedures and issues involved. *BJDC.* 30, 35-46.

GREENBERG, J.H. 1966: *Language Universals*. The Hague: Mouton.

GREENBLATT, S.H. 1973: Alexia without agraphia or hemianopia: anatomical analysis of an autopsied case. *Brain* 96, 307-16.

GREENE, J. 1972: *Psycholinguistics*. Harmondsworth, Penguin.

GRODZINKSI, Y. and SHAPIRO, L.P. 1988: Two perspectives on the modularity of language. *Aphasiology*, 2, 295-8.

HALPERN, H. 1965: Effect of stimulus variables on dysphasic verbal errors. *Perceptual and Motor Skills* 21, 291-8.

—1965b: Effects of stimulus variables on perseveration of dysphasic subjects. *Perceptual and Motor Skills* 20, 421-9.

—1972: *Adult Aphasia*. Indianapolis: Bobbs-Merrill.

HARRIS, M. and COLTHEART, M. 1986: *Language Processing in Children and Adults*. London: Routledge and Kegan Paul.

HATFIELD, F.M. and WALTON, K. 1975: Phonological patterns in a case of aphasia. *Language and Speech* **18**, 341-57.

HEAD, H. 1926: *Aphasia and Kindred Disorders of Speech, Vols. 1 & 2*, London: Cambridge University Press.

HEALY, A.F. 1974: Separating item from order information in short term memory. *JVLVB* **13**, 644-55.

HÉCAEN, H. 1972: Studies of language pathology. In T.A. Sebeock (ed.), *Current Trends in Linguistics* **9**, The Hague: Mouton.

HÉCAEN, H. and DUBOIS, J. 1971: La neurolinguistique. In G.E. Perren and J.L.M. Trim (eds.)*Applications of Linguistics*, London: Cambridge University Press.

HÉCAEN, H. and GOLDBLUM, M.C. 1972: Etudes neurolinguistiques sur l'aphasie sensorielle—recherches de formes particulières. In P. de Francisco (ed.), *Dimensions de la Psiquiatria Contemporanea Libro Homenaje al profeser Nieto*. Mexico: Ed. Fournier S.A.

HÉCAEN, H. and KREMIN, H. 1976: Neurolinguistic research on reading disorders resulting from left hemisphere lesions. In H. Whitaker and H.A. Whitaker (eds.) *Studies in Neurolinguistics, Vol. 2* New York: Academic.

HEILMAN, K.M., SAFRAN, A. and GESCHWIND, N. 1971: Closed head trauma and aphasia. *J. Neurology, Neurosurgery and Psychiatry* **34**, 265-9.

HEILMAN, K.M., SCHOLES, R. and WATSON, R.J. 1976: Defects of immediate memory in Broca's and conduction aphasia. *Brain and Language* **3**, 201-8.

HELD, J.P. 1975: The natural history of stroke. In S. Licht (ed.), *Stroke and its Rehabilitation*. New Haven, Connecticut: E. Licht.

HILDEBRANDT, N., CAPLAN, D. and EVANS, K. 1987: The man$_i$ left$_i$ without a trace: a case study of aphasic processing of empty categories. *Cognitive Neuropsychology* **4**, 257-302.

HOLLAND, A. 1980: *Communicative Abilities in Daily Living*. Baltimore: University Park Press.

—1982: Observing functional communication of aphasic adults. *JSHD.* **47**, 50-6.

HOLMES, J.M., MARSHALL, J.C. and NEWCOMBE, F. 1971: Syntactic class as a determinant of word-retrieval in normal and dyslexic subjects. *Nature* **234**, 418.

HOPPER, R., KOCH, S. and MANDELBAUM, J. 1986: Conversation analysis methods. In D.G. Ellis and W.A. Donoghue (eds.), *Contemporary Issues in Language and Discourse Processes*. London: Lawrence Erlbaum.

HÖRMANN, H. 1971: *Psycholinguistics*. Amsterdam: North Holland.

HOUSTON, S.H. 1972: *A Survey of Psycholinguistics*. Janua Linguarum Series Minor **98**. The Hague: Mouton.

HOWARD, D. 1986: Beyond randomised controlled trials: the case for effective case studies of the effects of treatment in aphasia. *BJDC* **21**, 89-102.

HOWES, D. 1964: Application of the word frequency concept to aphasia. In A.V.S. De Reuck and M. O'Connor (eds.), *Disorders of Language*. London: Churchill.

—1966: A word count of spoken English, *JVLVB* **5**, 572-604.

HUNT, E., LUNNEBERG, C. and LEWIS, J. 1975: What does it mean to be high verbal? *Cognitive Psychology* **7**, 194-227.

HYMES, D. 1971: Competence and performance in linguistic theory. In R. Huxley and E. Ingram (eds.), *Language Acquisition: models and methods*. New York: Academic.

JAFFRAIN, D. 1968: Contribution à l'étude de la réeducation des aphasiques à partir de l'approche linguistique du problème de l'aphasie. *Information Psychologique (Brussels)* **31/32**, 35-61.

JAKOBSON, R. 1955: *Aphasia as a linguistic topic*. Clarke University Monographs on Psychology and Related Disciplines, Worcester. Reprinted in *Roman Jakobson, Selected Writings, Vol. 2 Words and Language*, 1971. The Hague: Mouton.

—1964: Towards a linguistic typology of aphasia impairments. In A.V.S. De Reuck and M. O'Connor (eds.), *Disorders of Language*. London: Churchill.

—1968: *Child Language, Aphasia and Phonological Universals*. Janua Linguarum Series Minor **72**. The Hague: Mouton.

—1971: *Studies on Child Language and Aphasia*. Janua Linguarum. Series Minor **114**. The Hague: Mouton.

—1978: Aphasic disorders from a linguistic angle. In J.Kristeran, J.C. Milber and N. Ruwet (eds.), *Language, Discours, Société*. Paris: Editions du Seuil.

JOHNS, D.F. and DARLEY, F.L. 1970: Phonemic variability in apraxia of speech. *JSHR* **13**, 556-83.

JOHNSON-LAIRD, P.N. 1987: The mental representation of the meaning of words. *Cognition* **25**, 189-211.

JONES, E.V. 1986: Building the foundations for sentence production in a non-fluent aphasic. *BJDC* **21**, 63-82.

JONES, L.V. and WEPMAN, J.M. 1966: *A Spoken Word Count*. Chicago: Language Research Associates.

KATZ, J.J. and FODOR, J.A. 1963: The structure of a semantic theory. *Language* **39**, 170-210.

KAY, J., LESSER, R. and COLTHEART, M. in preparation: *The Psycholinguistic Assessment of Language Processing in Aphasia*. London: Lawrence Erlbaum.

KEAN, M.L. 1979: Agrammatism: a phonological deficit? *Cognition*, **7**, 69-84.

KENT, G.H. and ROSANOFF, A.J. 1910: A study of association in insanity. *American Journal of Insanity* **67**, 37-96, 317-90.

KERSCHENSTEINER, M., POECK, K., HUBER, W. and STACHOWIAK, F.J. 1975: Die Untersuchung auf Aphasie. *Aktuelle Neurologie* **2**, 151-57.

KERTESZ, A. 1982: *The Western Aphasia Battery*. New York: Grune and Stratton.

KIMURA, D. 1973: The asymmetry of the human brain. *Scientific American*, March.

KIMURA, D. and ARCHIBALD, Y. 1974: Motor functions of the left hemisphere. *Brain* **97**, 337-50.

KINSBOURNE, M. and WARRINGTON, E.K. 1963: Jargon aphasia. *Neuropsychologia* **1**, 27-37.

KISS, G.R. 1973: *An Associative Thesaurus of English and its Structure*. Medical Research Council Report, April (mimeographed).

KOLK, H., VAN GRUNSVEN, M. and KEYSER, A. 1985: On parallelism between production and comprehension in agrammatism. In M.L. Kean (ed.) *Agrammatism*. New York: Academic.

KREINDLER, A., CALVAREZO, C. and MIHAILESCU, L. 1971: Linguistic analysis of one case of jargon aphasia. *Revue Roumaine de Neurologie* **8**, 209-28.

KREINDLER, A. and FRADIS, A. 1971: *Performances in Aphasia*. Paris: Gouthier-Villers

KREINDLER, A., MIHAILESCU, L. and WEIGL, I. 1974: Aphasic performances to syntagms. *Revue Roumaine de Neurologie et Psychiatrie* **11**, 227-42.

KREMIN, H. and GOLDBLUM, M.C. 1975: Etude de la comprehension syntaxique chez les aphasiques. *Linguistics* **154/5**, 31-46.

KUČERA, H. and FRANCIS, W.N. 1967: *Computational analysis of present-day American English*. Providence, RI: Brown University Press.

LABOV, W. 1965: *The Social Stratification of English in New York City*. Washington: Center for Applied Linguistics.

LAKOFF, R. 1972: Language in context. *Language* **48**, 907-27.

LANDAUER, R.K. and MEYER, D.E. 1972: Category size and semantic-memory retrieval. *JVLVB* **11**, 539-49.

LANE, H.L and MOORE, D.J. 1962: Reconditioning a consonant discrimination in an aphasic: an experimental case history. *JSHD* **29**, 232-43.

LANSDELL, H. 1973: Effect of neurosurgery on the ability to indentify popular word associations. *J. Abnormal Psychology* **81**, 255-8.

LEBRUN, Y. 1967: Linguistic analysis of two cases of emissive aphasia. *J. Neurological Sciences* **4**, 271-7.

—1970: On the so-called patterning of language dissolution in aphasia. *Actes du x<sup>e</sup> Congrès Int. des Linguistes*, Bucharest.

—1987: *New trends in the study of acquired aphasia in children.* Paper presented at Conference of the PanHellenic Association of Specialists in Speech and Language, Athens.

LEBRUN, Y., BRUYSSENS, E. and HENNEAUX, J. 1973: Phonetic aspects of anarthria. *Cortex* **9**, 126-53.

LEBRUN, Y. and HOOPS, R. '1974: *Intelligence and Aphasia.* Amsterdam: Swets and Zeitlinger.

LEBRUN, Y., LENAERTS, M., GOIRIS, K. and DEMOL, O. 1969: Aphasia and the concept of the phoneme. *Logopedie en Foniatrie* **41**, 127-35.

LECOURS, A.R. 1974: Le cerveau et le langage. *L'Union Méd. du Canada* **103**, 232-263.

—1975: Methods for the description of aphasic transformations of language. In E.H. Lenneberg and E. Lenneberg (eds.), *Foundations of Language Development, Vol. 2.* New York: Academic.

LECOURS, A.R. and CAPLAN, D. 1975: Review of S. Blumstein 'A phonological investigation of aphasic speech', *Brain and Language* **2**, 237-54.

LECOURS, A.R., DORDAIN, G. and LHERMITTE, F. 1970: Recherches sur le langage des aphasiques: I. Terminologie neurolinguistique. *Encéphale* **59**, 520-546.

LECOURS, A.R. and LHERMITTE, F. 1969: Phonemic paraphasias: linguistic structures and tentative hypotheses. *Cortex* **5**, 193-228.

—1972: Recherches sur la langage des aphasiques, 4: analyse d'un corpus de néologisms. *L'Encéphale* **61**, 295-315.

—1976: The 'pure form' of the phonetic disintegration syndrome (pure anarthria): anatomo-clinical report of a historical case. *Brain and Language* **3**, 88-113.

LECOURS, A.R. and ROUILLON, F. 1976: Neurolinguistic analysis of jargon aphasia and jargonagraphia. In H. Whitaker and H.A. Whitaker (eds.), *Studies in Neurolinguistics, Vol. 2.* New York: Academic.

LECOURS, A.R. and VANIER-CLEMENT, M. 1976: Schizophasia and jargonaphasia. *Brain and Language* **3**, 516-65.

LEECH, G. 1969: *Towards a Semantic Description of English.* London: Longman.

—1974: *Semantics.* Harmondsworth: Penguin.

LEHRER, A. 1974: *Semantic Fields and Lexical Structure.* Amsterdam: North-Holland.

LEISCHNER, A. and FRADIS, A. 1974: Die Asymbolien. *Forschritte der Neurologie, Psychiatrie und Ihrer Grenzgebiete* 42, 264-79.

LENNEBERG, E.H. 1973: The neurology of language *Daedalus* **102**, 115-33.

—1975: The concept of language differentiation. In E.H. Lenneberg and E. Lenneberg (eds.), *Foundations of Language Development, Vol. 1.* New York: Academic.

LESSER, R. 1973: Word association and availability of response in an aphasic subject. *J. Psycholinguistic Research* **2**, 355-67.

—1974: Verbal comprehension in aphasia: an English version of three Italian tests. *Cortex* **10**, 247-63.

—1976a: Verbal and non-verbal memory components in the Token Test. *Neuropsychologia* **14**, 79-85.

—1976b: *Lexical-semantic impairment after right-hemisphere damage?* Paper presented at European Brain and Behaviour Workshop, London.

—1979: Turning tokens into things: linguistic and mnestic aspects of the initial sections of the Token Test. In F. Boller and M. Dennis (eds.), *Auditory Comprehension: Clinical and Experimental Studies with the Token Test.* New York: Academic.

—1984: Sentence comprehension and production in aphasia: an application of lexical grammar. In F.C. Rose (ed.) *Advances in Neurology, Vol. 42: Progress in Aphasiology.* New York: Raven.

—1987: Cognitive neuropsychological influences on aphasia therapy *Aphasiology* **1**, 189-200.

—in press a: Language in the brain: neurolinguistics. In N. Collinge (ed.) *Encyclopaedia of Language*. London: Croom Helm.

—in press b: Intervention in aphasia. In M. Leahy (ed.) *Disorders of Communication: The Science of Intervention*. London: Taylor and Francis.

—in press c: Some issues in the neuropsychological rehabilitation of anomia. In X. Seron and G. Deloche (eds.) *Cognitive Approaches in Neuropsychological Rehabilitation*. Hillsdale: Lawrence Erlbaum.

LESSER, R. and MILROY, L. 1987: Two frontiers in aphasia therapy. *Bulletin of the College of Speech Therapists* **420**, 1-4.

LESSER, R.P. and LÜDERS, H., MORRIS, H.H., DINNER, D.S., KLEM, G., HAHN, J. and HARRISON, M. 1986: Electrical stimulation of Wernicke's area interferes with comprehension. *Neurology* **36**, 658-63.

LEVINSOHN, J. 1969: The investigation of the disintegration of phonemic discrimination on a perception and production level in adults with aphasia *J. South African Logopedic Society* **16**, 48-72.

LEVY, C.B. and TAYLOR, G.L. 1968: *Transformational complexity and comprehension in adult aphasics*. Paper presented at ASHA Convention. Denver.

LEVY, J. 1974a: Psychobiological implications of bilateral asymmetry. In S.J. Dimond and J.G. Beaumont (eds.), *Hemispheric Function in the Human Brain*. London: Elek.

—1974b: Cerebral asymmetries as manifested in split-brain man. In M. Kinsbourne and W.L. Smith (eds.), *Hemispheric Disconnection and Cerebral Function*. Springfield: Thomas.

LHERMITTE, F., DEROUESNÉ, J. and LECOURS, A.R. 1971: Contribution à l'étude des troubles sémantiques dans l'aphasie. *Revue Neurologique* **125**, 81-101.

LHERMITTE, F., LECOURS, A.R. and BERTEAUX, D. 1969: Activation and seriation of linguistic units in aphasic transformations. In L.D. Proctor (ed.), *Biocybernetics of the Central Nervous System*. Boston: Little Brown.

LIBERMAN, A., 1974: The specialization of the language hemisphere. In F.G. Schmitt and F.G. Worden (eds.), *The Neurosciences: third study Program*. Cambridge, Mass.: MIT.

LICHT, S. 1975: *Stroke and its Rehabilitation*. New Haven, Connecticut: E. Licht.

LINEBARGER, M.C., SCHWARTZ, M.F. and SAFFRAN, E.M. 1983: Sensitivity to grammatical structure in so-called agrammatic patients. *Cognition* **13**, 361-392.

LONIE, J. and LESSER, R. 1983: Intonation as a cue to speech act identification in aphasic and other brain-damaged patients. *Int. J. Rehab.*, **6**, 512-3.

LOONEN, M.C.B. and VAN DONGEN, H.R. in press: Acquired childhood aphasia: course and action. *Brain*.

LOW, A.A. 1931: A case of agrammatism in the English language. *Archives of Neurology and Psychiatry* **25**, 556-69.

LUBINSKI, R., DUCHAN, J. and WEITZNER-LIN, B. 1980: Analysis of breakdowns and repairs in aphasic adult communication. In R. Brookshire (ed.) *Clinical Aphasiology Conference Proceedings*. Minneapolis BRK.

LURIA, A.A. 1964: Factors and forms of aphasia. In A.V.S. De Reuck and M. O'Connor (eds.), *Disorders of language*. London: Churchill.

—1966: *Higher Cortical Functions in Man*. London: Tavistock.

—1970: *Traumatic Aphasia*. The Hague: Mouton.

—1973: *The Man with a Shattered World: History of a brain wound*. London: Cape.

—1975a: Two kinds of disorders in the comprehension of grammatical constructions. *Linguistics* **154/5**, 47-56.

—1975b: Basic problems of language in the light of psycholinguistics and neurolinguistics. In E. Lenneberg and E. Lenneberg (eds.), *Foundations of Language Development, Vol. 2*. New York: Academic.

—1976: *Basic Problems of Neurolinguistics*. Janua Linguarum Series Maior **73**. The Hague: Mouton.

—1977: On quasi-aphasic speech disturbances in lesions of the deep structures of the brain. *Brain and Language* **4**, 432-59.

LURIA, A.R. and HUTTON, J.T. 1977: A modern assessment of the basic forms of aphasia. *Brain and Languiage* **4**, 129-51.

LURIA, A.R. and KARASSEVA, T.A. 1968: Disturbances of auditory speech memory in focal lesions of the deep regions of the left temporal lobe. *Neuropsychologia* **6**, 97-104.

LURIA, A.R. and SIMERNITSKAYA, E.G. 1977: Note: Interhemispheric relations and the functions of the minor hemisphere. *Neuropsychologia* **15**, 175-8.

LURIA, A.R. and VINOGRADOVA, O.S. 1959: An objective investigation of the dynamics of semantic systems *B.J. Psych.* 50, 89-105.

LYONS, J. 1969: *Introduction to Theoretical Linguistics*. London: Cambridge University Press.

McCARTHY, R. and WARRINGTON, E.K. 1985: Category specificity in an agrammatic patient: the relative impairment of verb retrieval and comprehension. *Neuropsychologia* **23**, 709-27.

McCAWLEY, J.D. 1968: The role of semantics in grammar. In E. Bach and R.T. Harms (eds.), *Universals in Linguistic Theory*. New York: Holt, Rinehart and Winston.

McFIE, J. 1975: *Assessment of Organic Intellectual Impairment*. London: Academic.

McGLONE, J. 1982: Sex differenes in human brain organization: a critical survey. *The Behavioral and Brain Sciences* **3**, 215-227.

McMAHON, M.K.C. 1972a: Modern linguistics and aphasia, *BJDC* **7**, 54-63.

MARATSOS, M.P. 1974: Children who get worse at understanding the passive: a replication of Bever. *J. Psycholinguistic Research* **3**, 65-74.

MARCIE, P. 1967: Analyse de la structure des phrases dans des énoncés d'aphasiques de conduction. *Langages* **5**, 37-48.

MARIE, P. 1906: The third left frontal convolution plays no special role in the function of language. In M.F. Cole (1971), *Pierre Marie's Papers on Speech Disorders*. New York: Academic.

MARIN, O.S.M. and SAFFRAN, E. 1975: Agnosic behaviour in anomia: a case of pathological verbal dominance. *Cortex* **11**, 83-9.

MARSHALL, G.R. and COFER, C.N. 1963: Associated indices as measures of word relatedness: a summary and comparison of ten methods. *JVLVB* **1**, 408-21.

MARSHALL, J.C. and NEWCOMBE, F. 1966: Syntactic and semantic errors in paralexia. *Neuropsychologia* **4**, 169-76.

—1973: Patterns of paralexia: a psycholinguistic approach. *J. Psycholinguistic Research* **2**, 175-99.

MARSHALL, J.C., NEWCOMBE, F. and HOLMES. J.M. 1978: Lexical memory: a linguistic approach. In R.A. Kennedy and A.L. Wilkes (eds.), *Studies in Long Term Memory*. New York: Academic.

MARSHALL, M., NEWCOMBE, F. and MARSHALL, J.C. 1970: Word finding difficulties in dysphasics. In G.B. Flores D'Arcais and W.J.M. Levelt (eds.), *Advances in Psycholinguistics*. Amsterdam: North Holland.

MARTIN, A.D. 1974: Some objections to the term 'apraxia of speech'. *JSHD* **39**, 53-64.

MARTIN, A.D. and RIGRODSKY, S. 1974: An investigation of phonological impairment in aphasia. Part I and Part II (Distinctive feature analysis of phoneme commutation errors in aphasia). *Cortex* **10**, 317-28, 329-46.

MARTIN, A.D., WASSERMAN, N.H., GILDEN, L., GERSTMAN, L. and WEST, J.A. 1975: A process model of repetition in aphasia: an investigation of phonological and morphological interactions in aphasic error. *Brain and Language* **2**, 434-450.

MARUSZEWSKI, M. 1975: *Language, Communication and the Brain*. Janua Linguarum Series Maior **80**, The Hague: Mouton.

MESULAM, M.M. 1982: Slowly progressive aphasia with generalized dementia. *Ann. Neurol.* **11**, 592-8.

METTER, E.J. 1987: Neuroanatomy and physiology of aphasia: evidence from positron emission tomography. *Aphasiology* **1**, 3-33.

MEYER, D.E., SCHVANEVELDT, R.W. and RUDDY, M.G. 1972: *Activation of lexical memory*. Paper presented to Psychonomic Society, St Louis.

—1974: Loci of contextual effects on visual word-recognition. In P. Rabbit (ed.), *Attention and Performance, Vol. 5*. New York: Academic.

MEYERSON, R. and GOODGLASS, H. 1972: Transformational grammars of aphasic patients. *Language and Speech* **15**, 40-50.

MICELI, G., MAZZUCCHI, A., MENN, L. and GOODGLASS, H. 1983: Contrasting cases of Italian agrammatic aphasia without comprehension disorder. *Brain and Language*, **19**, 65-97.

MICELI, G., SILVERI, M.C., NOCENTINI, U. and CARAMAZZA, A. 1988: Patterns of dissociation in comprehension and production of nouns and verbs. *Aphasiology*, **2**, 351-8.

MIHAILESCU, L. 1970: *La fréquence des phonemes individuels et des groupes biphonematiques chez les aphasiques*. Actes du x^e Congres Int. des Linguistes, Bucharest.

MIHAILESCU, L., BOTEZ, M.I. and KREINDLER, A. 1970: Decoding of correct and wrong word stress in aphasic patients. *Revue Roumaine de Neurologie* **7**, 65-74.

MIHAILESCU, L., VOINESCU, I. and FRADIS, A. 1967: Relative phoneme frequency in aphasics. *Revue Roumaine de Neurologie* **4**, 81-99.

MIHAILESCU, L., WEIGL, I., WEIGL, E. and KREINDLER, A. 1972: Performance in aphasics at conceptual and operational words used singly or within syntagms. *Revue Roumaine de Neurologie* **9**, 181-95.

MILBERG, W. 1988: Information processing deficits and aphasia. *Aphasiology* **2**, 359-62.

MILLER, G.A. 1969: A psychological method to investigate verbal concepts. *J. Math. Psych.* **6**, 169-91.

—1972: English verbs of motion: a case study in semantics and lexical memory. In A.W. Melton and E. Martin (eds.), *Coding Processes in Human Memory*. Washington: Winston.

MILLER, K.M. 1970: Free-association responses of English and Australian students to 100 words from the Kent-Rosanoff Word Association Test. In L. Postman and C. Keppel (eds.), *Norms of Word Association*. New York: Academic.

MILNER, B. 1971: Interhemispheric differences in the localization of psychological processes in man. *British Medical Bulletin* **27**, 272-7.

MILROY, L. 1985: What a performance! Some problems with the competence-performance distinction. *Australian J. Ling.* **51**, 1-17.

MILROY, L. 1987: *Observing and Analyzing Natural Language*. Oxford: Blackwell.

MOHR, J.P. 1976: Broca's area and Broca's aphasia. In H. Whitaker and H.A. Whitaker (eds.), *Studies in Neurolinguistics, Vol. 1*. New York: Academic.

MONRAD-KROHN, G.H. 1974a: The prosodic quality of speech and its disorders. *Acta Psychiatrica et Neurologica Scandinavia* **22**, 255-69.

—1974b: Dysprosody or altered 'melody of language'. *Brain* **70**, 405-15.

—1963: The third element of speech, prosody and its disorders. In L. Halpern (ed.), *Problems of Dynamic Neurology*. Jerusalem: Hebrew University.

MORTON, J. 1970: A functional model for memory. In D. Norman (ed.), *Models of Human Memory*. New York: Academic.

MOSCOVITCH, M. 1973: Language and the cerebral hemispheres: reaction time studies and their implications for models of cerebral dominance. In P. Pliner, L. Kramis and T. Alloway (eds.), *Communication and Affect*. New York: Academic.

MÖSSNER, A. and PILCH, H. 1971: Phonematik-syntaktische Aphasie. *Folia Linguistica* **5**, 394-409.

MUIR, J. 1972: *A Modern Approach to English Grammar*. London: Batsford.

NAESER, M.A. 1974: *The relationship between phoneme discrimination, phoneme picture perception and language comprehension in aphasia*. Paper presented to American Academy of Aphasia, Virginia.

—1988: Some effects of subcortical white matter lesions on language behaviour in aphasia. *Aphasiology* **2**, 363-8.

NEBES, R.D. 1974: Dominance of the minor hemisphere in commisurotomized man for the perception of part-whole relationships. In M. Kinsbourne and W.L. Smith (eds.), *Hemispheric Disconnection and Cerebral Function*. Springfield: Thomas.

—1975: The nature of internal speech in a patient with aphemie. *Brain and Language* **2**, 489-97.

NEEDHAM, E.C. and SWISHER, L.. 1972: A comparison of three tests of auditory comprehension for adult aphasics. *JSHD* **37**, 123-31.

NEWCOMBE, F. and MARSHALL, J.C. 1967: Immediate recall of 'sentences' by subjects with unilateral cerebral lesions. *Neuropsychologia* **5**, 329-34.

—1972: Word retrieval in aphasia. *Int. J. Ment. Health* **1**, 38-45.

NEWMAN, J.E., LOVETT, M.W. and DENNIS, M. 1986: The use of discourse analysis in neurolinguistics: some findings from the narratives of hemicorticate adolescents. *Topics in Language Disorders* **7**, 31-44.

NOLL, J.D. and HOOPS, H.R. 1967: Aphasic grammatical involvement as indicated by spelling ability. *Cortex* **3**, 419-32.

OBLER, L.K. and MENN, L. 1988: Agrammatism: the current issues. *Journal of Neurolinguistics* **3**, 63-76.

OJEMANN, G.A. 1983: Brain organization for language from the perspective of electrical stimulation mapping. *The Behavioral and Brain Sciences*, **2**, 189-230.

OMBREDANE, A. 1951: *L'Aphasie et l'Elaboration de la Pensée Explicite*. Paris: Presse Universitaire de France.

ORGASS, B., POECK, K. and KERSCHENSTEINER, M. 1974; Das Verständnis für Nomina mit spezifischer Referenz bei aphasischen Patienten. *Zeitschrift für Neurologie* **206**, 95-102.

OSCAR-BERMAN, M., ZURIF, B.B. and BLUMSTEIN, S. 1975: Effects of unilateral brain damage on the processing of speech sounds. *Brain and Language* **2**, 345-55.

OSGOOD, C.E. 1960: The cross-cultural generality of visual-verbal-synesthetic tendencies. *Behavioural Sciences* **5**, 146-69.

OSGOOD, C.E. and MIRON, M.S. 1963: *Approaches to the Study of Aphasia*. Urbana: University of Illinois Press.

OXBURY, J.M. 1976: Diseases of the central nervous system: treatment of stroke. *British Medical Journal* **4**, 450-52.

OXBURY, J.M., CAMPBELL, D.C. and OXBURY, S.M. 1974: Unilateral spatial neglect and impairments of spatial analysis and visual perception. *Brain* **97**, 551-64.

OXBURY, J.M., OXBURY, S.M. and HUMPHREY, N.K. 1969: Varieties of colour anomia. *Brain* **92**, 847-60.

PAAP, K.R. 1975: Theories of speech perception. In D.W. Massaro (ed.), *Understanding Language*. New York: Academic.

PAIVIO, A. 1971: *Imagery and Verbal Processes*. New York: Holt, Rinehart and Winston.

PALMER, F.R. 1976: *Semantics, a new outline*. London: Cambridge University Press.

PANAGOS, J.M. and KING, R.R. 1975: Self and mutual speech comprehension by deviant and normal speaking children. *JSHR* **18**, 653-62.

PARISI, D. and PIZZAMIGLIO, L. 1970: Syntactic comprehension in aphasia. *Cortex* **6**, 204-15.

PATTERSON, K.E. and MARCEL, A.J. 1977: Aphasia, dyslexia and the phonological coding of written words. *Q.J. Exp. Psych.* **29**, 307-18.

PENN, C. 1985: The Profile of Communicative Appropriateness: a clinical tool for the assessment of pragmatics. *The South African Journal of Communicative Disorders* **32** 18-23.

PERECMAN, E. 1984: Spontaneous translation and language mixing in a polyglot aphasic. *Brain and Language* **23**, 43-63.

PETERSEN, S.E., FOX, P.T., POSNER, M.I., MINTUN, M. and RAICHLE, M.E. 1988: Positron emission tomographic studies of the cortical anatomy of single-word processing. *Nature* **331** 585-9.

PEUSER, G. 1976: Der Drei-Figuren-Test: ein neues Verfahren zur qualitativen und quantitativen Bestimmung von Sprachverständnisstörungen. In G. Peuser (ed.), *Interdisciplinäre Aspekte der Aphasieforschung*. Cologne: Rheinland Verlag.

PICK, A. 1973: *Aphasia* translated by J.W. Brown. Springfield: Thomas.

PILCH, H. 1972: A linguistic view of aphasia. *Language Sciences* April 6-12.

PIZZAMIGLIO, L. and APPICCIAFUOCO, A. 1971: Semantic comprehension in aphasia. *J.Com. Dis.* **3**, 280-88.

PIZZAMIGLIO, L. and PARISI, D. 1970: Studies on verbal comprehension in aphasia. In G.B. Flores D'Arcais and W.J.M. Levelt (eds.). *Advances in Psycholinguistics*. Amsterdam: North-Holland.

PIZZAMIGLIO, L., PARISI, D. and APPICCIAFUOCO, A. 1968: Development of tests of verbal comprehension in aphasics and children. In J.W. Black and E.G. Jancosek (eds.), *Proceedings of Conference on Language for Aphasics*. Ohio State University (mimeographed).

PIZZAMIGLIO, L., MAMMUCARI, A. and RAZZANO, C. 1985: Evidence for sex differences in brain organization in recovery from aphasia. *Brain and Language* **31**, 109-21.

POECK, K., HARTJE, W., KERSCHENSTEINER, M. and ORGASS, B. 1973: Sprachverständnisstörungen bei aphasischen und nicht-aphasischen Hirnkranken. *Deutsche Medizinische Wochenschift* **98**, 139-47.

POECK, K. and HUBER, W. 1977: Note: to what extent is language a sequential activity? *Neuropsychologia* **15**, 359-63.

POECK, K. and STACHIOWIAK, F.J. 1975: Farbennungestörungen bei aphasischen und nichtaphasischen Hirnkranken. *J. Neurology* **209**, 95-102.

POECK, K. and LUZZATTI, C. in press: Slowly progressive aphasia in three patients: the problem of accompanying neuropsychological deficit. *Brain*.

PONCET, M., DEGOS, C., DELOCHE, G. and LECOURS, A.R. 1972: Phonetic and phonemic transformations in aphasia. *Int. J. Ment. Health* **1**, 45-54.

PORCH, B., 1967: *The Porch Index of Communicative Ability*. Palo Alto: Consulting Psychologists Press.

POSTMAN, L. and KEPPEL, G. 1970: *Norms of Word Association*. New York: Academic.

PRIBRAM, K. 1971: *Languages of the Brain*. Englewood Cliffs, Prentice Hall.

PRING, T. 1986: Evaluating the effects of speech therapy for aphasics: developing the single case methodology. *BJDC* **21**, 103-15.

PRINZ, P. 1980: A note on requesting strategies in adult aphasics. *Journal of Communication Disorders* **13**, 65-73.

PRUTTING, C.A. and KIRCHNER, D.M. 1987: A clinical appraisal of the pragmatic aspects of language. *JSHD* **52**, 105-19.

QUIRK, R., GREENBAUM, S., LEECH, G.N. and SVARTVIK, J. 1972: *A Grammar of Contemporary English*. London: Longman.

RACY, A., OSBORN, M.A., VERN, B.A. and MOLINARI, G.F. 1980: Epileptic aphasia. *Archives of Neurology*, **37**, 419-22.

REES, N.S. 1973: Auditory processing factors in language disorders: the view from Procrustes' bed. *JSHD* **38**, 304-15.

RIEGEL, K.F. and RIEGEL, R.M. 1961: Prediction of word recognition thresholds on the basis of stimulus parameters. *Language and Speech* **4**, 157-70.

RINNERT, C. and WHITAKER, H.A. 1973: Semantic confusions by aphasic patients. *Cortex* **9**, 56-81.

ROBINSON, G.M. and SOLOMON, D.J. 1974: Rhythm is processed by the speech hemisphere. *J. Exp. Psych.* **102**, 508-11.

ROCHFORD, G. 1971: A study of naming errors in dysphasic and in demented patients. *Neuropsychologia* **9**, 437-43.

—1974: Are jargon dysphasics dysphasic? *BJDC* **9**, 34-44.

ROCHFORD, G. and WILLIAMS, M. 1962: Studies in the development and breakdown of the use of names. I: The relationship between nominal dysphasia and the acquisition of vocabulary in childhood. II: Experimental production of naming disorders in normal people. *J. Neurology, Neurosurgery and Psychiatry* **25,** 222-23.

—1963: III: Recovery from nominal dysphasia. *J. Neurology, Neurosurgery and Psychiatry* **26,** 377-81.

—1965: IV: The effects of word frequency. *J. Neurology, Neurosurgery and Psychiatry* **28,** 407-13.

ROSENBAUM, D.H., SIEGEL, M., BARR, W.B. and ROWAN, A.J. 1986: Epileptic aphasia. *Neurology* **36,** 811-5.

ROSENBEK, J.C., WERTZ, R.T. and DARLEY, F.L. 1973: Oral sensation and perception in apraxia of speech and aphasia *JSHR* **16,** 22-36.

SABOURAUD, O., GAGNEPAIN, J. and CHATEL, M. 1971: Qu'est ce que l'anarthrie? *Presse Medicale* **79,** 675-80.

SABOURAUD, O., GAGNEPAIN, J. and SABOURAUD, A. 1965: Aphasie et linguistique. *Le Revue du Practicien* **15,** 2335-45.

SAFFRAN, E.M. and MARIN, O.S.M. 1977: Reading without phonology: evidence from aphasia. *Q.J. Exp. Psych.* **29,** 515-25.

SAFFRAN, E.M., BERNDT, R.S. and SCHWARTZ, M.F. 1987: *The quantitative analysis of agrammatic production: procedure and data.* Paper presented at British Aphasiology Society Conference, Newcastle Upon Tyne.

SAFFRAN, E.M. and SCHWARTZ, M.F. 1988: 'Agrammatic' comprehension it's not. *Aphasiology* **2,** 389-94.

SAFFRAN, E.M., SCHWARTZ, M.F. and MARIN, O. 1980: The word order problem in agrammatism: production. *Brain and Language* **10,** 263-80.

SARNO, M.T. 1975: Disorders of communication in stroke. In S. Licht (ed.), *Stroke and its Rehabilitation.* Connecticut: E. Licht.

SARNO, M.T., BUONAGURO, A. and LEVITA, E. 1985: Gender and recovery from aphasia after stroke. *J. Nerv. Ment. Dis.* **173,** 605-9.

SASANUMA, S. 1974: Note: Kanji versus Kana processing in alexia with transient agraphia, a case report. *Cortex* **10,** 89-97.

—1975: Kana and Kanji processing in Japanese aphasics. *Brain and Language* **2,** 369-83.

SASANUMA, S. and FUJIMURA, O. 1971: Selective impairment of phonetic and non-phonetic transcriptions of words in Japanese aphasic patients: Kana versus Kanji retrieval of words in Japanese aphasic patients' recognition and writing. *Cortex* **7,** 1-18.

—1972: An analysis of writing errors in Japanese aphasic patients: Kanji versus Kana loanwords. *Cortex* **8,** 265-82.

SASANUMA, S., TATSUMI, I.F., KIRITAMI and FUJISAKI, H. 1973: Auditory perception of signal duration in aphasic patients. *Annual Bulletin of the Research Institute of Logopedics and Phoniatrics* **7,** 65-72.

SATZ, P. and BULLARD-BATES, C. 1981: Acquired aphasia in children. In M.T. Sarno (ed.) *Acquired Aphasia.* New York: Academic.

SCHACTER, D.L., McANDREWS, M.P. and MOSCOVITCH, M. 1988: Access to consciousness: dissociations between implicit and explicit knowledge in neuropsychological syndromes. In L. Weiskrantz (ed.) *Thought without Language.* London: Oxford University Press.

SCHAEFFER, B. and WALLACE, R. 1970: The comparison of word meanings. *J. Exp. Psych.* **86,** 144-52.

SCHLANGER, B.B., SCHLANGER, P. and GERSTMAN, L.J. 1976: The perception of emotionally toned sentences by right hemisphere damaged and aphasic subjects. *Brain and Language* **3,** 396-403.

SCHNEIDER, W. 1987: Connectionism: is it a paradigm shift for psychology? *Behavior Research Methods, Instruments and Computers* **19,** 73-83.

SCHNIZTER, M.L. 1971: *Generative phonology: evidence from aphasia.* PhD thesis, University of Rochester.

—1974: Aphasiological evidence for five linguistic hypotheses. *Language* **50**, 300-315.

—1976: The role of phonology in linguistic communication: some neurolinguistic considerations. In H. Whitaker and H.A. Whitaker (eds.), *Studies in Neurolinguistics, Vol. 1.* New York: Academic.

—1978: The phonology of aphasia: a reply. *Pola* 18-19.

—1979: The aphasia paradigm, a key to the competence-performance distinction. In M. Studemund (ed.), *Reader zur Psycholinguistik.*

SCHNITZER, M.L. and MARTIN, J.E. 1974: *Sequential constraint impairment in aphasia: a case study. Brain and Language* **1**, 283-92.

SCHUELL, H.R. 1950: Paraphasia and paralexia *JSHD* **15**, 291-306.

—1965: *The Minnesota Test for the Differential Diagnosis of Aphasia.* Minneapolis: University of Minnesota Press.

SCHUELL, H.R., JENKINS, J.J. and JIMINEZ-PABON, E. 1964: *Aphasia in Adults.* New York: Harper and Row.

SCHUELL, H.R., JENKINS, J.J. and LANDIS, L. 1961: Relationships between auditory comprehension and word frequency in aphasia. *JSHR* **4**, 30-36.

SCHVANEVELDT, R.W. and MEYER, D.E. 1973: Retrieval and comparison processes in semantic memory. In S. Kornblum (ed.), *Attention and Performance, Vol. 4.* New York: Academic.

SCHVEIGER, P. 1968: Sur la pathologie de la dérivation et de l'intonation. *Cahiers de Linguistique Theorique et Appliquée* **5**, 219-20.

SCHWARTZ, M.F. 1987: Patterns of speech production deficit within and across aphasia syndromes: application of a psycholinguistic model. In M. Coltheart, G. Sartori and R. Job (eds.), *The Cognitive Neuropsychology of Language.* London: Lawrence Erlbaum.

SCHWARTZ, D. and HALPERN, H. 1973: Effect of body-image stimuli on verbal errors of dysphasic subjects. *Perceptual and Motor Skills* **36**, 994.

SEFER, J.W. 1973: A case study demonstrating the value of aphasia therapy. *BJDC* **8**, 99-104.

SEFER, J.W. and HENRIKSON, E. 1966: Relationships between word association and grammatical classes in aphasia. *JSHR* **9**, 529-41.

SELLS, P. 1985: *Lectures on contemporary syntactic theories.* Stanford: Center for the Study of Language and Information.

SEMMES, J. 1968: Hemispheric specialization: a possible clue to mechanism. *Neuropsychologia* **6**, 11-26.

SHALLICE, T. and WARRINGTON, E.K. 1975: Word recognition in a phonemic dyslexic patient. *Q. J. Exp. Psych* **27**, 187-99.

SHANKWEILER, D. and HARRIS, K.S. 1966: An experimental approach to the problem of articulation in aphasia. *Cortex* **2**, 277-92.

SHATTUCK-HUFNAGEL, S. 1979: Speech errors as evidence for a serial-ordering mechanism in sentence production. In W.E. Cooper and E.C.T. Walker (eds.) *Sentence Processing.* Hillsdale: Lawrence Erlbaum.

SHEWAN, C.M. 1969: *An investigation of auditory comprehension in adult aphasic patients.* Paper presented at ASHA Conference.

—1976: Error patterns in auditory comprehension of adult aphasics. *Cortex* **12**, 325-36.

SHEWAN, C.M. and CANTER, C.J. 1971: Effects of vocabulary, syntax and sentence length on auditory comprehension in aphasic patients. *Cortex* **7**, 209-26.

SIEGEL, G.M. 1959: Dysphasic speech responses to visual word stimuli. *JSHR* **2**, 152-60.

SKINNER, C., WIRZ, S., THOMPSON, I. and DAVIDSON, J. 1984: *The Edinburgh Functional Communication Profile.* Buckingham: Winslow.

SMITH, A. 1974: Dominant and non-dominant hemispherectomy. In M. Kinsbourne and W.L. Smith (eds.), *Hemispheric Disconnection and Cerebral Function.* Springfield: Thomas.

SMITH, M.D. 1974a: On the understanding of some relational words in aphasia. *Neuropsychologia* **12**, 371-84.

—1974b: Note: operant conditioning of syntax in aphasia. *Neuropsychologia* **12.** 403-5.

SMITH, N.V. 1974: The acquisition of phonological skills in children. *BJDC* **9,** 17-23.

SPARKS, R., HELM, N. and ALBERT, M. 1974: Aphasia rehabilitation resulting from melodic intonation therapy. *Cortex* **10,** 304-16.

SPARKS, W.R. and HOLLAND, A.L. 1976: Method: melodic intonation therapy for aphasia. *JSHD* **41,** 287-97.

SPERRY, R.W. 1974: Lateral specialization in the surgically separated hemispheres. In F.O. Schmitt and W.G. Worden (eds.), *The Neurosciences: Third Study Program.* Cambridge, Mass.: MIT.

SPREEN, O. 1968: Psycholinguistic aspects of aphasia. *JSHR* **11,** 467-80.

—1973: Psycholinguistics and aphasia: the contribution of Arnold Pick. In H. Goodglass and S. Blumstein (eds.), *Psycholinguistics and Aphasia.* Baltimore: Johns Hopkins.

SPREEN, O. and BENTON, A.L. 1969: *Neurosurgery Center Comprehensive Examination for Aphasia.* University of Victoria, BC.

SPREEN, O., and WACHAL, R.S. 1973: Psycholinguistic analysis of aphasic language: Theoretical formulations and procedures. *Language and Speech* **16,** 130-46.

STACHIOWIAK, F-J., HUBER, W., POECK, K. and KERSCHENSTEINER, M. 1977: Text comprehension in aphasia. *Brain and Language* **4,** 177-95.

STOREY, P. 1976: Depression after strokes. *Chest, Heart and Stroke Journal* **1,** 14-17.

STRUB, R.L. and GARDNER, H. 1974: The repetition defect in conduction aphasia: mnestic or linguistic? *Brain and Language* **1,** 241-55.

TAYLOR, J. 1958: *Selected writings of John Hughlings Jackson, Vol. 2.* London: Staples Press.

TAYLOR, M. 1953: *Functional Communication Profile.* New York University Medical Center.

—1965: A measurement of functional communication in aphasia. *Archives of Physical Medicine and Rehabilitation* **46,** 101-7.

TEIXERA, L.A., DEFRAN, R.H. and NICHOLS, A.C. 1974: Oral stereognostic differences between apraxics, dysarthrics, aphasics, and normals. *J. Com. Dis.* **7,** 213-25.

THORNDIKE, E.L. and LORGE, I. 1944: *The Teacher's Word Book of 30,000 Words.* New York: Teachers College Press.

TRAILL, A. 1970: Transformational grammar and the case of an Ndebele-speaking aphasic. *J. South Africa Logopedic Society* **17,** 48-66.

TROST, J. 1970: *A descriptive study of verbal apraxia in patients with Broca's aphasia.* PhD thesis, Northwestern University.

TROST, J. and CANTER, G.J. 1974: Apraxia of speech in patients with Broca's aphasia: a study of phoneme production accuracy and error patterns. *Brain and Language* **1,** 63-80.

TSVETKOVA, L.S. 1976: Sur les mécanisms des troubles de la répétition et de la comprehension du langage dans l'aphasie acoustico-mnestique. *Neuropsychologia* **14,** 343-52.

TZORTZIS, C. and ALBERT, M. 1974: Impairment of memory for sequences in conduction aphasia. *Neuropsychologia* **12,** 355-66.

ULATOWSKA, H., DOYEL, A., STERN, R., HAYNES, S. and NORTH, A. 1983: Production of procedural discourse in aphasia. *Brain and Language* **18,** 315-41.

ULATOWSKA, H., FREEDMAN-STERN, R., DOYEL, A., MALACUSO-HAYNES, S. and NORTH, A. 1983: Production of narrative discourse in aphasia. *Brain and Language* **19,** 317-34.

ULLMANN, S. 1956: The concept of meaning in linguistics. *Archivum Linguisticum* **8,** 12-20.

VAN LANCKNER, D. and FROMKIN, V.A. 1973: Hemisphere specialization for pitch and 'tone': evidence from Thai. *J. Phonetics* **1,** 101-9.

VIGNOLO, L.A. 1964: Evolution of aphasia and language rehabilitation: a retrospective exploratory study. *Cortex* **1,** 344-67.

VOINESCU, I. 1971: Syntactic complexity in aphasics. *Revue Roumaine de Neurologie* **8,** 69-80.

VON STOCKERT, T.R. 1972: Recognition of syntactic structure in aphasic patients. *Cortex* **8**, 323-54.

—1974: Ein neues Konzept zum Verständis der cerebralen Sprachtsörungen. *Nervenarzt* **45**, 94-7.

VON STOCKERT, T.R. and BADER, L. 1976: Some relations of grammar and lexicon in aphasia. *Cortex* **12**, 49-60.

WACHAL, R.S., SPREEN, O. and GOSSE, A. 1973: *Grammatical Analysis of Free Speech Samples: Manual of Instructions for Classification and Coding.* University of Victoria, BC.

WAGENAAR, E., SNOW, C. and PRINS, R. 1975: Spontaneous speech of aphasic patients: a psycholinguistic analysis. *Brain and Language* **2**, 281-303.

WALLESCH, C-W. and WYKE, M. 1985: Language and the subcortical nuclei. In S. Newman and R. Epstein (eds.) *Current Perspectives in Dysphasia.* Edinburgh: Churchill Livingstone.

WALSH, H. 1974: On certain practical inadequacies of distinctive feature systems. *JSHD* **39**, 32-43.

WARDHAUGH, R. 1985: *How Conversation Works.* Oxford: Blackwell.

WARRINGTON, E.K. 1969: The selective impairment of semantic memory. *J. Exp. Psych.* **27**, 635-57.

WARRINGTON, E.K. and SHALLICE, T. 1969: The selective impairment of auditory verbal short-term memory. *Brain* **92**, 885-96.

WARRINGTON, E.K. and TAYLOR, A. 1973: The contribution of the right parietal lobe to object recognition. *Cortex* **9**, 152-64.

WARRINGTON, E.K. and McCARTHY, R. 1987: Categories of knowledge: further fractionation and an attemped integration. *Brain*, **110**, 1273-96.

WEIDNER, W.E. and LASKY, E.Z. 1976: The interaction of rate and complexity of stimulus on the performance of adult aphasic subjects. *Brain and Language* **3**, 34-70.

WEIGL, E. 1961: The phenomenon of temporary deblocking in aphasia. *Zeitschrift für Phonetische Sprachwissenschaft und Kommunikationsforschung* **14**, 337-61.

—1970a: A neuropsychological contribution to the problem of semantics. In M. Bierwisch and E.E. Heidolph (eds.), *Progress in Linguistics.* The Hague: Mouton.

—1970b: Neuropsychological studies of the structure and dynamics of semantic fields with the deblocking method. In A. Greimas *et al.* (eds.), *Sign, Language, Culture.* Janua Linguarum Series Maior **1**, The Hague: Mouton.

WEIGL, E. and BIERWISCH, M. 1970: Neuropsychology and linguistics: topics of common research. *Foundations of Language* **6**, 1-18.

WEIGL, I. and MIHAILESCU, L. 1973: Interdependence between the syntactic context and its constituents. *Revue Roumaine Neurologie* **10**, 123-31.

WEINREICH, U. 1966: Explorations in semantic theory. In T.A. Sebeok (ed.), *Current Trends in Linguistics 3. Theoretical Foundations.* The Hague: Mouton.

WEINSTEIN, E.A. 1964: Affections of speech with lesions of the non-dominant hemisphere. In D. Rioch and E.A. Weinstein (eds.), *Disorders of Communication.* Baltimore: Williams and Wilkins

WEINSTEIN, E.A. and KELLER, N.J.A. 1963: Linguistic patterns of misnaming in brain injury. *Neuropsychologia* **1**, 79-90.

WEINSTEIN, E.A. and PUIG-ANTICH, J. 1974: Jargon and its analogues. *Cortex* **10**, 75-83.

WEINTRAUB, S., MESULAM, M.M. and KRAMER, L. 1981: Disturbances of prosody: a right hemisphere contribution to language. *Arch. Neurol.* **38**, 742-4.

WEISENBERG, T. and McBRIDE, K. 1935: *Aphasia.* New York: Commonwealth Fund.

WEPMAN, J.M. 1958: *Auditory Discrimination Test.* Chicago: Language Research Associates.

—1972: Aphasia therapy: a new look. *JSHD* **37**, 203-14.

—1976: Aphasia: language without thought or thought without language? *Asha* March 131-6.

WEPMAN, J.M., BOCK, R., JONES, L. and VAN PELT, D. 1956: Psycholinguistic study of aphasia: A revision of the concept of anomia. *JHSD* **21**, 468-77.

WEPMAN, J.M. and JONES, L.V. 1964: Five aphasias: A commentary on aphasia as a regressive linguistic phonomenon. *Research Publications of the Association for Research in Nervous and Mental Diseases* **42**, 190-123.

—1966: Studies in aphasia: classification of aphasic speech by the noun-pronoun ratio. *BJDC* **1**, 46-54.

WERNICKE, C. 1908: The symptom-complex of aphasia. In A. Church (ed.), *Disorders of the Nervous System*. New York: Appleton.

WHITAKER, H.A. 1970: Linguistic competence: evidence from aphasia. *Glossa* **4**, 46-53.

—1971a: *On the Representation of Language in the Human Brain*. Edmonton: Linguistic Research.

—1971b: Neurolinguistics. In W.O. Dingwall (ed.), *A Survey of Linguistic Science*. University of Maryland, College Park.

—1976: Disorders of speech production mechanisms. In E.C. Carterette and M.P. Friedman (eds.), *Handbook of Perception, Vol. 7. Language and Speech*. New York: Academic.

WHITAKER, H.A. and NOLL, J.D. 1972: Some linguistic parameters of the Token Test. *Neuropsychologia* **10**, 395-404.

WHITAKER, H.A. and SELNES, O.A. 1975: *Anatomic variations in the cortex: individual differences and the problem of the loci of language functions*. Paper presented at Conference on the Origins and Evolution of Language and Speech.

WHITAKER, H.A. and WHITAKER, H. 1972: Linguistic theory and speech pathology. *J. Minnesota Speech and Hearing Assocation* **11**, 51-6.

WHITAKER, H.A. and WHITAKER, H.A. 1978: Language disorders. In H.D. Brown and R. Wardhaugh (eds.), *A Survey of Applied Linguistics*. Ann Arbor: University of Michigan Press.

WIEGEL-CRUMP, C. and KOENIGSKNECHT, R. 1973: Tapping the lexical store of the adult aphasic: Analysis of the improvement made in word retrieval skills. *Cortex* **9**, 410-17.

WILLCOX, M., DAVIS, G.A. and LEONARD, L. 1978: Aphasics' comprehension of contextually conveyed meaning. *Brain and Language* **6**, 362-77.

WILLMES, K., POECK, K., WENIGER, D. and HUBER, W. 1983: Facet Theory applied to the construction and validation of the Aachen Aphasia Test. *Brain and Language* **18**, 257-76.

WILKINS, A.J. 1971: Conjoint frequency, category size and categorization time. *JVLVB* **10**, 382-5.

WOODS, B.T. and CAREY, S. 1979: Language deficits after apparent clinical recovery from childhood aphasia. *Ann. Neurol.* **6**, 405-9.

WYKE, M. 1962: An experimental study of verbal associations in dysphasic subjects. *Brain* **85**, 679-86.

WYKE, M. and HOLGATE, D. 1973: Colour naming defects in dysphasic patients—a qualitative analysis. *Neuropsychologia* **11**, 451-61.

YAMADORI, A. 1975: Ideogram reading in alexia. *Brain* **98**, 231-8.

YAMADORI, A. and ALBERT, M.L. 1973: Word category in aphasia. *Cortex* **9**, 112-25.

ZAIDEL, E. 1976: Auditory vocabulary in the right hemisphere following brain bisection and hemidecortication. *Cortex* **12**, 191-211.

—1977: Unilateral auditory language comprehension on the Token Test following cerebral commissurotomy and hemispherectomy. *Neuropsychologia* **15**, 1-18.

ZATORSKI, R.J. and LESSER, R. 1981: Notes and discussion: the lexicon and sentence generation in aphasia. *Brain and Language* **13**, 185-90.

ZINGESER, L.B. and BERNDT, R.S. 1988: Grammatical class and context effects in a case of pure anomia: implications for models of language processing. *Cognitive Neuropsychology* **5**, 473-516.

ZURIF, E.B. and CARAMAZZA, A. 1976: Psycholinguistic structures in aphasia: studies in syntax and semantics. In H. and H.A. Whitaker (eds.), *Studies in Neurolinguistics, Vol. 1*.

New York: Academic.

ZURIF, E.B., CARAMAZZA, A., and MYERSON, R. 1972: Grammatical judgements of agrammatic aphasics. *Neuropsychologia* **10,** 405-18.

ZURIF, E.B., CARAMAZZA, A., MYERSON, R. and GALVIN, J. 1974: Semantic feature representations for normal and aphasic language. *Brain and Language* **1,** 167-87.

ZURIF, E.B., GREEN, E., CARAMAZZA, A. and GOODENOUGH, C. 1976: Grammatical judgements of aphasic patients: sensitivity to functors. *Cortex* **12,**183-6.

ZURIF, E.B. 1980: Language mechanisms: a neuropsychological perspective. *American Scientist* **68,** 305-11.

# Index

Cole & Whurr Journals of related interest

# THE BRITISH JOURNAL OF DISORDERS OF COMMUNICATION

The British Journal of Disorders of Communication is an academically rigorous and intellectually challenging journal which presents the latest clinical and theoretical research and is a principal forum for the discussion of the entire range of communication disorders. The journal contains a representative and balanced selection of articles, with contributions from North America, Australasia and Continental Europe, as well as the UK. Among the leading articles published in recent issues are:
August 1987: Duncan & Gibbs - Acquisition of Syntax in Panjabi and English
December 1987: Gibbon and Hardcastle - Articulatory Description and Treatment of 'lateral /S/' using Electropalatography: A Case Study
April 1988: Perry - Surgical Voice Restoration following Laryngectomy: The Tracheo-oesophageal fistula technique (Singer-Blom)
August 1988: Bryan - Assessment of Language Disorders after Right Hemisphere Damage; Lebrun - Language and Epilepsy: A Review

The journal is owned by the College of Speech Therapists, and the Editor is Elspeth McCartney of Glasgow University and Jordanhill College. Issues are published three times a year and annual volumes are of up to 500 pages.

ISSN: 0007 098X

# THE BRITISH JOURNAL OF EXPERIMENTAL AND CLINICAL HYPNOSIS

This is the Journal of the British Society of Experimental and Clinical Hypnosis, a learned society which brings together appropriately qualified medical professionals who have a legitimate reason for using hypnosis in their work and who share a scientific interest in the research and practical application of hypnosis. The journal provides a forum for the critical discussion of ideas, theories, findings, procedures and social policies associated with the topic of hypnosis. It also disseminates information on all aspects of theory, research and practice. A book review section is included.

ISSN:0265 1033

Please send for the Cole & Whurr catalogue.

**Cole & Whurr Ltd**
**19b Compton Terrace, London N1 2UN**
**01-359 5979**